Understanding Alzheimer's Disease

Understanding Alzheimer's Disease

Edited by **Joshua Barnard**

New Jersey

Published by Foster Academics,
61 Van Reypen Street,
Jersey City, NJ 07306, USA
www.fosteracademics.com

Understanding Alzheimer's Disease
Edited by Joshua Barnard

International Standard Book Number: 978-1-63242-415-0 (Hardback)

Contents

Preface

The purpose of the book is to provide a glimpse into the dynamics and to present opinions and studies of some of the scientists engaged in the development of new ideas in the field from very different standpoints. This book will prove useful to students and researchers owing to its high content quality.

Over 6 million Europeans, out of which more than a quarter of people are over the age of 85 and 10% are over the age of 65, have been affected by Alzheimer's Dementia (AD). Given the steady aging of European societies, cognitive decline and dementia have grown into a crucial health problem with a great socioeconomic effect on patients, their caregivers and families, society, and national health care systems. The number of people with dementia is estimated to double by 2030 and further increase by 2050. There is a critical requirement for creative methods to boost understanding of pathological events that would transform into the establishment of successful prevention or new treatment techniques. Advancements in comprehending pathological events in AD have been achievable by employing cell cultures, genetically modified organisms and animal models that do not have the complexity of events happening in humans. This book provides the latest therapy strategies incorporated to treat the disease and some clinical presentations & prevention methods are also elucidated.

At the end, I would like to appreciate all the efforts made by the authors in completing their chapters professionally. I express my deepest gratitude to all of them for contributing to this book by sharing their valuable works. A special thanks to my family and friends for their constant support in this journey.

Editor

Therapy

Animal Assisted Therapy and Activities in Alzheimer's Disease

Sibel Cevizci, Halil Murat Sen, Fahri Güneş and Elif Karaahmet

Additional information is available at the end of the chapter

1. Introduction

Animal-Assisted Therapy (AAT) or *Pet Therapy* is a supportive goal-oriented intervention which is mainly result from human and animal interaction. [1]- [6] In this treatment process, a health professional/patients' doctor have to determine which animal model should be accompanied with a specific clinical goal. This interventions can be followed by physical therapists, neurologist, psychiatrist, veterinary public health specialists, psychologist, occupational therapists, provided that they have taken a certification in AAT. In addition, all therapy processes should be followed by patients' doctor according to the suggestions of AAT specialist.

Although there are so many approach about the effect mechanism of AAT, it is known that the human and animal interaction is the basis for all of them. The positive-constructive bond result from between human and animal interaction is the key point to initiate the effect mechanism of AAT. This curative effect starts to work four basic mechanism including psychological stimulation, emotional, playing, and physical according to the Ballarini. [4] However all of these mechanisms are different therapy ways, they can become interpenetrate with each others. The important point is that, it is supposed that the psychosomatic effects which give rise to curative features of AAT occurs when these mechanisms start to work. All of the mechanism together revealed that psychosomatic effects of human-animal bond and interaction in people taking an AAT and AAA. [5], [6]

Lafrance et al., reported that patients' social and verbal behaviors have been improved in a presence of a therapy dog. [7] Nathans et al., revealed that Animal Assisted Therapy can be used for improving anhedonia in patients with schizophrenia. In addition, they have found that AAT can be beneficial for rehabilitation of life quality and psycho-social behaviors. [8]

Different researchers have reported that AAT should be considered planning of the treatment of individual with dementia. [1], [9]- [12]

The interaction between an animal and human result in an increase neurochemicals initiating a decrease in blood pressure and relaxation. This relationship may be beneficial for ameliorating agitate behavior and psychological symptoms of dementia. In another study, it has been reported that aquarium assisted therapy may be beneficial for increasing eating behavior of aged people living in a nursing home. [10] Richeson revealed that AAT can be increase social interactions by initiating decrease the agitate behaviors of patients with dementia. [12] Kongable et al., observed that a therapy dog increased patients' some social behaviors such as smile, laugh, look, touch, verbalization. [13]

In aged people, AAT are used for ameliorating agitate behaviors, psychological, occupational, social and physical disorders especially in Alzheimer and Dementia. [14]- [20] People with Alzheimer may have an easier time decoding the simple repetitive, non-verbal actions of a dog. Animals can act as transitional objects, allowing people to first establish a bond with them and then extend this bond to people. Most of the study results revealed that AAT especially dog therapy had an "calming effect" on the patients with dementia and Alzheimer disease. [15]- [17], [20] This effect can be helpful as a communication link during therapy sessions and also decrease agitation behaviors. It is well known that incidence of aggression, agitation, social withdrawal, depression, and psychotic disorders are growing problems in Alzheimer disease for special care units, staff and family members of patients. Furthermore, environmental factors in nursing home or other health care units have been become increasingly forcible barrier for therapy of Alzheimer disease. In this conditions, AAT and other animal activities may be helpful to cope with these difficulties by presenting a different aspect.

AAT should be more commonly used in the world through increasing awareness of public health services about beneficials of companion animal and activities. Especially, AAT can be used for improving health disorders of aged people with physical-mental and social disabilities such as Alzheimer, dementia, aphasia, anxiety, depression, stres, schizophrenia, and feeling of loneliness, quality of life. An aquarium assisted therapy may be a good starting point to learn about benefits and facilities of AAT in developing countries like Turkey which have more lower the socio-economic groups than the developed countries.

Main principle of AAT is based on using psychosomatic effects, which appear as results of biological-physical-chemical changes during human and animal interactions. [4] Feeding animals or being together with animals cause these effects to appear, and play an important role in recovery of mental, social and physical health. [21] The strength of bonding between humans and animals has been revealed in a survey study, which is conducted on 14 veterinarians and 117 patients in Ontario. In the study, patients, whose pets are died, have received a survey to define causes and effects of their worries by a phone call or e-mail. Of 30% of participants has been observed to have severe worries. [22] This strong bonding between humans and animals can also affect physical and mental health, and sometimes death or loss of an animal can be so effective that it can change a subject's life. [23] Dog, horse and dolphin are the most commonly preferred animal species in animal assisted therapy.

There are also studies indicating that keeping an animal has positive effects on the community health. [24] Heady et. al. reported that AAT caused decreasing national health costs. [25] Governments have been recently realized the significance of interaction between humans and animals as well as the contributions into human health, life quality and economy. Many countries have passed laws, which are a new understanding to allow keeping animals in apartments for rent, so as to support pet owners. Positive measures are taken in many European countries to keep pets in houses by laws. [26] AAT is to benefit from animal companionship during a targeted therapy in order to facilitate achievement of optimum results in patients, and to support the therapy. It provides very positive effects like providing adaptations of subjects to stressful situations and hospital environments; decreasing anxiety, stress, pain and blood pressure; increasing mobility and muscle activity. It has been shown that guiding animals increase physical activity, help in prevention of some moods like loneliness and depression, improve daily life activities and provide a social support by increasing the life quality. [27]- [29]

2. Benefits of animal companionship for therapy from past to present

Close relationships between humans and animals are way back to the prehistoric ages. By using DNA techniques, it has been demonstrated that dogs might have been domesticated 100,000 years ago. [30] Animals have been used to improve emotional and functional conditions of humans since ancient Greeks. Ancient Greeks have used dog drawings in their therapeutic temples, and they have provided melancholic people to ride on horses so as to get rid of their diseased souls. These applications have been used later also by Romans. [31] A dog showing the way to a blind man is drawn on armor in Pompeii historical ruins. [32]

The first studies, which have shown animal assistance in therapy, were performed to recover behaviors of mentally ill people in 1792 in York Retreat in United Kingdom by using farm animals. [3] Florence Nightingale defined the significance of assisting animals for therapy as: "Especially during treatment of a patient with a chronic illness, a small pet is a perfect friend for the patient". [32]

Dogs were used in rehabilitation after the World War I, in the first half of the 20th century. To improve moods of American army officers, who experienced depression related to the war, dogs were given to them to keep in company. [33] In the same period, thousands of dogs were trained under a program to support blinded soldiers in Germany. In 1931, "Guiding Dogs Society" was established for blind people. Currently, dogs are being trained in order to support people with hearing problems; to alert people with seizures before the symptoms are started; and to support people with severe physical problems.

Similar applications have been widely spread all over the world, so they have helped thousands of people with disabilities to live freely. Lane et. al. have reported that this ability of dogs was very amazing, and this social support that they have provided for people they have accompanied was very significant. [34]

Since 1980s, animal assisted therapies, which have been performed by planning and an experienced team, have been shown to improve social functions and to be beneficial especially in elderly people, so studies about this issue have been supported. [35]- [37] Therefore, when it was 1990s, study results of many articles are published from different populations. [28], [29], [38]- [40] Sable explained in the manuscript how, especially dogs and cats, could contribute into well being of family members, with whom they lived all their lives, emotionally and socially. [39]

As mentioned before, the first scientific studies indicating effects of human and animal interactions have been conducted in the second half of 20th century. UK originated Society for Companion Animal Studies (SCAS) is established in 1979, whereas the international organization, named International Association of Human-Animal Interaction Organization (IA-HAIO) is established in 1990. IAHAIO is an affiliation of the World Health Organization, and it functions as a conductor organ among non-governmental organizations and other affiliations. The most marked point in the studies belonging to 2000s is that animal assisted therapy has been used against specific diseases, and evaluation of human-animal interaction results. [1], [23], [41]- [44]

Current patient healthcare methods, which are developing and containing evidence based interventions, are faced with some problems. Along with conventional treatments, complementary and adjuvant treatments are also included in these methods. Animal assisted therapy (AAT) is discussed as a supportive treatment approach with positive effects on life quality and health. [45]

3. Action mechanism in animal assisted therapies

Gagnon et. al. defined animal assisted therapy as a clinical intervention method, which has aimed to establish natural and improving bonding between humans and animals, and is applied for both preventive and therapeutic requirements. [46] Animal assisted therapy (AAT) can be applied through different action mechanisms in respect with the disease type and individual characteristics. Five factors directing the mechanism are psychological impulse, emotional, physical and playing mechanisms. [4] Although these mechanisms are defined separately, they cannot be considered independent from each other for functioning and developing of psychosomatic effects. The most important point in the treatment is human-animal interaction. This interaction constitutes a strong emotional background. It has been reported result benefits would depend on the strength of the emotional interactions.

In another words, confident, positive and sedative bonding between a human and an animal can trigger beneficial mechanisms by affecting secretions of adrenaline (epinephrine) and other corticosteroid hormones or stress hormones (like cortisol etc.); decreasing arterial blood pressure, cardiac and respiratory rates. Emotional, psychological impulse, playing and physical mechanisms used in AAT applications cause psychosomatic effects.

Understanding of "play" principle is quite important in animal assisted therapy. Ballarini reported that activities like "entertainment" and especially "laughing" are parts of the bonding between humans and animals. When an ill person plays with a cat or laughs at a dog's behavior, an increase in the healing potential of that illness is initiated. As playing increases mobility, it is a good physical activity source. [4] Haubenhofer and Kirchengast measured cortisol levels in saliva of dogs, which were involved in animal assisted interventions and therapies to investigate their physiological reactions. Cortisol levels, which were monitored during therapy sessions in the earlier time periods of day, were reported to be higher than those measured after the therapy and in the control periods. The study results showed that therapeutic work was physiologically activating for the dogs. [47] At this point, it may be considered that these physiologically changes occurred in dogs can result in positive reactions in humans during animal assisted therapies and activities. But, further research is needed to indicate whether these positive effects related to the animal assisted therapies or not.

We have already mentioned that action mechanism of AAT is based on positive-healing bonding, which has occurred by human-animal interaction, and psychological, emotional, playing and physical mechanisms, which have caused physical and biochemical reactions by activation of this bonding. [4], [46] Key structures activating these mechanisms in patients should be structured according to mainly four theories. These are touching, biophilia hypothesis, learning and cognitive theories. [48] In animal assisted therapy applications, all types of applications, which are performed according to these four theories, can provide various benefits.

Touching theory provides a special and continuous bonding between patient and animal at the first contact. The aim of this bonding is generally due to searching for closeness and tendency to preserve this closeness instinctively. It is normal that such a bonding occurs between an Alzheimer patient and a therapy dog. Because, may be, this is the first time that the patient has met another living organism without any prejudice, without verbal communication and agitated behaviors, and which has accepted him/her as he/she is. In this situation, patient firstly feels comfortable, and a trained dog will allow the patient to direct to itself first by expanding its limits, and allow the patient to touch it. Generally this initial contact in therapies is started with patient directing to the dog and touching it. During therapy period in this comfortable-caring treatment environment, many supportive benefits for clinical treatment compliance (being the leading one), relatives of patients, and healthcare personnel have been achieved.

Another important concept in therapies is *biophilia hypothesis*. As it has been mentioned in this review before, this concept defends that there is an instinctive, strong bonding between humans and all other living organisms, and both sides are in need of his strong bonding in order to survive. According to biophilia concept (short definition may be enthusiasm for life) human beings get in contact with the environment and all living creatures around genetically due to the human nature. This symbiotic relationship was started in the past, and continued in the present by contacting and keeping dogs, cats (the leading animals), other farm animals. As feeling of ownership has affected humans negatively in time, animals have been the mainly damaged side of this relationship. Especially animals, which we are calling currently domesticated, have moved away from their natural environments, and instead of living with humans, or accompanying humans, they have got under protection of humans. All other living creatures that human being as not felt close to himself, or could not domesticate or has not get under protection have remained as "Undomesticated-Wild". The reasons why we mention these philosophical approaches is the context of animal assisted therapies especially ethically, are applications, which are performed with animal companionship, and we would very much emphasize to use "living with the company of animals" term rather than "pet ownership" or "keeping an animal". Thus, "living with the company of animals" will be developed. May be this approach will help to develop the awareness of "living with somebody/living creature that is ill" rather than "having an ill relative". Then, experiencing the pure form of animal-human interaction at the beginning, and providing patient and his/her relatives to share this humane environment may reveal many positive effects, which we have not known or defined yet.

Learning theory, which is a model in psychology, defends that human beings give various responses to his/her surroundings by the learning principle. In AAT, the learning principle of the patient is triggered in a more human way; so a patient with Alzheimer's disease can show some behaviors that he or she has started to forget, without the degree of forgetting, in the same way again, or can show some behaviors for longer times without forgetting. For example, while feeding fish in the aquarium, their eating desire may be increased or they remember eating behavior and eat some food; while feeding a dog, they may start to use hand skills, so that these will help them to improve slightly their daily life activities etc. *This interaction with animals may be perceived as a more human approach than verbal reminding of healthcare personnel and/or patient's relatives or verbal commands of caregivers what to do. While healthcare personnel and/ or patient caregivers can be under intensive stress and may unintentionally pronounce these commands at higher and sharp voice tones, and they may even say/behave in agitated ways for patients.* Therefore, animal assisted therapies and activities can be a good supportive way in long term therapy and care for individuals with chronic diseases like Alzheimer's disease. *Cognitive theory*, which is another model in psychology, tries to explain human behaviors by investigating how human beings gain, process, and store the knowledge. Main headings in cognitive approach, which investigates perception of knowledge, processing of knowledge, and switching into behaviors, are perception language, attention, memory, problem solving, decision making-judging and intelligence.

As animals do not have any expectations and demands from humans at their first contacts, patients feel self-confidence, and they may feel that everything is under their controls. [48] Therefore, animals do not react like us when they meet a healthy or ill person. We, humans, tend to perceive, remember, shape up, judge with the previously learned concepts, and even show verbal-physical behaviors, when we first meet a healthy or ill person or any living being. This situation is quickly sensed and perceived by the opposite side. When a dog meets a blind, limb or amnestic person in the street, it will behave as if it has met a healthy individual. However, when we meet people with health problems in the street, we define them as "he has got no arm!", "he is blind!", "Is he a lunatic?", "ill person", and we imply our thoughts sometimes with words or sometimes with our behaviors. Due to these reasons, animal assisted therapies naturally eradicate negative conditions like these, and they provide a more humane surrounding for therapies of subjects with chronic diseases; they support them; they increase adaptation potentials of patients and their relatives to difficult therapy periods, and they improve their life qualities. After all, we should remembered that the aforementioned paragraphs are theoretical concepts which try to comprise biology, sociology, psychology and philosophy to explain some of the effects AAT on humans in general, not only for patients with Alzheimer's disease.

4. Fields of Animal Assisted Therapies (AAT)

According to medical studies and field screenings, it is evident that AAT has relaxing and supportive effects on humans. Recoveries obtained in some diseases through these positive interactions are listed in Table 1. [49], [34]- [39], [50] , [51]

Decreased anxiety and depression
Increased self-esteem
Increased impulse for communication
Decreased blood pressure
Increase in required motivation for recovery
Decrease in analgesic requirement in some patients, who have had previous operations
Improvement in communication with other patients or hospital personnel

Table 1. Main improvements observed in AAT applied subjects

This supportive therapy with various services is being provided to more than 35000 patients in more than 100 healthcare service units in San Francisco. Subjects mainly benefited from these services are as follows: *Children treated in pediatric clinic; AIDS patients; patients, who require acute care and physical rehabilitation services; children with conduct disorder and physical problems; subjects staying at hospitals (patients, their relatives and hospital personnel), patients with mental diseases.* Public health organizations currently provide various services with dogs suitable for therapies. Samples for some application fields of AAT are given in Table 2 regarding human health improvement and development. [4], [52]

As Ballarini has mentioned, AAT is no longer a mysterious application, but currently it has become a treatment option, which is applied for supportive aims, and has resulted in positive outcomes in many diseases. In recent years, AAT has gained more attention all over the world, and it is being preferred as a complimentary and supportive method to improve life quality and health in some therapies, during which various problems have arisen. [45], [53], [54] Therefore, many studies have been performed to establish its scientific background, and different AAT models are being developed. Dolphin assisted therapy is one of these, and it is employed as an adjunctive method in various diseases (Table 3). [55], [56] During therapies, it has been observed that dolphins have tried to communicate with ill subjects by increasing their sound levels. [57]

For psychological training

In children with poor or underdeveloped socialization attitudes,

In conduct disorders,

In children with low academic success and low self-esteem

To decrease hostile behaviors

In jails

In mental institutions with convicts

In reformatory schools

Psychiatric conditions

Mild or moderate autism

In treatment and prevention of depression symptoms in old people

Anxiety

Neuro-psychological tension

Medical interventions

In recovery periods of diseases

Arterial hypertension

Cardiopathies

Chronic muscle-nervous system diseases

Different motor disorder therapies and rehabilitation

Table 2. Application fields of AAT

Autism
Down syndrome
Rett syndrome
Depression (non-endogenous type)
Neurotic disorder
Brain trauma (without cramp syndrome)
Brain paralysis (without cramp syndrome)
Cerebral palsy in children
Childhood neurosis like fobby, enuresis and asthenia
Environmental conduct disorders
Support for post-coma treatment
Severe psychological and complex trauma
Cephalgia
Chronic fatigue syndrome
Delayed speech development
Delayed psychological development
Chronic diseases

Table 3. Some medical and mental health problems for application of dolphin therapy

5. AAT use in some chronic diseases

Since Alzheimer's disease is generally observed in elderly people, it may be concomitant with some other chronic diseases. Among these diseases, cardiovascular diseases are the leading ones. Conducted studies have indicated that systolic blood pressure and plasma triglyceride levels are lower in pet owner subjects when compared with the non-owners. [38] In Odendaal's study, neurochemicals (β-endorphin, oxytocin, prolactin, phenylacetic acid, dopamine, cortisol) related to drop down of blood pressure were evaluated between 18 subjects and 18 dogs before and after the positive interactions. Statistically significant data ($p<0.05$) have indicated that neurochemicals related to blood pressure are increased in both groups and attention behavior function is increased after AAT except cortisol (cortisol was low significantly in humans, but this decrease was not found to be significantly in dogs. [58] It has been reported in studies of another chronic disease, namely cancer, that AAT had positive effects both on patients and their relatives. [46], [59], [60] The positive effects are reported as decreased stress and anxiety; compliance with treatment and improvement in adaptation; relaxation; better nutrition; physical activity; socialization; participitating in new activities; verbalization of fright and concerns; decreased nervousness; increased feeling of happiness; thus improvement in life quality. [46], [60]

Similar results have been obtained in studies performed on disabled subjects. [61]- [64] Especially achieved improvements were increased non-verbal interactions, physical activities, and daily life activities leading to increased life quality. Although these studies have been performed commonly in children with widespread developmental disorders, it should also be considered that Alzheimer patients may have various disabilities, which would lower their life quality, so their daily life activities may be limited according to the stage and severity of disease. When evaluated in this aspect, animal assisted therapies will provide significant benefits.

In a study performed on AIDS patients, it has been reported that cat assisted therapy has supported patients' communications with their families and friends, and has provided prevention from the feeling of loneliness.

6. Psychological and psychiatric diseases

Animal assisted therapies are especially employed in hospitalized children and Alzheimer patients to decrease stress. Animal companionship is employed in anxiety, refusal of therapy, refusal of eating and decreasing other agitated behaviors, treatments of various psychological and psychiatric disorders o provide treatment compliance and to increase the life quality. Patients, who are hospitalized in rehabilitation centers are scheduled for weekly or monthly therapy programs with trained animals, so physical, emotional, social and cognitive benefit of AAT are used. It has been reported that blood pressure and cardiac rate are decreased, cortisol (stress hormone) is markedly decreased, and pain sensation is decreased.

Animal assisted therapy has been shown to be effective in patients with speech disorders like aphasia, schizophrenia and dementia (Table 4). [3], [7], [8], [12], [51]

Reference	Patients, study group	Pet therapy model	Results
Macauley BL, 2006[3]	Three men with aphasia from left-hemisphare strokes and during AAT therapy with a 8 year old neutered male Newfoundland dog participated into the study.	Dog therapy	Dog may act as an excellent catalyst to motivate the client to talk and provide an atmosphere of unconditional acceptance for the speech disorders and brain injuries.
LaFrance C et al, 2007[7]	A 61-year old male with non-fluent aphasia and a left cerebral vascular accident. A therapy dog was 5 year old tetriever.	Dog therapy	In condition with the dog and dog handler, it was found that both social verbal and non-verbal behaviors markedly increased in patient.
Nathans-Barel I et al, 2005[8]	Patients with hedonic tone of 10 chronic schizophrenia participated in 10 weekly sessions of AAT was compared to control group treated without animal.	Dog therapy	In AAT group, significant improvements of hedonic tone compared to control. It was observed that an increasing in use of leisure time and motivation.
Richeson N, 2003[12]	15 nursing home residents with dementia participated in a daily AAT for three weeks.	Dog therapy	Significant decrease in agitated behaviors and statistically significant increase in social interaction.
Kovács Z, 2004[51]	Seven schizophrenic patients living in a social institute participated into the study for 9 month treatment period. Each weekly therapeutic session was 50 min.	Dog therapy	AAT was found to be helpful in daily life activities and rehabilitation of schizophrenic patients. Significant improvement in domestic and health activities.

Table 4. Dog therapy models in aphasia, schizophrenia and dementia.

Nathan reported from his study that animal assisted therapy improved anhedonia in chronic schizophrenia patients. Anhedonia is one of the negative symptoms of dementia, and it is the main phenomenon related to poor social functionality and development of treatment resistance. In an active study performed with dogs, significant improvement has been observed in anhedonia in AAT group when compared with the controls. As a result of the study, it has been reported that animal assisted therapy might contribute in life quality and psychosocial rehabilitation of chronic schizophrenia patients.[8]

Antonioli and Reveley observed in their randomized, controlled study that depression symptoms were observed to be improved in the 2nd week of treatment in patients with mild-moderate depression. Antonioli responded the comment indicating that patient number was limited and study population was a specific group as this dolphin study has indicated that, according to "Biophilia" hypothesis, interaction between animals and humans could be beneficial in their natural environments. [65], [66] "Biophilia" term is first defined by psychologist Erich, and is based on "affection level, which is required for mental health and emotional well-being". [67] Kellert and Wilson improved biophilia concept, and stated that human health and well-being were related to interactions with the natural environments. [68]

7. How can a dog assisted therapy be beneficial for therapy in Alzheimer patients?

It may cause decreased agitation, improvement in the mood, and increased communication with the surrounding: Alzheimer patients may experience different clinical symptoms at different disease stages. Generally as the disease is progressed, they isolate themselves from their surroundings, family members, friends, healthcare personnel; they become quieter and less mobile. In this stage, an accompanying therapy dog may even become the only communication bridge to continue the interaction with their surroundings. Sometimes patients may end up the silence on a dog's touch or behaviors; they may smile, talk a few words, and even they may be involved more with their surroundings.

Indoor and outdoor safety problems are most commonly encountered problems in some patients. With the accompanying well-trained dog, the patient can feel more secure. Since the dog can estimate behaviors of the patient, it may warn the patient and his /her relatives and/or healthcare personnel before and/or during the behaviors. A guiding dog may prevent the patient, who would like to leave his/her surrounding (home or nursery home) without informing anybody, from many dangers he/she would be confronted with. When the patient come to the top of the ladder, the dog may inform the patient about his/her position, how he/she should act or what he/she should do next by barking or behaving differently non-verbally without agitating the patient. It may protect the patient while crossing the street. The dog guiding a patient, who will forget the way home or the address of his/her home, can lead the patient home safely and in good health.

Aquarium assisted therapy studies have revealed that eating habits of Alzheimer patients are improved by feeding fish. Moreover aquarium assisted activities improve hand skills as well as they increase socialization of patients. Various mood disorders like nervousness, agitation, unhappiness, very quietness, and loneliness may be observed in subjects with dementia, who live in nursery homes. Aquariums at nursery homes may attract attention of subjects in these crowded environments, they may provide relaxation and happiness for them as well as they may help people live in more humane environments by decreasing work load and stress also for relatives of patients and healthcare personnel. Aquariums may help all individuals to share the same environment with the underwater creatures.

AAT is especially effective in elderly subjects with cognitive disorders like Alzheimer disease. Patients with dementia usually experience various degrees of agitation mainly in the evening. This situation, known as "sundowning", is not only stressful for patients, but can also be challenging for the healthcare personnel. Even touching an animal may decrease anxiety during challenging evening hours, and increase calmness/well-being feelings.

It has been observed that responses have been achieved in patients with advanced dementia by animal assisted therapies. Some patients with dementia may develop better and easier communications with animals when compared with humans. A pet can listen to a patient with dementia without judging. In guiding dog visits in AAT program, dogs may allow patients to come near to them and play with them. It has been reported that dog assisted therapies may help these exercises to be happier and more motivating experiences in patients, who are recommended to take a walk. These patients are also reported to have improved life quality, and socialization desires when compared with patients, who have not kept or lived with animals.

A therapy dog provides the Alzheimer patient a unique communication and love bonding, which can be re-shaped according to the target whichever animal assisted therapy is required, and various physical, mental and social health benefits can be achieved. Fish, cat, dog, horse or tortoise may present human benefits, which we cannot presume for Alzheimer patients, and by supporting patients' treatment compliances, they provide that patient relatives and healthcare personnel serve under more positive conditions. To provide the most benefit from AAT or AAA, in especially dog therapies, "resident" or "visiting" models can be used together for patients with dementia and Alzheimer's disease. [14], [15], [18] It is not clearly explored which therapy model more useful than the other one. [9] In another review written by Williams and Jenkins reported that animal visitings to nursing-care units can provide various benefits including relaxation, improving of apathy and decreasing in agitation, aggression behavior and blood pressure for both patients and their caregivers, relatives. [18] According to the Churchill et al., a therapy dog can reduce some agitation behaviors of Alzheimer patients with especially sundown syndrome, and also help increasing social behaviors and calm down. [16]

Studies shown that environmental factors or changes in Alzheimer's disease special care units can be effect on patients' behavioral health outcomes including aggression, resident agitation, social withdrawal, depression, psychotic problems. [69], [70] That is why, treatment procedures should be planned and managed considering a balanced combination of pharmacologic, behavioral and environmental options in order to improve health, behavior and quality of life of patients with Alzheimer's disease. [70] It is important that physicians who are playing a key role in recognizing problems and arranging suitable treatment for their patients should consider alternative treatment options based on social and recreational interventions including meditation, validation therapy, reality orientation, reminiscence therapy, sensory interventions (therapeutic touch and massage therapy, aromatherapy, music therapy, dance therapy, light therapy, multisensory stimulation therapy), social contact (animal-assisted therapy, simulated presence therapy), exercise, art therapy and Montessori-based activities. [71], [72] In addition, most of the AAT studies have been focused on dog, cat and other small animal activities. It is not well-known that animal assisted therapies with farm animals may have positive effects on self-efficacy and coping ability among psychiatric patients. [73]

As displayed on Table 5, AAT especially dog therapies can be used successively as a preventive and interventional method in patients with Alzheimers' disease and dementia. Also, recent studies have shown that AAT may be beneficial to improve for various psychiatric diseases including Alzheimer, dementia, depression, anxiety, addiction, schizophrenia, autism spectrum disorder. [74]- [79]

Authors	Patients or study group	Pet therapy model	Results	Study design
Moretti F, et al. 2011	Over 84 age patients with dementia, depression and psychosis Pet group (n=10) Control group (n=11)	Dog therapy	Comparing to the control group, improvements as below was observed in the pet group: Decreasing of depression symptoms at 50% level and increasing 4.5 times in mini mental scores.	Methodological Study (6 weeks)
McCabe BW, et al. 2002	Patients with Alzheimer in a special care unit	Resident dog therapy in a special care unit	Significantly decreasing of problem behaviors at the end of the 4 weeks.	Methodological study (4 weeks)
Edwards NE and Beck AM, et al. 2002	62 patients with Alzheimer living a special care unit	Aquarium therapy used for improving nutrition intake behaviors	Since 2th weeks, nutritional intake behavior increased significantly and this increase kept on during 6 weeks. Over 16 week period, it was observed that patients had needed less nutritional supplements than baseline. Finally, authors indicated that dog therapy can provide health care cost savings (personal communication).	Methodological study (Follow-up) (6 weeks)
Fritz CL, et al. 1996	244 caregivers working with Alzheimer patients in Northern California. 124 caregivers contact with pets. 120 caregivers didn't contact with pets included into the control group.	Man and women contacted with pets regular (dog or cat)	It was observed that man who were attached to dogs scored better psychological health than men who had no pets. While, women less than 40 years old attached to cats were scored better some psychological health than women same aged and had no pets, women aged 40 to 59 years attached to dogs scored worse of life satisfaction and depression than women in the same age and had no pets.	Case-control study

Authors	Patients or study group	Pet therapy model	Results	Study design
Fritz CL, et al. 1995	64 Alzheimer patients living in a private nursing home.	Pet-therapy group: 34 patients contact with pets Control group: 34 patients didn't contact with pets.	It was observed that, verbal aggression and anxiety was reported less in patients exposed to companion animals than patients didn't exposed to pets.	Methodological study
Tribet J, et al. 2008	2 female and one male patients in a nursing home diagnosed with severe dementia.	A dog therapy used 15 times over 9 months. A therapy performed in the same place for 30 min, once a week.	Psychological benefits obtained from the study as follows: *Calming effect* was observed on the patients, which is this effect provided that communication link would be needed during therapy sessions. With the dogs' unconditional acceptance *increased patients' self-esteem* need to pateints felt theirselfs was in more secure environment. Addition, it was observed that their *social behaviours increased* by touching dog and its non-verbal communication.	Prospective-qualitative study
Kanamori M, et al. 2001	7 patients with senile dementia and 20 patients enrolled into the control group in an adult day care center.	AAT was used for 6 weeks. Before and after AAT was evaluated mini mental state, activities of daily living, behavioral pathology and salivary CgA.	The average mini mental state exam score was more higher than baseline, activities of daily living was more higher than baseline, behavioral pathology was more lower than baseline and finally salivary CgA was found to be decreasing tendency. Several methods can be used in order to show useful effects of AAT in patients with dementia as determined in this study by Kanamori M, et al.	Methodological study

Table 5. Animal Assisted Therapy Studies in patients with Alzheimer´s disease and other dementia

According to the literature, number of studies recommending animal assisted therapies in clinical and social medicine practices in elderly people with dementia, Alzheimer´s disease, ability losses, mental health problems and conduct disorders, cognitive problems, physical and functional health problems have been increased rapidly. [1-3], [63] Targeted acquisitions in AAT applications can be classified under five headings as social, psychological, training, physical and motivational. Moreover, what we expect from all applications in a patient with Alzheimer's disease are mainly physiological improvements, better focusing on environment, enabling physical contact, interaction with surroundings, improvements in nutritional behaviors, socialization, acceptance, motivation, increased physical activity, stress, decreased mood disorders like depression, and agitation, enjoying, and decreased feeling of loneliness.

8. Risks of AAT and Their managements

In USA, 60% of the population has at least one pet at home. Patients and animals participating in AAT require special care for prevention of zoonotic diseases, hypersensitivity reactions and injuries during visits. Therefore, the maximum benefit obtained from this therapy method depends on the multidisciplinary team work of a veterinarian specialist, a veterinarian public health specialist, a medical doctor, and an experienced therapist. [49], [80] Animal assisted therapy performed at treatment centers should always be performed following by a structured program, under the recommended guides, and targeted at the objectives of the program. [49] Hamsworth and Pizer reported after they investigated studies, which evaluated interactions with animals, and risk factors for zoonosis in immunocomprimised children, and guidelines that information obtained from specialists were not adequately evidence-based. Keeping an animal is beneficial for prevention and development of emotional and physical health. However, guidelines are also required to conduct treatments. [81]

Minimization of risks in such applications depends upon a careful planning with multidisciplinary approaches, written protocols, personnel training, documentation, and investigations. Veterinarian public health practices, which will be performed in this field, are important sources to keep risks endangering human and animal health at minimum levels. Especially veterinarians should choose the appropriate animal for therapy of each patient group according to temperament and behaviors of animals, perform the care for each animal, work for prevention of zoonotic diseases, and suggest an appropriate interaction model for the therapy. [32] Infection controlling policies and regulations should be obeyed in treatment and prevention of zoonotic diseases, so that animal assisted therapies will be more widespread. If measures for risk prevention are taken, then AAT applications can be performed safely. [82], [83]

In studies, where risk analyses have been performed, people interacting with pets have been observed to have benefits for their health. It has been reported from regions, where risks were not significantly high, controlled environmental conditions are provided especially in Europe and North America, potential benefits are reported in treatments with animals kept at home or at hospitals. Guidelines have been developed to limit infection risk during applications and to perform safe treatments. [84]- [86]

In addition to guidelines used during treatments, supportive units have also been established. Animal Assisted Crisis Response (AACR) unit is one of these. This unit provides services in how to struggle with the impending crises for assigned healthcare personnel, consultants and other trainers during animal assisted therapies. [87] Efficiency of these studies depends upon conductance of communication between the related units with a mutual language and a multidisciplinary approach. The most commonly encountered crises issues may be animal behavior, infection risk, and patient-trainer dispute.

Before starting animal assisted therapy and during its' all procedures, it is always remembered that AAT should be performed according to the guidelines in order to prevent risks including adverse reactions of patients, animals, physicians, caregivers, nurses, health personnels, and also relatives of patients, infectious diseases, bitings, etc. it is well clearly explained that AAT should be arranged, managed and performed by a specialist team including patients' physician, veterinary surgeon, psychologist, occupational therapist, expert caregivers, specialist nurses. Therefore, especially veterinary students should be trained about animal assisted therapies, activities and first of all human-animal bond during their undergraduate and postgraduate education. [88]- [91] At this point, according to the Timmins, a veterinary family practice conception can be helpful to understand and contribute human-animal bond from the theoretical framework into the practice for providing needs of patients. [92]

During applications, issues like increased work intensity of the personnel, zoonotic diseases, comfort and care of animals are considered. [93] These may be prevented by well-planned programming. [94] Disease risk can be easily prevented by regular animal health controls, and follow up of individuals. In developing countries like Turkey, animal assisted therapy is not practiced as a specialty filed, yet. Only limited services can be provided according to positive outcomes of human-animal interactions. But recently, an international project (Animals in Therapy Education) have been implemented for 2 years among different institutions from Turkey, Italy and France with financial supporting by European Union LLP Grundtvig Program for aged people. This project intends to design a collection of best practices related to implementation of pet therapy on aged people. As a result of this project will also ease the transfer of pet therapy practices through the comparison and the evaluation of different solutions adopted in the countries involved among partners from Italy, France and Turkey. [95]

9. Conclusion

In this present review, some information about what animal assisted therapies are, application fields, mechanism of action, sample applications for Alzheimer patients, and risk control in AAT, and some recommendations are suggested. It has been observed that this supportive therapeutic approach has been aimed at "complete well-being of individuals physically, socially and mentally as well as improvements of these well-being conditions", which is always emphasized in public health aspect. However, there are still some questions without clear answers, such as AAT is also effective in group therapies as it has been in individualized therapy; how temperament and other features of assisting animal should be. Whatever types the program is, temperaments of all animals should be tested; they should be examined by a veterinarian; and listening-learning training should be performed with patients.

When AAT is practiced according to guidelines, appropriate ethical principles, then it will be an effective supportive treatment option for improvement of human health, life quality, and especially preservation of health state of individuals. However, as it has been undertaken in this present review, it is believed that studies related to animal assisted therapies are required also in our country to evaluate its efficacies in different patient groups correctly.

Author details

Sibel Cevizci[1*], Halil Murat Sen[2], Fahri Güneş[3] and Elif Karaahmet[4]

*Address all correspondence to: cevizci.sibel@gmail.com

1 Canakkale Onsekiz Mart University, School of Medicine, Department of Public Health, Canakkale, Turkey

2 Canakkale Onsekiz Mart University, School of Medicine, Department of Neurology, Canakkale, Turkey

3 Canakkale Onsekiz Mart University, School of Medicine, Department of Internal Medicine, Canakkale, Turkey

4 Canakkale Onsekiz Mart University, School of Medicine, Department of Psychiatry, Canakkale, Turkey

References

[1] Laun, L. Benefits of pet therapy in dementia. Home Healthc Nurse (2003). , 21, 49-52.

[2] Sockalingam, S, Li, M, Krishnadev, U, et al. Use of animal-assisted therapy in the rehabilitation of an assault victim with a concurrent mood disorder. Issues Ment Health Nurs (2008). , 29, 73-84.

[3] Macauley, B. L. Animal-assisted therapy for persons with aphasia: A pilot study. J Rehabil Res Dev (2006). , 43, 357-366.

[4] Ballarini, G. Pet therapy Animals in Human Therapy. Conference Report. Acta Bio Medica (2003). , 74, 97-100.

[5] Cevizci, S, Erginöz, E, & Baltas, Z. A new assisted therapy concept for improving of mental health- Animal assisted therapy. Nobel Med (2009). , 5(1), 4-9.

[6] Cevizci, S, Erginöz, E, & Baltas, Z. Animal assisted therapy for improving human health. TAF Prev Med Bull (2009). , 8(3), 263-272.

[7]   LaFrance CGarcia LJ, Labreche J. The effect of a therapy dog on the communication skills of an adult with aphasia. J Commun Disord (2007). , 40(3), 215-224.

[8]   Nathans-barel, I, Feldman, P, Berger, B, et al. Animal-assisted therapy ameliorates anhedonia in schizophrenia patients. A controlled pilot study. Psychother Psychosom (2005). , 74(1), 31-35.

[9]   Filan, S. L, & Llewellyn-jones, R. H. Animal-assisted therapy for dementia: a review of the literature. Int Psychogeriatr (2006). , 18(4), 597-611.

[10] Edwards, N. E, & Beck, A. M. Animal-assisted therapy and nutrition in Alzheimer's disease. West J Nurs Res (2002). , 24(6), 697-712.

[11] Libin, A, & Cohen-mansfield, J. Therapeutic robocat for nursing home residents with dementia: preliminary inquiry. Am J Alzheimers Dis Other Demen (2004). , 19(2), 111-116.

[12] Richeson, N. Effects of animal-assisted therapy on agitated behaviors and social interactions of older adults with dementia. Am J Alzheimers Dis Other Demen (2003). , 18(6), 353-358.

[13] Kongable, L. G, Buckwalter, K. C, & Stolley, J. M. The effects of pet therapy on the social behavior of institutionalized Alzheimer's clients. Arch Psychiatr Nurs. (1989). , 3(4), 191-8.

[14] Perkins, J, Bartlett, H, Travers, C, & Rand, J. Dog-assisted therapy for older people with dementia: a review. Australas J Ageing. (2008). , 27(4), 177-82.

[15] Tribet, J, Boucharlat, M, & Myslinski, M. Animal-assisted therapy for people suffering from severe dementia. Encephale. (2008). , 34(2), 183-6.

[16] Churchill, M, Safaoui, J, Mccabe, B. W, & Baun, M. M. Using a therapy dog to alleviate the agitation and desocialization of people with Alzheimer's disease. J Psychosoc Nurs Ment Health Serv. (1999). , 37(4), 16-22.

[17] Mccabe, B. W, Baun, M. M, Speich, D, & Agrawal, S. Resident dog in the Alzheimer's special care unit. West J Nurs Res. (2002). , 24(6), 684-96.

[18] Williams, E, & Jenkins, R. Dog visitation therapy in dementia care: a literature review. Nurs Older People. (2008). , 20(8), 31-5.

[19] Kanamori, M, Suzuki, M, Yamamoto, K, Kanda, M, Matsui, Y, Kojima, E, Fukawa, H, Sugita, T, & Oshiro, H. A day care program and evaluation of animal-assisted therapy (AAT) for the elderly with senile dementia. Am J Alzheimers Dis Other Demen. (2001). , 16(4), 234-9.

[20] Cevizci, S. AAT in Turkiye. ATE: Animals in Therapy Education, European Community, LLP Grundtvig Program. Second Project Meeting, Istanbul, Turkiye, March (2011). , 3-4.

[21]   Friedmann, E, & Son, H. The human-companion animal bond: how human benefit. Vet Clin North Am Small Anim Pract (2009). , 39(2), 293-326.

[22]   Adams, C. L, Bonnett, B. N, & Meek, A. H. Predictors of owner response to companion animal death in 177 clients from 14 practices in Ontario. J Am Vet Med Assoc (2000). , 217(9), 1303-1309.

[23]   Clements, P. T, Benasutti, K. M, & Carmone, A. Support for bereaved owners of pets. Perspect Psychiatr Care (2003). , 39(2), 49-54.

[24]   Serpell, J. Beneficial effects of pet ownership on some aspects of human health and behaviour. Journal of the Royal Society of Medicine (1991). , 84, 717-720.

[25]   Headey, B, Grabka, N. A, F, Zheung, M, & Pets, R. and human health in Australia, China and Germany: evidence from three continents. 10th International IAHAIO Conference on Human-Animal Interactions. Glasgow, UK, (2004).

[26]   Bryant, I, & Mcbride, A. Pets, Policies and Tenants: Report on PATHWAY Housing provider 'Pet Policy' Survey. London, Dogs Trust. (2004).

[27]   Dembicki, D, & Anderson, J. Pet ownership may be a factor in improved health of the elderly. J Nutr Elder (1996). , 15(3), 15-31.

[28]   Raina, P, Waltner-toews, D, Bonnett, B, et al. Influence of companion animals on the physical and psychological health of older people: an analysis of a one-year longitudinal study. J Am Geriatr Soc (1999). , 47(3), 323-329.

[29]   Friedmann, E, & Thomas, S. A. Pet ownership, social support, and one-year survival after acute myocardial infarction in the Cardiac Arrhythmia Suppression Trial (CAST). Am J Cardiol (1995). , 76(17), 1213-1217.

[30]   Vila, C, Savolainen, P, Maldonado, J. E, et al. Multiple and ancient origins of the domestic dog. Science (1997). , 276, 1687-1689.

[31]   Rennie, A. The therapeutic relationship between animals and humans. SCAS Journal (1997). IX;, 1-4.

[32]   Ormerod, E. J. Edney ATB, Foster SJ, Whyham MC. Therapeutic applications of the human-companion animal bond. Veterinary Record (2005). , 157, 689-691.

[33]   Bustad, L. The role of pets in therapeutic programmes, historic perspectives. In The Waltham Book of Human-Animal Interaction: Benefits and Responsibility of Pet Ownership. Ed I. Robinson. Oxford, Pergamon Press. (1995). , 55-57.

[34]   Lane, D. R, Mcnicholas, J, & Collis, G. M. Dogs for the disabled: benefits to recipients and welfare of the dog. Applied Animal Behaviour Science (1998). , 59, 49-60.

[35]   Ryder, E. L. Pets and the elderly. A social work perspective. Vet Clin North Am Small Anim Pract (1985). , 15(2), 333-343.

[36] Beck, A. M. The therapeutic use of animals. Vet Clin North Am Small Anim Pract (1985). , 15(2), 365-75.

[37] Messent, P. R. Pets as social facilitators. Vet Clin North Am Small Anim Pract (1985). , 15(2), 387-393.

[38] Anderson, W. P, Reid, C. M, & Jennings, G. L. Pet ownership and risk factors for cardiovascular disease. Med J Aust (1992). , 157(5), 298-301.

[39] Sable, P. Pets, attachment, and well-being across the life cycle. Soc Work (1995). , 40(3), 334-341.

[40] Graf, S. The elderly and their pets. Supportive and problematic aspects and implications for care. A descriptive study. Pflege (1999). , 12(2), 101-111.

[41] Johnson, R. A, & Meadows, R. L. Older Latinos, pets, and health. West J Nurs Res (2002). , 24(6), 609-620.

[42] Shore, E. R, Douglas, D. K, & Riley, M. L. What's in it for the companion animal? Pet attachment and college students' behaviors toward pets. J Appl Anim Welf Sci (2005). , 8(1), 1-11.

[43] Neidhart, L, & Boyd, R. Companion animal adoption study. J Appl Anim Welf Sci (2002). , 5(3), 175-192.

[44] Wright, J. D, Kritz-silverstein, D, Morton, D. J, et al. Pet Ownership and Blood Pressure in Old Age. Epidemiology (2007). , 18(5), 613-618.

[45] Cole, K. M, & Gawlinski, A. Animal-assisted therapy: the human-animal bond. AACN Clin Issues (2000). , 11(1), 139-149.

[46] Gagnon, J, Bouchard, F, Landry, M, et al. Implementing a hospital-based animal therapy program for children with cancer: a descriptive study. Can Oncol Nurs J (2004). , 14(4), 217-222.

[47] Haubenhofer, D. K, & Kirchengast, S. Physiological arousal for companion dogs working with their owners in animal-assisted activities and animal-assisted therapy. J Appl Anim Welf Sci (2006). , 9(2), 165-172.

[48] Fine, A. H. Handbook on Animal-Assisted Therapy: Theoratical Foundations and Guidlines for Practice. Chapter 2. Kruger AK, Serpell JA. Animal-Assisted Interventions in Mental Health: Definitions and Theoretical Foundations. S: 0-12369-484-1Press, (2006). by Elsevier. http://www.scribd.com/doc/76130150/1/CHAPTER-1#page=40Access time: 03.06.2012], 21-38.

[49] Jofré, M L. Animal-assisted therapy in health care facilities. Rev Chilena Infectol (2005). , 22(3), 257-263.

[50] http://wwwsfspca.org/info_rack/aat.pdf

[51] Kovács, Z, Kis, R, Rózsa, S, & Rózsa, L. Animal-assisted therapy for middle-aged schizophrenic patients living in a social institution. A pilot study. Clin Rehabil (2004). , 18(5), 483-486.

[52] Niksa, E. The use of animal-assisted therapy in psychiatric nursing: the story of Timmy and Buddy. J Psychosoc Nurs Ment Health Serv (2007). , 45(6), 56-58.

[53] Connor, K, & Miller, J. Help from our animal friends. Nurs Manage (2000). , 31(7), 42-6.

[54] Connor, K, & Miller, J. Animal-assisted therapy: an in-depth look. Dimens Crit Care Nurs (2000). , 19(3), 20-26.

[55] Brensing, K, Linke, K, & Todt, D. Can dolphins heal by ultrasound? J Theor Biol (2003). , 225(1), 99-105.

[56] http://www.dolphinchildtherapy.com/index.asp?langid=70000&location=1#indikationen

[57] Akiyama, J, & Ohta, M. Increased number of whistles of bottlenose dolphins, Tursiops truncatus, arising from interaction with people. J Vet Med Sci (2007). , 69(2), 165-170.

[58] Odendaal, J. S. Animal-assisted therapy-Magic or medicine? J Psychosom Res. (2000). , 49(4), 275-80.

[59] Johnson, R. A, Meadows, R. L, Haubner, J. S, & Sevedge, K. Animal-assisted activity among patients with cancer: effects on mood, fatigue, self-perceived health, and sense of coherence. Oncol Nurs Forum (2008). , 35(2), 225-32.

[60] Sobo, E. J, Eng, B, & Kassity-krich, N. Canine visitation (pet) therapy: pilot data on decreases in child pain perception. J Holist Nurs. (2006). , 24(1), 51-7.

[61] Esteves, S. W, & Stokes, T. Social Effects of a Dog's Presence on Children with Disabilities. Anthrozoos (2008). , 21(1), 5-15.

[62] Yorke, J, Adams, C, & Coady, N. Therapeutic Value of Equine-Human Bonding in Recovery from Trauma. Anthrozoös (2008). , 21(1), 17-30.

[63] Lotan, M. Alternative therapeutic intervention for individuals with Rett syndrome. Scientific World Journal (2007). , 7, 698-714.

[64] Burrows, K. E, Adams, C. L, & Spiers, J. Sentinels of safety: service dogs ensure safety and enhance freedom and well-being for families with autistic children. Qual Health Res. (2008). , 18(12), 1642-1649.

[65] Basil, B, & Mathews, M. Human and animal health: strengthening the link: methodological concerns about animal facilitated therapy with dolphins. BMJ (2005).

[66] Antonioli, C, & Reveley, M. A. Randomised controlled trial of animal facilitated therapy with dolphins in the treatment of depression. BMJ (2005).

[67] Kellert, S. R. Kinship to mastery. Biophilia in human evolution and development. Washington DC:Island Press (1997). , 1997, 3-115.

[68] Kellert, S. R, & Wilson, E. O. Thebiophilia hypothesis. Washington DC: Island Press, (1993).

[69] Sloane, P. D, Mitchell, C. M, Preisser, J. S, Phillips, C, Commander, C, & Burker, E. Environmental correlates of resident agitation in Alzheimer's disease special care units. J Am Geriatr Soc. (1998). , 46(7), 862-9.

[70] Zeisel, J, Silverstein, N. M, Hyde, J, Levkoff, S, Lawton, M. P, & Holmes, W. Environmental correlates to behavioral health outcomes in Alzheimer's special care units. Gerontologist. (2003). , 43(5), 697-711.

[71] Teri, L, & Logsdon, R. Assessment and management of behavioral disturbances in Alzheimer's disease. Compr Ther. (1990). , 16(5), 36-42.

[72] Manepalli, J, Desai, A, & Sharma, P. Psychosocial-Environmental Treatments for Alzheimer's Disease. Primary Psychiatry. (2009). , 16(6), 39-47.

[73] Berget, B, Ekeberg, O, & Braastad, B. O. Animal-assisted therapy with farm animals for persons with psychiatric disorders: effects on self-efficacy, coping ability and quality of life, a randomized controlled trial. Clin Pract Epidemiol Ment Health. (2008).

[74] Rossetti, J, & King, C. Use of animal-assisted therapy with psychiatric patients. J Psychosoc Nurs Ment Health Serv. (2010). , 48(11), 44-8.

[75] Knisely, J. S, Barker, S. B, & Barker, R. T. Research on benefits of canine-assisted therapy for adults in nonmilitary settings. US Army Med Dep J. (2012). , 2012, 30-7.

[76] Bánszky, N, Kardos, E, Rózsa, L, & Gerevich, J. The psychiatric aspects of animal assisted therapy]. Psychiatr Hung. (2012). , 27(3), 180-90.

[77] Javelot, H, Antoine-bernard, E, Garat, J, Javelot, T, Weiner, L, & Mervelay, V. Snoezelen and animal-assisted therapy in dementia patients]. Soins Gerontol. (2012).

[78] Marcus, D. A. Complementary medicine in cancer care: adding a therapy dog to the team. Curr Pain Headache Rep. (2012). , 16(4), 289-91.

[79] Aoki, J, Iwahashi, K, Ishigooka, J, Fukamauchi, F, Numajiri, M, Ohtani, N, & Ohta, M. Evaluation of cerebral activity in the prefrontal cortex in mood [affective] disorders during animal-assisted therapy (AAT) by near-infrared spectroscopy (NIRS): A pilot study. Int J Psychiatry Clin Pract. (2012). , 16(3), 205-13.

[80] Hoff, G. L, Brawley, J, & Johnson, K. Companion animal issues and the physician. South Med J (1999). , 92(7), 651-659.

[81] Hemsworth, S, & Pizer, B. Pet ownership in immunocompromised children-a review of the literature and survey of existing guidelines. Eur J Oncol Nurs (2006). , 10(2), 117-27.

[82] Guay, D. R. Pet-assisted therapy in the nursing home setting: potential for zoonosis. Am J Infect Control (2001). , 29(3), 178-186.

[83] Brickel, C. M. The therapeutic roles of cat mascots with a hospital-based geriatric population: a staff survey. Gerontologist (1979). , 19, 368-372.

[84] Writing Panel of Working GroupLefebvre SL et al. Guidelines for animal-assisted interventions in health care facilities. Am J Infect Control (2008). , 36(2), 78-85.

[85] DiSalvo HHaiduven D, Johnson N, et al. Who let the dogs out? Infection control did: utility of dogs in health care settings and infection control aspects. Am J Infect Control (2006). , 34(5), 301-307.

[86] Brodie, S. J, Biley, F. C, & Shewring, M. An exploration of the potential risks associated with using pet therapy in healthcare settings. J Clin Nurs (2002). , 11(4), 444-456.

[87] Greenbaum, S. D. Introduction to working with Animal Assisted Crisis Response animal handler teams. Int J Emerg Ment Health. (2006). , 8(1), 49-63.

[88] Schaffer, C. B. Enhancing human-animal relationships through veterinary medical instruction in animal-assisted therapy and animal-assisted activities. J Vet Med Educ. (2008). , 35(4), 503-10.

[89] Sherman, B. L, & Serpell, J. A. Training veterinary students in animal behavior to preserve the human-animal bond. J Vet Med Educ. (2008). , 35(4), 496-502.

[90] Wensley, S. P. Animal welfare and the human-animal bond: considerations for veterinary faculty, students, and practitioners. J Vet Med Educ. (2008). , 35(4), 532-9.

[91] Ormerod, E. J. Bond-centered veterinary practice: lessons for veterinary faculty and students. J Vet Med Educ. (2008). , 35(4), 545-52.

[92] Timmins, R. P. The contribution of animals to human well-being: a veterinary family practice perspective. J Vet Med Educ. (2008). , 35(4), 540-4.

[93] Khan, M. A, & Farrag, N. Animal assisted activity and infection control implications in a healthcare setting. Journal of Hospital Infection (2000). , 46, 4-11.

[94] Jorgenson, J. Therapeutic uses of companion animals in health care. Journal of Nursing Scholarship (1997). , 29, 249-254.

[95] ATE: Animals in Therapy Educationhttp://www.forsas.it/ate/Sito%20Eng/Ate_en.pdfAccess time: 12.07.(2012).

Chapter 2

Potential Therapeutic Strategies to Prevent the Progression of Alzheimer to Disease States

Ester Aso and Isidre Ferrer

Additional information is available at the end of the chapter

1. Introduction

Alzheimer is an age-dependent neurodegenerative process distinct from normal aging and characterized morphologically by the presence of senile plaques and neurofibrillary tangles, which progress from the brain stem and inner parts of the temporal lobes to most the telencephalon.

Senile plaques are mainly composed of different species of fibrillar β-amyloid (Aβ), a product of the cleavage of the β-amyloid precursor protein (APP), and they are surrounded by dystrophic neurites, reactive astrocytes and microglia. Aβ fibrillar deposits also occur in diffuse plaques, subpial deposits and in the wall of the cerebral and meningeal blood vessels in the form of amyloid angiopathy. A substantial part of β-amyloid is not fibrillar but soluble and forms oligomers of differing complexity which are toxic to nerve cells.

Neurofibrillary tangles are mainly composed of various isoforms of tau protein, which is hyper-phosphorylated and nitrated. It has an altered conformation and is truncated at different sites through the action of a combination of several proteolytic enzymes giving rise to species of low molecular weight which are toxic to nerve cells. Abnormal tau deposition also occurs in the dystrophic neurites of senile plaques and within the small neuronal processes, resulting in the formation of neuropil threads.

The mechanisms of disease progression are not completely understood but Aβ initiates the pathological process in the small percentage of familial cases due to mutations in genes encoding APP, presenilin 1 and presenilin 2, the latter involved in the cleavage of APP, and potentiates tau phosphorylation in sporadic cases that represent the majority of affected individuals (β-amyloid cascade hypothesis). Moreover, Aβ act as a seed of new β-amyloid production and deposition under appropriate settings, and abnormal tau promotes the production and deposition of hyper-phosphorylated tau. Therefore, Aβ and hyper-phosphorylated tau promote the progression of the process and this may occur in an exponential way once these abnormal proteins are accumulated in the brain.

In addition to these pathological hallmarks, multiple alterations play roles in the degenerative process. Several genetic factors, such as apolipoprotein ε4 (APOE4), and external factors, such as vascular and circulatory alterations and repeated cerebral traumatisms, among others, facilitate disease progression in sporadic forms. Furthermore, metabolic components mainly, but not merely, associated with aging have a cardinal influence, including mitochondrial defects and energy production deficiencies, production of free radicals (oxidative and nitrosative reactive species: ROS and NOS) and oxidative and nitrosative damage, increased reticulum stress damage, altered composition of membranes, inflammatory responses and impaired function of degradation pathways such as autophagy and ubiquitin-proteasome system.

It has been proven that the degenerative process, at least the presence of neurofibrillary tangles, starts in middle age in selected nuclei of the brain stem and entorhinal cortex, and then progresses to other parts of the brain. Instrumental stages of Braak cover stages I and II with involvement of the entorhinal and transentorhinal cortices; stages II and IV also affect the hippocampus and limbic system together with the basal nucleus of Meynert; and stages V and VI involve the whole brain although neurofibrillary tangles are not found in selected regions such as the cerebellar cortex and the dentate gyrus. The distribution of senile plaques is a bit different as they first appear in the orbitofrontal cortex and temporal cortex and then progress to the whole convexity.

A concomitant decline in neuronal organization occurs most often in parallel with senile plaques and neurofibrillary tangles manifested as synaptic dysfunction and synaptic loss, and neuronal death and progressive isolation of remaining neurons.

An important observation is that about 80% of individuals aged 65 years have Alzheimer-related changes, at least at stages I-III, whereas only 5% have cognitive impairment and dementia. About 25% of individuals aged 85 years suffer from cognitive impairment and dementia of Alzheimer type. Stages I-IV are often silent with no clinical symptoms. Cognitive impairment and dementia usually occur at stages V and VI when the neurodegenerative process is very advanced. Importantly, the progression from stage I to stage IV may last decades, whereas the progression to stages V and VI is much more rapid. Therefore, Alzheimer is a well-tolerated degenerative process during a relatively long period of time, but it may have devastating effects once thresholds are crossed. Moreover, clinical symptoms may be complicated by concomitant vascular pathology.

Several attempts have been made to predict the evolution to disease states. Neuroimaging, including high resolution and functional magnetic resonance imaging, positron emission tomography and the use of relative selective markers of β-amyloid and tau deposition in the brain, together with reduced levels of Aβ and increased index of phospho-tau/total tau in the cerebrospinal fluid, are common complementary probes (biomarkers) in addition to the data provided by the neuropsychological examination. Unfortunately, these tests, at present, detect relatively advanced stages of the process in pathological terms.

It is very illustrating to visualize under the microscope how a brain at middle stages of the degenerative process has been working without apparent neurological deficits during life. The adaptive capacities of the brain in coping with current functions in spite of the decrepitude of composition and organization resulting from the chronic progression of the degenerative process are impressive.

Taking into consideration this scenario, it is compulsory to increase understanding of the first stages of the degenerative process and to act on selective targets before the appearance of clinical symptoms.

The present review is not a mere list of putative treatments of Alzheimer's disease (AD) but rather an approach to learning about observations made on experimental models and early stages of disease aimed at curbing or retarding disease progression on the basis of definite rationales. It is also our aim to encourage the consideration of Alzheimer as a degenerative process not necessarily leading to dementia [1]. This concept has important clinical implications as it supports early preventive measures in the population at risk (i.e. persons over 50 years) even in the absence of clinical symptoms.

2. Experimental therapeutic strategies to prevent Alzheimer progression to Alzheimer Disease (AD) states

Several reviews have focused on various aspects related to habits and dietary elements which may act as protective factors against AD, including physical and mental exercise, low caloric intake, various diets with low fat content, and vitamin complements [2, 3]. It is worth noting that neuropathological studies in old-aged individuals usually present combined pathologies, and combination of Alzheimer changes and vascular lesions are very common [4]. It is well documented that vascular pathology potentiates primary neurodegenerative pathology and that vascular factors may be causative of cognitive impairment and dementia [5]. Therefore, therapies geared to reduce vascular risk factors are also protective factors against AD clinical manifestations.

2.1. Targeting Aβ

Most of the current drug development for the prevention or treatment of AD is based on the β-amyloid cascade hypothesis and aims at reducing the levels of Aβ in the brain. Overproduction, aggregation and deposition of the Aβ peptide begin before the onset of symptoms and they are considered an essential early event in AD pathogenesis. Thus, targeting these early Aβ alterations is assumed to reduce the progression to disease states. The different strategies developed to achieve this objective include decreasing Aβ production through modulating secretase activity, interfering with Aβ aggregation, and promoting Aβ clearance.

2.1.1. Secretase-targeting therapies

APP is processed in the brain exclusively by three membrane-bound proteases, α-, β- and γ-secretase. Therefore, specifically modifying such enzyme activity should result in a reduction of Aβ production [6].

* *α-secretase activators*: α-secretase initiates the non-amyloidogenic pathway by cleaving APP within the Aβ sequence, thereby preventing the production of Aβ and producing a non-toxic form of APP derivative which is neuroprotective and growth- promoting [7]. Therefore, compounds that stimulate α-secretase activity could become an attractive strategy to reduce Aβ production. In fact, some indirect methods of promoting α-secretase activity, such as the stimulation of the protein kinase C (PKC) or Mitogen-activated protein kinases (MAPK) pathways, the use of α-7-nicotinic acetylcholine (ACh) receptor and 5-hydroxi-tryptamine (5-HT) receptor 4 agonists, and γ-aminobutyric acid A receptor modulators, result in α-secretase-mediated cleavage of APP and reduced Aβ levels *in vivo* [8]. However, the development of a direct activator of α-secretase as a drug treatment for AD seems premature because of the lack of knowledge about the consequences of chronic up-regulation of α-secretase-mediated cleavage on other substrates [6].

* *β-secretase inhibitors*: the β-secretase enzyme initiates the amyloidogenic pathway, cleaving APP at the amino terminus of the Aβ peptide. Further cleavage of the resulting carboxy-terminal fragment by γ-secretase results in the release of Aβ. β-secretase activity is specifically mediated by the β-site APP cleaving enzyme 1 (BACE1), which is also involved in the processing of numerous substrates in addition to APP. The research of drugs inhibiting BACE1 activity was encouraged by studies revealing that the expression of mutated BACE1 reduces amyloidogenesis and cognitive impairment in APP transgenic mice [9, 10]. The first generation of BACE1 inhibitors was peptide-based mimetics of the APP β-cleavage site. Unfortunately, these compounds exhibited some difficulties because of the large substrate binding site of BACE1 and because of the difficulty in crossing the blood–brain barrier (BBB) and penetrating the plasma and endosomal membranes to gain access to the intracellular compartments where endogenous BACE1 plays its function. Recently, non-peptide small-molecule BACE1 inhibitors have been reported to improve bioavailability and to lower cerebral Aβ levels in animal models of AD [11, 12]. However, the involvement of BACE1 in other important physiological processes raises concerns about minimizing the potential adverse effects derived from generalized BACE1 inhibition.

* *γ-secretase inhibitors (GSIs)*: γ-secretase is a complex composed of presenilin 1 and presenilin 2 (PS1 and PS2) forming the catalytic core and three accessory proteins, anterior pharynx-defective 1 (APH-1), nicastrin and presenilin enhancer protein 2 (PEN2). The γ-secretase complex displays a high degree of subunit heterogeneity and little is known about the physiological roles of the diverse complexes and how they process different trans-membrane substrates in addition to APP. This heterogeneity suggests that selective targeting of one particular subunit might be a more effective treatment strategy than non-selective γ-secretase inhibition [13]. Thus, removal of APH-1B and APH-1C isoforms in a mouse model of AD decreased Aβ plaque formation and improved behavioral deficits [14]. A number of orally bioavailable and brain-penetrating GSIs have been shown to decrease Aβ production

and deposition in APP mouse models and in humans [15-17]. However, target-based toxicity of GSIs has been a major obstacle to the clinical development of these compounds. In fact, two large Phase III clinical trials of *Semagacestat*, the only GSI extensively studied in AD, were prematurely interrupted because of the observation of detrimental cognitive and functional effects of the drug [18]. Several dozen γ-secretase substrates have been identified, including Notch1 trans-membrane receptor, which plays an important role in a variety of developmental and physiological processes by controlling cell fate decisions. To overcome these toxicity issues, pharmaceutical companies have been trying to develop a second generation of 'Notch-sparing' GSIs, which revealed beneficial effects in *in vitro* and in animal models of AD [19-21]. They are currently under clinical studies. Such 'Notch-sparing' GSIs have higher pharmacological selectivity than the first GSIs probably due to the distinct binding to the substrate docking site on γ-secretase of Notch and APP. Identification of several γ-secretase inhibitors has been reviewed elsewhere [22].

2.1.2. Aβ degrading enzymes

Almost 20 enzymes are currently known to contribute to Aβ degradation in the brain, although the most studied are two zinc metalloproteases, neprilysin (NEP) and insulin-degrading enzyme (IDE). NEP is one of the major Aβ-degrading enzymes in the brain [23] and NEP levels are decreased in the brain of AD and animal models [24, 25]. Lentiviral delivery of the NEP gene to the brain of AD transgenic mice reduced Aβ pathology [26]. A number of subsequent studies with NEP and other related peptidases such as endothelin-converting enzymes 1 and 2 (ECE-1 and ECE-2) further supported this observation [27]. Similarly, over-expression of IDE in neurons significantly reduces brain Aβ levels, prevents Aβ plaque formation and its associated cytopathology, and rescues the premature lethality present in these particular APP transgenic mice [28]. A growing body of evidence has been accumulated supporting the potential therapeutic properties of IDE in AD [29].

Other specific Aβ-cleaving proteases such as angiotensin-converting enzyme (ACE), matrix metalloproteinase-9 (MMP-9) and the serine protease plasmin, which have distinct sub-cellular localizations and differential responses to aging, oxidative stress and pharmacological agents, are also potential candidates to become novel therapeutic strategies for AD prevention and treatment [27].

Targeting the delivery of these compounds to the brain remains a major challenge. The most promising current approaches include peripheral administration of agents that enhance the activity of Aβ-degrading enzymes and direct intra-cerebral release of enzymes by convection-enhanced delivery. Genetic procedures geared at increasing cerebral expression of Aβ-degrading enzymes may offer additional advantages [30].

2.1.3. Decreasing Aβ aggregation

Compounds that suppress the aggregation or reduce the stability of Aβ oligomers may bind monomers in order to attenuate formation of both the oligomeric and senile plaque fibrillar Aβ constituents. One of the amyloid-binding drugs more extensively studied in animal models and AD patients is tramiprosate (3-amino-1-propanesulfonic acid; Alzhemed). Tramiprosate was effective in reducing Aβ polymerisation *in vitro*, inhibiting the formation of neurotoxic aggregates, and decreasing Aβ plaque formation in animal models [31]. However, recent phase III clinical trials did not produce any significant improvement in cognition in AD patients chronically treated with tramiprosate in spite of the significant reduction in hippocampus volume loss [32]. Similarly, some other compounds known to inhibit Aβ aggregation and fibril formation showed positive effects in animal and *in vitro* models of AD but failed to produce conclusive results in human clinical trials. This is the case with scyllo-inositol and PBT2. Scyllo-inositol inhibited cognitive deficits in TgCRND8 mice and significantly ameliorated disease pathology, even in animals at advanced stages of AD-like pathology, without interfering with endogenous phosphatidylinositol lipid production [33, 34]. Yet a phase II clinical trial failed in supporting or refuting a benefit of scyllo-inositol in mild to moderate AD patients [35]. PBT2 is a copper/zinc ionophore which targets metal-induced aggregation of Aβ. When given orally to two models of Aβ-bearing transgenic mice, PTB2 was able to markedly decrease soluble brain Aβ levels within hours and to improve cognitive performance within days [36]. These results correlated with a rapid cognitive improvement in AD patients in a recent phase IIa clinical trial [37], an observation that argues for large-scale testing of PBT2 for AD.

Another promising recent experimental approach is the use of dendrimers as agents interfering with Aβ fibrilization. Dendrimers are globular branched polymers, typically symmetric around the core with a spherical three-dimensional morphology. Their chemical structure allows dendrimers to couple to active amyloid species through hundreds of possible sites. Dendrimers have been shown to be able to modulate Aβ peptide aggregation by interfering in different ways with the polymerization process, including fibril breaking, inhibition of fibril formation and acceleration of fibril formation [38, 39]. However, some dendrimers assayed in amyloidogenic systems are toxic to cells. The development of non-toxic glycodendrimers, which reduce toxicity by clumping fibrils together [40], opens the possibility of using dendrimers with low intrinsic toxicity in AD. Additional difficulties in dendrimer administration involve the crossing of the BBB so as to reach their targets in the brain.

2.1.4. Facilitating Aβ clearance: Immunotherapy against Aβ

Active and passive immunotherapy against Aβ peptide has been explored as a therapeutic approach to stimulate the clearance of Aβ in the brain at the preclinical and clinical stages of the disease in animal models. Pioneering studies proved that vaccination of young APP transgenic mice using a synthetic aggregated form of Aβ$_{42}$ (AN-1792) effectively prevented Aβ plaque formation, neuritic dystrophy and astrogliosis in adult brains [41]. Subsequent studies further demonstrated improvement of memory loss in those APP transgenic mice vaccinated against Aβ [42, 43]. Different models, methods and ways of administration showed the beneficial effects of active and passive immunization in animal models of AD. Nevertheless, the phase II trial in humans was discontinued because of the occurrence of aseptic meningoencephalitis in a number of cases [44-46]. The cause of the meningoencephalitis was a concomitant T-cell-mediated autoimmune response [45, 46]. Moreover, several studies in APP transgenic mice have reported an increased risk of microhemorrhages at sites of cerebrovascular Aβ deposits [47]. Yet important conclusions were drawn from the studies in humans: immunization reduced the number of Aβ plaques and the number of dystrophic neurites, including tau phosphorylation around plaques, but not Aβ burden in blood vessels; however, immunization increased intracerebral levels of soluble Aβ [48-50].

New vaccines containing immunodominant B-cell epitopes of Aβ [51] and recognizing other Aβ residues [52, 53], and the use of passive immunization with deglycosylated antibodies [54] have demonstrated positive effects in the clearance of Aβ without causing inflammatory response or hemorrhages in animal models of AD [55]. These findings have prompted new clinical trials which are currently evaluating the toxicity and effectiveness of at least ten vaccines in mild-to-moderate AD patients worldwide [56]. While vaccines hold great hope as AD therapies, it is important to stress that immunization at pre-symptomatic stages is essential in order to avoid the irreversible brain damage occurring even at the early symptomatic stages [57].

2.2. Targeting tau

The interest in tau-related therapies is still emerging and very few clinical studies are underway, in part because of the difficulties encountered with anti-Aβ strategies that captured most efforts in the two last decades, but also because of the challenging identification of tractable therapeutic targets related to tau. Current research in the prevention of tau pathology developed in animal models of AD has resulted in some promising results [58]. Main rationales in tau pathology are based on: 1: inhibition of tau aggregation, 2: reduction of tau phosphorylation by inhibition of tau kinases or activation of phosphatases (including PP2a activity), 3: reduction of tau levels by increasing tau degradation or by using active immunization, and 4: stabilization of microtubule [59].

2.2.1. Inhibition of tau aggregation

Some compounds that are known to inhibit tau-tau interactions have been tested as agents aimed at slowing Alzheimer progression to disease states. Among them, phenothiaziazine methylene blue inhibits tau-tau interactions, is neuroprotective and is able to facilitate soluble tau clearance in a mouse model of human tauopathy [60, 61]. Moreover, phenothiaziazine methylene blue has shown beneficial effects in a phase II clinical trial conducted for one year [62]. Another promising inhibitor of tau aggregation is the immunosuppressant FK506, which exerts its beneficial effects in transgenic mice by directly binding tau to the FK506 binding protein 52 and by modulating microglial activation [63, 64].

However, some concerns araise from the use of tau aggregation inhibitors in that at least some tau aggregation inhibitors enhance the formation of potentially toxic tau oligomers [65].

2.2.2. Reduction of tau hyperphosphorylation

Kinases which participate in the phosphorylation of tau and phosphatases which dephosphorylate tau are clear putative therapeutic targets for AD [66]. The most widely studied tau kinases in AD pathogenesis are Glycogen synthase kinase 3 beta (GSK-3β) and Cyclin-dependent kinase (CDK5) [67, 68]. Several GSK-3β inhibitors, including lithium, aloisines, flavopiridol, hymenialdisine, paullones, and staurosporine, are under active investigation and development [69]. Lithium revealed some promising results when administered in transgenic mice expressing the P301L human 4R0N tau at pre-symptomatic stages; it improved behavior and reduced the levels of phosphorylation, aggregation and insoluble tau in transgenic mice [70]. However, several concerns have arisen in relation of the use of GSK-3β in the treatment of AD; these are based on the fact that lithium lacks specificity over GSK-3β activity and it has a narrow safety margin [71]. Moreover, GSK-3β acts on multiple metabolic pathways that are also impaired with unknown consequences after chronic treatment.

CDK5 inhibitors prevent Aβ-induced tau hyper-phosphorylation and cell death *in vitro* [72, 73]. A recent *in vivo* study further demonstrates that inhibition of CDK5 activates GSK-3β, which plays a more dominant role in overall tau phosphorylation than does CDK5 [74]. Thus, considering that CDK5 inhibitors might be unable to reverse abnormal hyper-phosphorylation of tau and treat neurofibrillary degeneration because of the interplay between CDK5 and GSK-3β, as well as the essential role played by CDK5 in multiple cell signaling pathways [75], the interest of such compounds as a tau-targeting therapy for AD is limited.

Another approach to reverse tau hyper-phosphorylation is up-regulation of tau phosphatases [66]. The major tau phosphatase, PP2A, is down-regulated in AD brain. In consequence, correcting PP2A levels is the primary target to be considered. Among the compounds known to reverse PP2A inhibition, memantine is the most outstanding because of the demonstrated clinical benefit in AD. In an animal model, memantine was able to reverse okadaic acid–induced PP2A inhibition and to prevent tau hyper-phosphorylation, restoring MAP2 expression [76]. Similarly, melatonin has also been shown to restore PP2A activity and reverse tau hyper-phosphorylation, both *in vitro* and in experimental animals [77]. One important concern in considering PP2A as a potential therapeutic target is that all protein phosphatases have much broader substrate specificities than protein kinases. Thus, more undesirable effects might be expected than when using kinase inhibitors [66]. A further intriguing point is that PP2A function and activity depend on multiple subunits and cofactors which are dysregulated in AD [78]. It is not clear how all these elements can be resolved to result in maintained balanced activity.

2.2.3. Reduction of tau levels

A potential alternative to modulate tau phosphorylation is reducing overall tau levels [58]. Experiments carried out in genetically-modified mice expressing reduced tau levels revealed diminished cognitive impairment and Aβ-induced neuronal damage [79-81]. An alternative method to reduce tau levels could is by targeting molecules that regulate the expression or clearance of tau. Tau can be degraded via the ubiquitin-proteasome system and the lysosomal pathways. Reduction of the levels of the tau ubiquitin-ligase CHIP increases the accumulation of tau aggregates in JNPL3 mice, suggesting that increasing the expression of CHIP could result in reduced tau levels [82]. Acetylation of tau inhibits its degradation [83], alters its microtubule binding, and enhances aggregation [84]. Thus, the combination of tau acetylation inhibition and ubiquitination-proteasome enhancement might produce a synergy that lowers the levels of pathogenic tau species.

Tau degradation can also be enhanced by immunization. Active immunization targeting phosphorylated tau reduces filamentous tau inclusions and neuronal dysfunction in JNPL3 transgenic mice [85, 86]. Moreover, recent studies have raised the possibility of modulating tau pathology by passive immunization revealing reduced behavioral impairment and tau pathology in two transgenic models of taupathies [87].

2.2.4. Microtubule stabilizers

Since microtubule disruption occurs in several models of AD and is associated with tau dysfunction, microtubule stabilizers have been assayed in preclinical and clinical trials for AD [88]. The anti-mitotic drug paclitaxel prevents Aβ-induced toxicity in cell culture [89], as well as axonal transport deficits and behavioral impairments in tau transgenic mice [90]. Unfortunately, paclitaxel is a P-glycoprotein substrate and it has very low capacity to cross the BBB, making it unsuitable for the treatment of human tauopathies. Epothilone D, which has better BBB permeability, improves microtubule density and cognition in tau transgenic mice [91]. Finally, the peptide NAP stabilizes microtubules and reduces tau hyper-phosphorylation [92]. NAP can be administered intra-nasally and has shown promising results in a phase II clinical trial [93].

2.3. Oxidative stress

Several pieces of evidence demonstrate that oxidative stress precedes other hallmarks of the neurodegenerative process in human brains and animal models of AD, including Aβ deposition, NFT formation, and metabolic dysfunction and cognitive decline. It plays a functional role in the pathogenesis of the disease [94-100]. These findings sustain the possibility of using anti-oxidants in the prevention and treatment of Alzheimer [101, 102]. Several studies in AD transgenic mouse models support the potential beneficial effect of antioxidant compounds as preventive drugs.

2.3.1. Naturally-occurring anti-oxidants

Several nutritional antioxidants such as resveratrol, curcumin, epigallocatechin gallate, L-acetyl-carnitine, RRR-α-tocopherol (vitamin E) and ascorbic acid (vitamin C) have been tested to counteract oxidative stress-induced brain damage in AD.

- *Resveratrol* is a polyphenolic compound found in grapes, berries and peanuts with well known anti-oxidant, anti-cancer, anti-inflammatory and estrogenic activities. *In vitro* and animal experiments reveal that resveratrol protects against Aβ toxicity by promoting the non-amyloidogenic cleavage of APP, thus enhancing the clearance of Aβ peptides by promoting their degradation through the ubiquitin-proteasome system, as well as reducing neuronal damage by decreasing the expression of inducible nitric oxide synthase (iNOS) and cyclooxigenase 2 (COX-2), and the pro-apoptotic factors Bax and c-Jun N-terminal kinase (JNK). Moreover, the capacity of resveratrol to induce the over-expression of sirtuins, proteins having a role in cell survival, probably contributes to its neuroprotective effect [103, 104].

- *Curcumin* is a polyphenolic compound present in the rhizome of *Curcuma longa*, commonly used as a spice to color and flavor food, which has anti-inflammatory, anti-carcinogenic and anti-infectious properties. The first evidence of a protective role of curcumin in AD was derived from epidemiological studies based on populations subjected to a curcumin-enriched diet. Additionally, *in vitro* studies have shown that curcumin protects neurons from Aβ toxicity whereas the use of AD transgenic mouse models show that curcumin suppresses inflammation and oxidative damage as well as accelerating the Aβ rate of clearance and inhibiting Aβ aggregation. Curcumin is considered a bi-functional anti-oxidant because it is a direct scavenger of oxidants as well as a long-lasting protector promoting the expression of cytoprotective proteins through the induction of Nrf2-dependent genes [105, 106]. Regrettably, no significant improvement in cognitive function between placebo and curcumin-treated groups has been observed in the only two clinical trials carried out until now [107].

- *Epigallocatechin gallate (EGCG)* is a polyphenolic flavonoid encountered in green tea. Human epidemiological and animal data suggest that tea may decrease the incidence of dementia and AD. EGCG has been demonstrated to exert its neuroprotective activity by reducing Aβ production and inflammation, and increasing mitochondrial stabilization, iron chelation and ROS scavenging [108]. However, to date no clinical trials have been performed to verify whether EGCG neuroprotective/neurorestorative actions can be successfully translated into human beings.

- *Acetyl-L-Carnitine (ALC)* is a natural compound found in red meat whose biological role is to facilitate the transport of fatty acids to the mitochondria. Thus, the main mechanism of action of ALC is the improvement of mitochondrial respiration, which allows the neurons to produce the necessary ATP to maintain normal membrane potential. Yet ALC is neuro-protective through a variety of additional effects, including an increase in protein kinase C activity and modulation of synaptic plasticity by counteracting the loss of NMDA receptors in the neuronal membrane and by increasing the production of neurotrophins [105]. Moreover, ALC reduces Aβ toxicity in primary cortical neuronal cultures by increasing both heme-oxygenase 1 (HO-1) and heat-shock protein 70 (Hsp70) expression, probably through transcription factor Nrf2. In two clinical studies, ALC administered for one year significantly reduced cognitive decline in early-onset AD patients [109, 110] thus sustaining the potential use of ALC in AD prevention and treatment at early stages.

- *RRR-a-tocopherol (Vitamin E)* is probably the most important lipid-soluble natural antioxidant in mammalian cells. Most vegetable oils, nuts and some fruits are important dietary sources of vitamin E. The interest in evaluating its potential beneficial properties in AD is also sustained by its known ability to cross the BBB and to accumulate in the central nervous system. Deficiency in the α-tocopherol transfer protein mediating vitamin E activity induces an increase in brain lipid peroxidation, earlier and more severe cognitive dysfunction, and increased Aβ deposits in the brain of Tg2576 mice; this phenotype was ameliorated with vitamin E supplementation [111]. However, although epidemiological studies have demonstrated that increasing the intake of fruit and vegetables rich in vitamins prevents or retards the onset of AD, clinical trials for vitamin E treatment have revealed paradoxical results: whereas vitamin E supplementation partially prevents the memory loss associated with the progression of the disease in some cases, the same treatment was detrimental in others [112].

• *Ascorbic acid (Vitamin C)* is an essential nutrient since it acts as a cofactor in elemental enzymatic reactions, but in contrast to most of organisms, humans are not able to synthesize ascorbic acid. The main dietary source of vitamin C is fresh fruit and vegetables. The main interest in vitamin C for the treatment of neurodegenerative processes is related to its potent anti-oxidant properties. Some studies have revealed that vitamin C supplementation reduces oxidative stress, and mitigates Aβ oligomer formation and behavioral decline, but it did not decrease plaque deposition in AD mouse models [113, 114]. Despite epidemio-logical studies reporting reduced prevalence and incidence of AD in consumers of vitamin supplements [115], meta-analyses revealed the risks of chronic consumption of high doses of vitamin C thus discouraging its routine use in AD. [116]

• *Egb76* is a standardized *Ginkgo biloba* extract already approved in some countries as symptomatic treatment for dementia although the evidence for its effectiveness remains inconclusive [117]. However, Egb761 has anti-oxidant properties, inhibits Aβ oligomeriza-tion *in vitro*, reduces impaired memory and learning capacities and enhances hippocampal neurogenesis in AD transgenic mice [118]. For these reasons, *Ginkgo biloba* extract is currently under evaluation as a preventive drug in AD.

In spite of the experimental evidence of beneficial effects of natural anti-oxidants in cultured cells and transgenic models, clinical studies have demonstrated only minimal effect in humans probably due to the bioavailability and pharmacokinetics of these substances [102, 105]. What's more, a slight acceleration in cognitive decline has been observed in patients treated for 16 weeks with a cocktail of natural antioxidants [119].

2.3.2. Mitochondrial antioxidants

In contrast to other antioxidants, those designed to target the free radical damage to mito-chondria provide greater therapeutic potential.

• *Lipoic acid (LA)* is a naturally-occurring precursor of an essential cofactor of many mitochondrial enzymes, including pyruvate dehydrogenase and alpha-ketoglutarate dehydrogenase, which is found in almost all foods. LA has been shown to present a variety of properties that can interfere with pathogenic processes of AD. LA increases ACh production, stimulates glucose uptake, protects against Aβ toxicity, chelates redox-active transition metals, scavenges reactive oxygen species (ROS) and induces anti-oxidant protective enzymes probably through the activation of the transcription factor Nrf2. Via the same mechanisms, down-regulation of redox-sensitive inflammatory processes is also achieved [120]. Data from cell culture and animal models suggest that LA can be combined with other dietary anti-oxidants to synergistically decrease oxidative stress, inflammation, Aβ levels, and thus provide a combined benefit in the treatment of AD. However, clinical benefits after LA administration were quite small in patients with mild or moderate dementia [121].

- *N-acetyl-cysteine (NAC)* is a precursor of glutathione (GSH), the most abundant endogenous anti-oxidant. NAC acts itself as an anti-oxidant by directly interacting with free radicals, as well as by increasing GSH levels. NAC protects against $A\beta$-induced cognitive deficits by decreasing the associated oxidative stress and related neuroinflammation, but also by activating anti-apoptotic signaling pathways in neuronal cultures [122]. Late-stage AD patients supplemented with NAC over a period of six months showed significantly improved performance in some cognitive tasks, although levels of oxidative stress in peripheral blood did not differ significantly from untreated patients [123].

- *Coenzyme Q_{10} (CoQ$_{10}$)* is a small electron-carrier of the respiratory chain with anti-oxidant properties due to its role in carrying high-energy electrons from complex I to complex II during oxidative phosphorylation. CoQ$_{10}$ and its analogues, idebenone and mitoquinone (or MitoQ), have been widely used for the treatment of mitochondrial disorders, as well as for the treatment of Friedreich's ataxia, and they are also being tested in other neurodegenerative disorders such as amyotrophic lateral sclerosis, and Huntington's, Parkinson's and Alzheimer's diseases [124]. CoQ$_{10}$ reduces oxidative stress damage and $A\beta$ plaque burden, and ameliorates behavioral performance in mouse models of AD [125, 126]. However, CoQ$_{10}$ presents two major weaknesses. First, the function of the enzyme is entirely dependent on the electron transport chain (ETC) which is usually damaged in AD mitochondria. Second, CoQ$_{10}$ does not efficiently cross the BBB when administered systemically, being unable to directly protect neurons from damage. Consequently, CoQ$_{10}$ derivatives such as MitoQ, which is a more soluble compound able to penetrate the BBB and that does not depend on ETC, are seen to offer more promising results [127].

2.4. Inflammation

There is a general consensus that neuroinflammation is a prominent feature in AD with activated microglia being one of the main manifestations. Neuroinflammation is a complex process that has both beneficial effects, in terms of maintaining brain homeostasis after various kinds of insults, and detrimental effects when sustained chronically [128]. This latter situation is what occurs in AD, in which neuroinflammation is driven by different mechanisms including $A\beta$ production and plaque formation, tau pathology, oxidative stress, and autocrine and paracrine release of cytokines and other inflammatory molecules which contribute to a feed-forward spiral favoring the self-propagation of neuroinflammation.

Early epidemiological studies suggesting that long-term use of antiinflammatories might reduce the risk for developing AD [129] prompted several studies designed to evaluate the preventive properties of non-steroid anti-inflammatory drugs (NSAIDs). The main NSAID mechanism of action is to inhibit the activity of cyclooxigenase-1 and -2 (COX-1 and COX-2) which are the enzymes responsible of the production of prostaglandins and other inflammatory agents [130]. The administration of the NSAID ibuprofen at early stages of the pathological process resulted in the reduction of the $A\beta$ burden, dystrophic neurites and activated microglia in at least three different AD transgenic models [131-134]. Another study indicated that ibuprofen was effective even in older mice once lesions are well established [135]. Other NSAIDs such as indomethacin and nimuselide exhibit milder effects compared to ibuprofen in the Tg2576 mice [136, 137]. In contrast, the selective COX-2 inhibitor celecoxib failed to reduce the inflammatory burden and, even worse, increased the $A\beta_{42}$ levels when administered to young Tg2576 mice [138].

In spite of the promising results in animal models and the data from retrospective human epidemiological studies identifying long-term use of NSAIDs as being protective against AD, prospective clinical trials have not confirmed the efficiency of this group of drugs in the amelioration of symptoms and in the progression of AD [139].

Other anti-inflammatory agents such as trifusal have been shown to be beneficial in certain AD transgenic mice models [140].

2.5. Energetic failure: Metabolic deficiency and mitochondrial impairment

Several findings indicate that brain glucose hypometabolism, deficient bioenergetics and mitochondrial dysfunction precede clinical symptoms in AD [1, 141-143]. The energetic failure observed even in the prodromal phase of the Alzheimer process is thought to be produced by the combination of mitochondria dysfunction, alteration of energy metabolism at pore-mitochondrial level, and increase in energetic demands of altered nerve cells. Thus, strategies to improve brain energy supply and to preserve mitochondrial functions becomes relevant in the prevention of progression to disease states [1, 144-146].

2.5.1. Metabolic deficiency

The primary fuel for the brain under normal conditions is glucose, whereas the energetic contribution made by fatty acids is minor. Therefore, facilitation of energy metabolism and energy availability has been assayed in animal models and AD by facilitating glucose metabolism and shifting towards the use of alternative fuels.

- *Targeting reduced glucose metabolism*: Reduction in the utilization of glucose in AD [147] can be due to several causes including deficient insulin signaling, impairment in glucose transport mechanisms and dysfunction in glucolysis. Preclinical studies in animal models of AD have revealed some beneficial effects of anti-diabetic treatments. Thus, the use of the insulin sensitizer rosiglitazone, an activator of peroxisome-proliferator-activated receptor gamma (PPARγ) receptor, resulted in the rescue of behavioral deficits and insulin responsiveness in Tg2576 mice [148, 149]. Similarly, exendin-4, an antidiabetic agent that stimulates the insulin signaling pathway through activation of glucagon-like peptide -1 (GLP1) receptors, shows beneficial effects in AD, and reduces brain soluble Aβ levels, amyloid plaque burden, and cognitive impairment in treated APP/PS1 transgenic mice [150, 151]. Therefore, it seems that the positive effects of targeting insulin signaling in AD are related to the role played by insulin receptor in memory formation, inflammation and Aβ neuroprotective effects rather than to the facilitation of glucose transport into the brain [149, 150]. This hypothesis seems also to be supported by a recent study revealing that insulin did not ameliorate the disruption of energetic homeostasis induced by Aβ oligomers in cultured neurons [152]. In the end, clinical trials designed to test whether PPARγ agonists could be beneficial in AD patients provided negative results [153].

- *Shift to alternative energy source*: Under metabolically challenging conditions neurons can utilize acetyl-CoA generated from ketone body metabolism, produced distally in the liver or locally in the brain by glial cells. In this way, ketone bodies can bypass defects in glucose metabolism and enter the tricarboxylic acid cycle in the mitochondria of neurons as a source of ATP. The use of ketogenic diets reduces Aβ40 and Aβ42 levels in young AD transgenic mice [154] and enhances mitochondrial bioenergetic capacity, reducing Aβ generation and increasing mechanisms of Aβ clearance in a mouse model of AD [155]. The ketogenic compound AC-1202 administered in patients with AD has shown a significant improvement in some cognitive parameters more notable in individuals APOE4(-) [156]. Another possible alternative source of ATP is creatine. Preliminary studies have shown that creatine has protective effects against Aβ *in vitro* [157] and against injury *in vivo* by maintaining ATP levels and mitochondrial function [158], suggesting a potential therapeutic effect of creatine supplementation in AD.

2.5.2. Mitochondrial dysfunction

In addition to the already discussed antioxidant compounds, other potential drugs targeting mitochondrial dysfunction in AD are available. Several findings point towards a role for Aβ toxicity in the mitochondrial dysfunction found in AD.

The progressive Aβ accumulation in mitochondria is associated with diminished enzymatic activity of respiratory chain complexes (III and IV) and reduction in the rate of oxygen consumption, contributing to cellular dysfunction in AD [159]. Aβ in mitochondria binds to Aβ-binding alcohol dehydrogenase (ABAD) to block ABAD activity, increasing the production of ROS, reducing the mitochondrial membrane potential and the activity of the respiratory chain complex IV, and ultimately leading to a decrease in ATP levels [160]. In fact, double transgenic mice over-expressing mutated APP and ABAD exhibit exaggerated oxidative stress and memory impairment [160]. Therefore, compounds designed to block Aβ-ABAD interactions are considered putative therapeutic agents in AD. In line with this hypothesis, a recent study has shown that AG18051, a novel small ABAD-specific compound inhibitor, partially blocked the Aβ-ABAD interaction, prevented the Aβ42-induced down-regulation of ABAD activity and protected cultured neurons against Aβ42 toxicity by reducing Aβ42-induced impairment of mitochondrial function and oxidative stress [161]. Furthermore, the introduction of an ABAD-decoy peptide into transgenic APP mice reduces Aβ-ABAD interaction and protects against Aβ-mediated mitochondrial toxicity [162].

Another line of research suggests that drugs that activate ATP-sensitive potassium (K_{ATP}) channels present in the mitochondrial inner membrane exhibit therapeutic potential in the treatment of AD, as K_{ATP} channels are activated when cellular ATP levels fall below a critical value thereby reducing excitability so as to maintain ion homeostasis and preserve ATP levels [163]. Long-term administration of diazoxide improves neuronal bioenergetics, suppresses Aβ and tau pathologies, and ameliorates memory deficits in the 3xTgAD mouse model of AD [164].

Finally, another potential drug in the treatment of AD that acts on mitochondrial pathways is latrepirdine, also known as Dimebon™ [165]. Latrepirdine reduces Aβ-induced mitochondrial impairment and increases the threshold of inductors to mitochondrial pore transition, making mitochondria more resistant to lipid peroxidation and increasing neuronal survival *in vitro* [166-168]. The interest in developing latrepirdine as a drug against AD is also supported by its multiple potential mechanism of action apart from mitochondrial effects, including anti-excitotoxic agent, inhibitor of AChE, channel-regulatior and neurotrophic stimulator [165]. A preliminary clinical trial revealed that latrepirdine was safe and well tolerated, and significantly improved the clinical course of the disease in patients with mild-to-moderate AD [169]. Current phase III clinical trials are already being conducted [165].

2.6. Neurotransmitter dysfunction

The alteration of several transmitter systems is assumed to trigger both cognitive and neuropsychiatric symptoms in AD. A number of *post-mortem* studies indicate that neurotransmitter systems are not uniformly affected in AD. Thus, while cholinergic, serotonergic and glutamatergic deficits are present at relatively early stages of AD, dopaminergic and GABAergic systems appear to be affected later [170].

2.6.1. Cholinergic system

A large body of evidence has shown that basal forebrain cholinergic neurons are vulnerable to AD leading to a progressive cholinergic denervation of the cerebral neocortex [171, 172]. Taking into account the involvement of this system in the cognitive processing of memory and attention, the current attempts in cholinergic therapy in AD are justified [172, 173]. The various cholinergic strategies include the use of ACh precursors, inhibitors of cholinesterases, muscarinic and nicotinic agonists, and ACh releasers, in addition to the rescue of cholinergic function by nerve growth factor (NGF) which is reviewed in section 2.8.

- *ACh precursor.* Animal studies report that choline and lecithin increased the production of brain ACh which argues for their use in the treatment of cholinergic deficits in AD. However, evidence from randomized trials did not sustain this hypothesis [174].

- *Cholinesterase inhibitors (ChEIs).* Physostigmine, tacrine and derivatives donepezil, galantamine and rivastigmine have been tested in AD patients during the last three decades. Their therapeutic properties have been profusely reviewed [172, 175-177] and for this reason a detailed revision of ChEIs is beyond the scope of this chapter. Nevertheless, it is worth briefly indicating additional mechanisms of action of these compounds beyond inhibition of cholinesterases, including increase of nicotinc ACh receptor expression, facilitation of APP processing and attenuation of Aβ-induced toxicity [173, 178]. In spite of the fact that their efficacy has been proved in several clinical trials, only approximately 50% of patients respond positively. This limited effect of ChEIs on cognitive decline, together with the occurrence of undesirable side-effects such as diarrhea, nausea, insomnia, fatigue and loss of appetite, reduces the therapeutic capacities of ChEIs.

- *Muscarinic receptor 1 agonist.* The cholinergic deficiency in AD appears to be mainly pre-synaptic. Thus, the pharmacological stimulation of the post-synaptic M1 muscarinic receptors, which are preserved until late stages of AD, may balance the degeneration of pre-synaptic cholinergic terminals unable to properly synthesize and release ACh [173]. In fact, the selective M1 agonist AF267B reduces memory impairment, Aβ42 levels, and tau hyper-phosphorylation in AD triple transgenic mice [179], corroborating some early studies *in vitro* [180, 181]. This selective agonist is currently under clinical evaluation for safety and tolerability and a number of other M1 agonists are being investigated [173].

- *Nicotinic agonists.* Preclinical studies in animal models and some pilot studies in AD have shown that the activation of pre-synaptic nicotinic ACh receptors may reduce cognitive impairment by increasing ACh release and may have beneficial effects on Aβ metabolism [182, 183]. Thus, chronic nicotine treatment results in a significant reduction in plaque burden and in cortical Aβ concentrations in Tg2575/PS1-A246E mice [184]. However, nicotine exacerbates tau pathology in 3xTg-AD mice [185]. These apparently contradictory results may be due to the presence of several subtypes of nicotinic receptors, the activation of which may have disparate effects in AD. Therefore, more specific nicotine agonists are needed to act exclusively on determinate subtypes of nicotinic receptor [186]. In this line, α7 nAChR gene delivery into mouse hippocampal neurons leads to functional receptor expression and improves spatial memory-related performance and hyperphosphorylation of tau [187]. Regarding α4β2 nicotinic receptor, the selective agonist cytisine inhibits Aβ cytotoxicity in cortical neurons [188].

- *ACh releasers.* Facilitation of ACh release can be achieved with depolarizing agents of the cholinergic neurons acting via potassium-channel blockade as happens with linopirdine and analogues [189] or by the blockade of the pre-synaptic inhibitory M2 muscarinic receptor via specific antagonists [190, 191]. However, clinical trials using linopirdine did not demonstrate effectiveness in improving cognitive function [192]. On the other hand, certain selective M2 antagonists, such as SCH-57790 and SC-72788, restore memory impairments in animal models that mimic to some extent the cholinergic failure in AD [193]. It must be kept in mind that the potential benefit of M2 antagonists is limited because of the progressive pre-synaptic cholinergic degeneration in AD and because of the possible side-effects derived from the blockade of peripheral M2 receptors including cardiac M2 receptors.

2.6.2. Glutamatergic system

Low concentrations of Aβ oligomers are able to activate certain glutamate receptors including NMDA receptors. The activation of NMDA receptors may increase glutamate activity, raise intracellular Ca2+ concentration and promote excitotoxicity and neuronal damage [194, 195]. Another process contributing to the excessive glutamate activity in AD is the impairment of glial cells to remove glutamate form the synaptic cleft possibly due to the action of free radicals on the glutamate transporter 1 (GLT-1) [196]. Glutamatergic activation, in turn, may disrupt synaptic plasticity promoting long term depression (LTD) and inhibiting long term potentiation (LTP) of 2-amino-3-(5-methyl-3-oxo-1,2-oxazol-4-yl)propanoic acid (AMPA) receptor-mediated synaptic transmission [197]. The associated persistent reduction in the number of functional synaptic AMPA receptors reduces fast excitatory transmission and eventually triggers spine retraction and synaptic loss [198]. Moreover, glutamate receptors are not only involved in the process of Aβ-mediated synaptic dysfunction but also play important roles in Aβ production [199, 200].

Based on these observations, several studies have been designed in an attempt to correct glutamatergic dysfunction in AD, including the modulation of both AMPA and NMDA receptors [201]. First attempts were carried out with AMPAKines [202], which are drugs that prolong the action of glutamate on AMPA receptors by increasing their sensitivity. Interestingly, AMPAKines proved effective in restoring cognitive deficits in aging rats [203, 204]. These compounds were tested in AD patients [205]. The modulation of the NMDA receptor was assessed via the glycine co-agonist site in rats with disrupted glutamatergic temporal systems resulting in improved learning and memory [206]. Preliminary clinical studies suggested some promising effects in AD [207] but full-scale trials have not yet been initiated.

The most relevant glutamatergic strategy against AD is the non-competitive NMDA antagonist memantine [201, 208], which has succeeded in clinical trials in moderate and severe AD as reviewed in detail elsewhere [209, 210]. Several studies performed in animal models of AD corroborate the beneficial properties of memantine as a symptomatological and neuroprotective treatment in AD [211-215]. Nevertheless, memantine has no benefits in cases with mild AD [216] suggesting that this drug is not a good choice for preventing the progression to disease states.

2.6.3. Serotonergic system

Loss of serotonergic nerve terminals in AD was described several years ago [217, 218]. Although the suggested serotonergic dysfunction was initially related almost exclusively with the neuropsychiatric symptoms of AD, including anxiety, irritability, fear and depression, recent studies have demonstrated that serotonin signaling also plays an important role in cognition and in the development of Aβ and tau pathologies [219].

Antidepressant compounds, acting through serotonin signaling, result in cognitive improvements and reduce the levels of Aβ and tau pathology in animal models of AD [220, 221]. Similar compounds reduce amyloid burden in humans [221]. Additional serotonergic compounds that are currently being investigated in AD are 5-hydroxytryptamine (5-HT or serotonin) receptors: 5-HT_1 and 5-HT_6 antagonists, and 5-HT_4 agonists. The 5-HT_{1A} antagonist lecozotan (SRA-333) enhances cognition in primates and is now being tested in AD [222-224]. The pro-cognitive effects of 5-HT_{1A} antagonists are probably due to the facilitation of glutamategic and cholinergic transmission after reduction of the inhibitory effects of serotonin. Similarly, 5-HT_6 antagonists improve cognitive performance in animal models and human beings by modulating multiple neurotransmitter systems [225]. These properties mark 5-HT_6 antagonists as potential symptomatic drugs in AD. In addition, 5-HT_4 receptor agonists are neuroprotective, modulating the production of Aβ, and have the property of ameliorating cognitive deficits [226, 227].

2.7. Synaptic dysfunction

Synaptic dysfunction and failure are processes that occur early in the Alzheimer process and progress during the course of the disease from an initially reversible functionally-responsive stage of down-regulated synaptic function to stages irreversibly associated with degeneration.

These alterations are manifested early as impaired metabotropic glutamate receptor/phospholipase C signaling pathway [230] and up-regulation of adenosine receptors in the frontal cortex in AD [231].

The initial reversible stages are important targets for protective treatments to slow progression and preserve cognitive and functional abilities [232, 233]. *In vivo* and *in vitro* studies have demonstrated that high levels of Aβ impair structural and functional plasticity of synapses by affecting the balance between excitation and inhibition and contributing to the destabilization of neuronal networks, eventually causing synaptic loss [234]. Two main designs have been proposed to antagonize synaptic plasticity-disrupting actions of Aβ oligomers in preclinical AD: maintenance of the structure and fluidity of the lipid membranes forming the synaptic buttons, and stimulation of synaptic plasticity by neurotrophic factors.

Minor changes in the fluidity of phospholipidic membranes might have an important impact on the function of synapses by influencing neurotransmitter receptor activity. In fact, AD brains exhibit altered lipid composition of lipid rafts, key membrane microdomains that facilitate the transfer of substrates and protein-protein and lipid-protein interactions, as a result of the abnormally low levels of n-3 long-chain polyunsaturated fatty acids, mainly docosahexaenoic acid (DHA), increasing viscosity and energy consumption and contributing to synaptic dysfunction [142, 235]. Abnormal lipid raft composition may also modify the activity of key enzymes that modulate the cleavage of APP to form toxic Aβ. Thus, the preservation of adequate membrane composition has become an alternative way to prevent the deleterious effect of Aβ at the synapses. DHA is a major lipid constituent of synaptic end-sites and its delivery is a prerequisite for the conversion of nerve growth cones to mature synapses [236]. Numerous epidemiological studies have highlighted the beneficial influence of DHA on the preservation of synaptic function and memory capacity in aged individuals or after Aβ exposure, whereas DHA deficiency is presented as a risk factor for AD [237]. Moreover, a number of studies have reported the beneficial effects of dietary DHA supplementation on cognition and synaptic integrity in various AD models [238]. According to thes evidence, DHA, which can be synthesized or obtained directly from fish oil, appear to be one of the most valuable diet ingredients whose neuroprotective properties contribute to preventing AD.

Cytidine 5'-diphosphocholine, CDP-choline, or citicoline is an essential intermediate in the biosynthetic pathway of structural phospholipids in cell membranes, particularly phosphatidylcholine. Chronic administration has been beneficial in patients with mild cognitive impairment [239].

Another emerging potential line to preserve synaptic function is the targeting of scaffolding proteins that modulate neurotransmitter receptor activity at the synapses. Scaffolding proteins stabilize post-synaptic receptors at the spines in close proximity to their intracellular signaling proteins, phosphatases and kinases, thereby facilitating signal-transduction cascades. Evidence from *in vitro* cell and animal models of AD indicates that reductions in the post-synaptic density membrane-associated guanylate kinase (PSD-MAGUK) proteins are linked to synaptic dysfunction that might trigger plastic changes at early stages of the Alzheimer process [240]. However, specific molecules that affect interactions between scaffolding proteins and neurotransmitter receptors are still in development and further research is necessary to evaluate their potential benefit in AD.

2.8. Neurotrophic factors

Neurotrophins represent a family of proteins that play a pivotal role in the mechanisms underlying neuronal survival, differentiation, modulation of dendritic branching and dendritic spine morphology as well as synaptic plasticity and apoptosis [241]. All the members of the neurotrophin family, including NGF, brain-derived neurotrophic factor (BDNF) and neurotrophins 3 to 7, transduce their biological effects by interacting with two types of cell surface receptors, the tyrosine kinase receptor (Trk) and the p75 pan-neurotrophin receptor (p75^{NTR}) [241]. Other growth factor families also related to synaptic plasticity include the cytokine family of growth factors, the transforming growth factor-β (TGFβ) family, the fibroblast growth factor family and the insulin-like growth factor family. Evidence accumulated during recent years suggests that targeting neurotrophic factor signaling can retard nerve cell degeneration and to some extent preserve synaptic function. The most studied neurotrophic factors in AD are NGF, BDNF and TGFβ1.

- *NGF*: Mature basal forebrain cholinergic neurons are highly dependent on the availability of NGF for the maintenance of their biochemical and morphological phenotype, and for survival after lesions or variegated insults [242, 243]. For this reason, exploitation of NGF activity on cholinergic neurons may provide an attractive therapeutic option for preventing cholinergic cell degeneration in AD. Levels of proNGF, the precursor form of NGF, are highly elevated in AD brains and animal models, a feature that may be associated with a reduced conversion to NGF and augmented degradation of mature NGF. These combined effects have been interpreted as causative of cholinergic atrophy in AD [244]. A role for Aβ peptide in the induction of such NGF altered metabolism has been described [245]. Minocycline, a second-generation tetracycline antibiotic known to potentiate NGF activity, is able to normalize proNGF levels and to reverse the increased activity of the NGF-degrading enzyme matrix metalloproteinase 9, as well as to increase the expression of iNOS and microglial activation, leading to improved cognitive behavior in a transgenic mouse model of AD [245]. Yet a disturbing finding is the demonstration of AD proNGF when compared to proNGF of control individuals [246-248]. Whether this abnormal form of AD-related proNGF has any impact on the pathogenesis of AD needs further investigation. Another putative therapy is the use NGF, but NGF does not readily cross the BBB and requires intra-cerebroventricular infusion to reach targeted brain areas. Pilot clinical trials were discontinued because of the side-effects of NGF infusions [249]. Therefore, the development of NGF therapy is constrained by the need to achieve adequate concentrations in the relevant brain areas with susceptible target neurons while preventing unwanted adverse effects in non-target regions or cells. Alternative strategies that are currently under development include gene therapy and nasal delivery of recombinant forms of NGF, the use of small molecules with NGF agonist activity, NGF synthesis inducers, NGF processing modulators, and proNGF antagonists [250].

- *BDNF*: This neurotrophin is normally produced in the cerebral cortex with high levels in the entorhinal cortex and hippocampus in adulthood [241]. BDNF levels are reduced in the cerebral cortex and hippocampus in AD [251-254]. Several studies have shown beneficial effects of BDNF in animal models of AD [255]. For instance, sustained BDNF gene delivery using viral vectors after disease onset resulted in elevated BDNF levels in the entorhinal cortex and hippocampus which were associated with improvement in learning and memory, and with restoration of most genes altered as a result of mutant APP expression in that specific transgenic mice model [256]. Similar results were obtained in a different mouse model of AD, and in aged rats and primates by using distinct BDNF delivery systems [256, 257]. It is worth pointing out that BDNF did not change β-amyloid plaque density in any case suggesting that the therapeutic effects of BDNF occur independently of direct action on APP processing. However, the multiple variegated effects of BDNF on neuronal function also raise the hypothetical possibility that unintended adverse effects of BDNF may limit its clinical efficacy in AD [256]. An additional point must be considered; BDNF signaling pathway is also altered in AD as TrkB expression is reduced and truncated TrkB is highly expressed in astrocytes at least in advanced stages of the disease [251]. Therefore, regarding BDNF function in AD, there is not only an alteration in the expression of BDNF but also an impaired downstream pathway that may corrupt the signal of the trophic factor acting on inappropriate receptors. Preliminary clinical trials are currently in progress to evaluate the safety and efficacy of BDNF.

- *TGFβ1*: Astrocytes and microglia are the major sources of TGF-β1 in the injured brain [258, 259]. Impaired TGF-β1 signaling has been demonstrated in AD brain, particularly at the early phase of the disease; this is associated with Aβ pathology and neurofibrillary tangle formation in animal models [260]. Reduced TGF-β1 seems to induce microglial activation [259] and ectopic cell-cycle re-activation in neurons [261]. Several drugs may induce TGF-β1 release by glial cells, including estrogens [262], mGlu2/3 agonists [263], lithium [264], the antidepressant venlafaxine [265] and glatiramer, which is a synthetic amino acid co-polymer currently approved for the treatment of multiple sclerosis [266]. All of them have neuroprotective effects in different *in vitro* and *in vivo* models of AD pathology [260]. Additionally, small molecules with specific TGF-β1-like activity are being developed as neuroprotectors [267].

A final point must be considered. A generalized sprouting is produced around β-amyloid deposits in senile plaques in both humans and in animal models [268-270]. The reasons for such sprouting are not well defined but amyloid species may play a trigger role. In any case, trophic factors might increase aberrant sprouting at the senile plaques through receptors expressed at these localizations.

2.9. Autophagy

Autophagy is a catabolic process occurring in all cell types in which the machinery of the lysosome degrades cellular components such as long-lived or damaged proteins and organelles. Thus, a failure of autophagy in neurons results in the accumulation of aggregate-prone proteins that might exacerbate neurodegenerative process [271, 272]. Autophagy is also implicated in the accumulation of altered mitochondria and polymorphous inclusions in the dystrophic neurites around amyloid plaques [273-278].

Indeed, autophagic dysfunction is implicated in the progression of Alzheimer from the earliest stage, when a defective lysosomal clearance of autophagic substrates and impaired autophagy initiation occurs and leads to massive buildup of incompletely digested substrates within dystrophic axons and dendrites [279]. The pharmacological induction of 'preserved' autophagy might enhance the clearance of intracytoplasmic aggregate-prone proteins and therefore ameliorate pathology [272]. Attempts to restore more normal lysosomal proteolysis and autophagy efficiency in mouse models of AD pathology have revealed promising therapeutic effects on neuronal function and cognitive performance, demonstrating the relevance of the failure of autophagy in the pathogenesis of AD, and the potential of autophagy modulation as a therapeutic strategy. Autophagy induction with the mTOR-inhibiting drug rapamycin in young mice resulted in a reduction in Aβ plaques, NFT and cognitive deficits in the adulthood in two different models of AD [280-283]. Interestingly, rapamycin did not alter any of those parameters when administered in old animals once the pathology was established, highlighting the importance of early treatmenting in the disease progression [282]. However, the kinase mTOR plays an important role in multiple signaling pathways apart from negatively regulating autophagy [284]. Therefore, rapamycin treatment is also a putative inducer of undesirable side-effects. Other drugs including lithium, sodium valproate and carbamazepine acting have ben proved to induce autophagy through the inhibition of of inositol monophosphatase in an mTOR-independent pathway [285]. These compunds reveal positive effects by reducing the accumulation and toxic effects of aggregation-prone proteins in cell models as well as by protecting against neurodegeneration in *in vivo* models of Huntington's disease [286]. Further research is needed to learn whether they can also be useful tools in the treatment of AD.

2.10. Multi-target treatments

Considering the multifactorial etiology of AD, and the numerous and complex pathological mechanisms involved in the progression of the disease, it is quite reasonable that treatments targeting a single causal or modifying factor may have limited benefits. Therefore, growing interest is focused on therapeutic agents with pleiotropic activity, which will be able to target, in parallel, several processes affected in AD [287, 288]. Several compounds already mentioned in the previous sections fulfill these properties, such as DHA which presents anti-inflammatory, anti-oxidant, neuroprotective and anti-tau phosphorylation properties apart from the modulation of synaptic membrane composition [289], and curcumin, which in addition to anti-oxidant properties also exhibits anti-inflammatory and Aβ- and tau-binding properties [106]. Similarly, rosiglitazone and dimebon are known to produce beneficial effects through insulin receptor signaling modulation and mitochondrial protection [153, 165]. Other multi-target potential treatments currently under development for AD are based on the use of the following compounds:

- *Caffeine*: This is one of the most consumed psychoactive drugs which mainly acts blocking adenosine receptors 1 and 2 [290, 291]. In addition, caffeine reduces amyloid burden in animal models of AD [292, 293]. Epidemiological studies in humans have also shown protection against cognitive decline [294-296].

- *Estrogen*: This steroid hormone is known to play an important role in neuronal survival, mitochondrial function, neuroinflammation and cognition, with important neuroprotective effects [297-299]. Some of the neuroprotective actions mediated by estrogens are related to the insulin-like growth factor-1 (IGF-1) signaling pathway [300]. Several studies in animal models of AD have revealed therapeutic properties of estrogen against the progression of the disease. For instance, the treatment of ovariectomized 3xTg-AD mice with estrogen resulted in prevention of the increased Aβ accumulation and worsening memory performance induced by the depletion of sex steroid hormones [301]. Clinical and epidemiological studies in AD support the beneficial effets of estrogens [302]. However, a critical factor for success in estrogen therapy for AD is the age at the initiation of the treatment; the efficacy of estrogens is greatest in younger women and in women who initiated the estrogen therapy at the time of menopause [303].

- *Cannabinoids*: The natural compounds derived from *Cannabis sativa* or synthetic compounds acting on endogenous cannabinoid system have emerged as potential agents against several neurodegenerative processes [305]. Cannabinoids offer a multi-faceted approach for the treatment of AD as the stimulation of the widely brain-expressed cannabinoid receptors provides neuroprotection against Aβ [305, 306] and reduces neuroinflammation [306-308] and tau phosphorylation [306, 309] in AD-like transgenic mice. In addition, cannabinoids support brain repair mechanisms by augmenting neurotrophin expression and enhancing neurogenesis [310]. Moreover, cannabinoids are able to reduce Aβ-dependent oxidative stress [311] and Aβ-mediated lysosomal destabilization related to apoptosis [312]. In addition, some cannabinoids are able to inhibit acetylcholinesterase activity [313]. It is worth stressing that molecular achievements of cannabinoids are accompanied by cognitive improvement and reduction of several degenerative markers in two different animal models of AD [306, 308]. Examination of the potential beneficial effects of chronic administration of low doses of cannabinoids with little psychotropic effect at early stages of the degenerative process in humans seems very promising.

- *Erythropoietin (EPO) and derivatives*: EPO is effective in neuroprotection against ischemia and traumatic brain injury [314]. In addition, animal studies reveal that EPO both reduces tau phosphorylation through modulation of PI3K/Akt-GSK-3beta pathway [315] and protects against Aβ-induced cell death through anti-oxidant mechanisms [316]. An additional characteristic of EPO that confers potential utility in AD is the specific effect on cognition: EPO enhances hippocampal LTP and memory by modulating plasticity, synaptic connectivity and activity of memory-related neuronal networks [317]. In spite of these benefits, chronic administration of EPO is problematic because of the concomitant excessive erythropoiesis. In this sense, some new derivatives of EPO that do not bind to the classical EPO receptor (carbamylated EPO) or that have such a brief half-life in the circulation that they do not stimulate erythropoiesis (asialo EPO and neuro EPO) have demonstrated neuroprotective activities without the potential adverse effects on circulation associated with EPO [318]. Therefore, these new compounds are considered as potential treatments in AD.

- *Statins*: Evidence has accumulated that a high cholesterol level may increase the risk of developing AD and that the use of statins to treat hyper-cholesterolemia is useful in treating and preventing AD [319]. Statins reduce the production of cholesterol and isoprenoid intermediates. These isoprenoids modulate the turnover of small GTPase molecules that are essential in numerous cell-signaling pathways, including vesicular trafficking and inflammation [320]. Thus, statins reduce the production of Aβ by disrupting secretase enzyme function and by curbing neuroinflammation in experimental models of AD [321, 322].

- *Ladostigil* is a dual acetylcholine-butyrylcholineesterase and brain selective monoamine oxidase (MAO)-A and -B inhibitor *in vivo*. Interest in this compound in AD treatment research is sustained by the potential increase in brain cholinergic activity properties but also by the capacity of ladostigil to prevent gliosis and oxidative-nitrosative stress damage. Moreover, ladostigil has been demonstrated to possess potent anti-apoptotic and neuroprotective properties *in vitro* and in various neurodegenerative animal models including AD transgenic mice [323]. These neuroprotective activities involve regulation of APP processing, activation of protein kinase C and mitogen-activated protein kinase signaling pathways, inhibition of neuronal death markers, prevention of the fall in mitochondrial membrane potential, up-regulation of neurotrophic factors, and anti-oxidative activity.

- *Huperzine A* is an extract of the Chinese plant *Huperzia serrata*. Huperzine A is a selective potent inhibitor of AChE [324]. In addition, some studies have shown that huperzine A may shift APP metabolism towards the non-amyloidogenic α-secretase pathway [325]. In addition, huperzine A reduces glutamate-induced cytotoxicity by antagonizing cerebral NMDA receptors [326]. Finally, huperzine A reverses or attenuates cognitive deficits in some animal models of AD [325]. Large-scale, randomized, placebo-controlled trials are necessary to establish the role of huperzine A in the treatment of AD [327].

- *Phytochemicals* as curcumin, catechins and resveratrol beyond their antioxidant activity are also involved in antiamyloidogenic, anti-inflammatory mechanisms and inhibitors of NFkappaB [328-330].

- *Celastrol* is another compound whicha appears to have multiple functions as anti-inflammatory, anti-oxidant and reductor of amyloouid via BACE 1 [331, 332].

3. Concluding remarks

Main targets of therapeutic intervention at early stages of Alzheimer are summarized in Figure 1. Based on the presently available data several conclusions can be drawn. Combination therapies with drugs targeting different pathological factors or the use of multi-target compounds appear to be the most effective strategy in the treatment of the neurodegenerative process in Alzheimer. Most potential experimental therapies exhibit the highest efficiency when applied during the pre-symptomatic phase of the disease. Therefore, it is essential to develop diagnostic tools to detect Alzheimer at early stages. Moreover, considering that Alzheimer, as a degenerative process not necessarily leading to dementia, affects a large percentage of individuals in the sixth decade of life, it would be wise to introduce habits and low-cost, safe treatments to prevent the progression of Alzheimer early in life, as occurs in artheriosclerosis, to transform AD into a chronic, incomplete and non-devastating disease thereby allowing for normal life in the elderly.

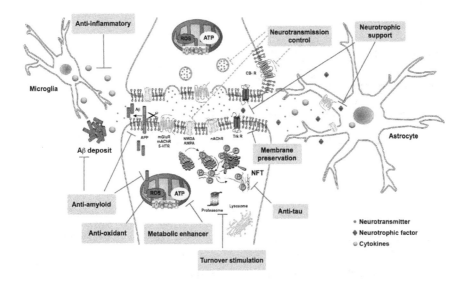

Figure 1. Schematic representation of the main cellular targets that are currently under development to prevent or retard the progression of Alzheimer to disease states. Most of the experimental approaches are designed to block or mitigate (red lines) pathological events occurring at the earliest stages, including abnormal Aβ and tau aggregation, chronic inflammatory responses, and oxidative stress damage. Other strategies (blue lines) aim at stimulating the metabolism to reduce Alzheimer's energetic failure as well as to promote intrinsic mechanisms that protect or repair cellular damage, including synaptic plasticity, preservation of the lipid membrane composition, and the promotion of damaged protein and organelle turnover. Therapeutic approaches based on the modulation of neurotransmission (green dashed lines) are designed to bypass deficient cholinergic neurotransmission whereas other compounds aim to block glutamatergic excitotoxicity. Considering the complex scenario of the Alzheimer neurodegenerative process, multi-target therapies applied at early stages of the disease appear to be the most effective strategy.

In addition to these general conclusions, several points deserve a particular comment. Recognition of the genotypic background, clinical and neuropathological subtypes and different pace of clinical manifestations is important to refine personalized treatments [333-335]. This includes modifications of the treatment as Alzheimer is not a mere accumulation of defects but rather a combination of deficiencies and plastic changes that imply shifts in molecular pathways with disease progression. Drugs and treatments beneficious at first stages of the degenerative process may be harmful at advanced stages. Special effort must be put into practice to learn about the combination of drugs at which determinate time for every particular individual.

Acknowledgements

Parts of the work used in this review were supported by the project BESAD-P (Instituto Carlos III), Mutua Madrileña and Agrupación Mútua. We wish to thank T. Yohannan for editorial assistance.

Author details

Ester Aso and Isidre Ferrer*

*Address all correspondence to: 8082ifa@gmail.com

Institut de Neuropatologia, Hospital Universitari de Bellvitge, Universitat de Barcelona, CIBERNED, Spain

References

[1] Ferrer I. Defining Alzheimer as a common age-related neurodegenerative process not inevitably leading to dementia. Prog Neurobiol. 2012; 97: 38-51.

[2] Petot GJ, Friedland RP. Lipids, diet and Alzheimer disease: an extended summary. J Neurol Sci. 2004; 226: 31-3.

[3] Luchsinger JAQ, Tang Noble JM, Scarmeas N. Diet and Alzheimer's disease. Curr Neurol Neurosci Rep. 2007; 7: 366-72.

[4] Kovacs GG, Alafuzoff I, Al-Sarraj S, Arzberger T, Bogdanovic N, Capellari S, Ferrer I, Gelpi E, Kövari V, Kretzschmar H, Nagy Z, Parchi P, Seilhean D, Soininen H, Troakes C, Budka H. Mixed brain pathologies in dementia: the brainNet Europe consortium experience. Dementia. 2008; 26: 343-50.

[5] Ferrer I. Cognitive impairment of vasxcular origin: Neuropathology of cognitive impairment of vascular origin. J Neurol Sci. 2010; 299-339-49.

[6] De Strooper B, Vassar R, Golde T. The secretases: enzymes with therapeutic potential in Alzheimer disease. Nat Rev Neurol. 2010; 6: 99-107

[7] Ring S, Weyer SW, Kilian SB, Waldron E, Pietrzik CU, Filippov MA, Herms J,Buchholz C, Eckman CB, Korte M, Wolfer DP, Müller UC. The secreted beta-amyloid precursor

protein ectodomain APPs alpha is sufficient to rescue the anatomical, behavioral, and electrophysiological abnormalities of APP-deficient mice. J Neurosci. 2007; 27: 7817-26.

[8]   Bandyopadhyay S, Goldstein LE, Lahiri DK, Rogers JT. Role of the APP non-amyloidogenic signaling pathway and targeting alpha-secretase as an alternative drug target for treatment of Alzheimer's disease. Curr Med Chem. 2007; 14: 2848-64.

[9]   Laird FM, Cai H, Savonenko AV, Farah MH, He K, Melnikova T, Wen H, Chiang HC, Xu G, Koliatsos VE, Borchelt DR, Price DL, Lee HK, Wong PC. BACE1, a major determinant of selective vulnerability of the brain to amyloid-beta amyloidogenesis, is essential for cognitive, emotional, and synaptic functions. J Neurosci. 2005; 25:11693-709.

[10] McConlogue L, Buttini M, Anderson JP, Brigham EF, Chen KS, Freedman SB, Games D, Johnson-Wood K, Lee M, Zeller M, Liu W, Motter R, Sinha S. Partial reduction of BACE1 has dramatic effects on Alzheimer plaque and synaptic pathology in APP Transgenic Mice. J Biol Chem. 2007; 282: 26326-34.

[11] Hills ID, Vacca JP. Progress toward a practical BACE-1 inhibitor. Curr Opin Drug Discov Devel. 2007; 10: 383-91.

[12] Rajendran L, Schneider A, Schlechtingen G, Weidlich S, Ries J, Braxmeier T, Schwille P, Schulz JB, Schroeder C, Simons M, Jennings G, Knölker HJ, Simons K. Efficient inhibition of the Alzheimer's disease beta-secretase by membrane targeting. Science. 2008; 320: 520-3.

[13] Serneels L, Van Biervliet J, Craessaerts K, Dejaegere T, Horré K, Van Houtvin T, Esselmann H, Paul S, Schäfer MK, Berezovska O, Hyman BT, Sprangers B, Sciot R, Moons L, Jucker M, Yang Z, May PC, Karran E, Wiltfang J, D'Hooge R, De Strooper B. gamma-Secretase heterogeneity in the Aph1 subunit: relevance for Alzheimer's disease. Science. 2009; 324: 639-42.

[14] Serneels L, Dejaegere T, Craessaerts K, Horré K, Jorissen E, Tousseyn T, Hébert S, Coolen M, Martens G, Zwijsen A, Annaert W, Hartmann D, De Strooper B. Differential contribution of the three Aph1 genes to gamma-secretase activity in vivo. Proc Natl Acad Sci U S A. 2005; 102:1719-24.

[15] Dovey HF, John V, Anderson JP, Chen LZ, de Saint Andrieu P, Fang LY, Freedman SB, Folmer B, Goldbach E, Holsztynska EJ, Hu KL, Johnson-Wood KL, Kennedy SL, Kholodenko D, Knops JE, Latimer LH, Lee M, Liao Z, Lieberburg IM, Motter RN, Mutter LC, Nietz J, Quinn KP, Sacchi KL, Seubert PA, Shopp GM, Thorsett ED, Tung JS, Wu J, Yang S, Yin CT, Schenk DB, May PC, Altstiel LD, Bender MH, Boggs LN, Britton TC, Clemens JC, Czilli DL, Dieckman-McGinty DK, Droste JJ, Fuson KS, Gitter BD, Hyslop PA, Johnstone EM, Li WY, Little SP, Mabry TE, Miller FD, Audia JE. Functional gamma-secretase inhibitors reduce beta-amyloid peptide levels in brain. J Neurochem. 2001; 76: 173-81.

[16] Abramowski D, Wiederhold KH, Furrer U, Jaton AL, Neuenschwander A, Runser MJ, Danner S, Reichwald J, Ammaturo D, Staab D, Stoeckli M, Rueeger H, Neumann U,

Staufenbiel M. Dynamics of Abeta turnover and deposition in different beta-amyloid precursor protein transgenic mouse models following gamma-secretase inhibition. J Pharmacol Exp Ther. 2008; 327: 411-24.

[17] Bateman RJ, Siemers ER, Mawuenyega KG, Wen G, Browning KR, Sigurdson WC, Yarasheski KE, Friedrich SW, Demattos RB, May PC, Paul SM, Holtzman DM. A gamma-secretase inhibitor decreases amyloid-beta production in the central nervous system. Ann Neurol. 2009; 66: 48-54.

[18] Schor NF. What the halted phase III γ-secretase inhibitor trial may (or may not) be telling us. Ann Neurol. 2011; 69: 237-9.

[19] Netzer WJ, Dou F, Cai D, Veach D, Jean S, Li Y, Bornmann WG, Clarkson B, Xu H, Greengard P. Gleevec inhibits beta-amyloid production but not Notch cleavage. Proc Natl Acad Sci USA. 2003; 100:12444-9.

[20] Mayer SC, Kreft AF, Harrison B, Abou-Gharbia M, Antane M, Aschmies S, Atchison K, Chlenov M, Cole DC, Comery T, Diamantidis G, Ellingboe J, Fan K, Galante R, Gonzales C, Ho DM, Hoke ME, Hu Y, Huryn D, Jain U, Jin M, Kremer K, Kubrak D, Lin M, Lu P, Magolda R, Martone R, Moore W, Oganesian A, Pangalos MN, Porte A, Reinhart P, Resnick L, Riddell DR, Sonnenberg-Reines J, Stock JR, Sun SC, Wagner E, Wang T, Woller K, Xu Z, Zaleska MM, Zeldis J, Zhang M, Zhou H, Jacobsen JS. Discovery of begacestat, a Notch-1-sparing gamma-secretase inhibitor for the treatment of Alzheimer's disease. J Med Chem. 2008; 51: 7348-51.

[21] Borgegard T, Juréus A, Olsson F, Rosqvist S, Sabirsh A, Rotticci D, Paulsen K,Klintenberg R, Yan H, Waldman M, Stromberg K, Nord J, Johansson J, Regner A,Parpal S, Malinowsky D, Radesater AC, Li T, Singh R, Eriksson H, Lundkvist J. First and second generation γ-secretase modulators (GSMs) modulate amyloid-β (Aβ) peptide production through different mechanisms. J Biol Chem. 2012; 287:11810-9.

[22] D'Onofrio G, Panza F, Frisardi V, Solfrizzi V, Imbimbo BP, Paroni G, Cascavilla L, Seripa D, Pilotto A. Advances in the identification of γ-secretase inhibitors for the treatment of Alzheimer's disease. Expert Opin Drug Discov. 2012; 7: 19-37.

[23] Shirotani K, Tsubuki S, Iwata N, Takaki Y, Harigaya W, Maruyama K, Kiryu-Seo S, Iwata H, Tomita T, Iwatsubo T, Saiudo TC. Neprilysin degrades both amyloid beta peptides 1-40 and 142 most rapidly and efficiently among thiorphan- and phosphoramidon-sensitive endopeptidases. J Biol Chem. 2001; 276: 21895-901.

[24] Iwata N, Takaki Y, Fukami S, Tsubuki S, Saido TC. Region-specific reduction of A beta-degrading endopeptidase, neprilysin, in mouse hippocampus upon aging. J Neurosci Res. 2002; 70: 493-500.

[25] Wang DS, Iwata N, Hama E, Saido TC, Dickson DW. Oxidized neprilysin in aging and Alzheimer's disease brains. Biochem Biophys Res Commun. 2003; 310: 236-41.

[26] Marr RA, Rockenstein E, Mukherjee A, Kindy MS, Hersh LB, Gage FH, Verma IM, Masliah E. Neprilysin gene transfer reduces human amyloid pathology in transgenic mice. J Neurosci. 2003; 23: 1992-6.

[27] Nalivaeva NN, Beckett C, Belyaev ND, Turner AJ. Are amyloid-degrading enzymes viable therapeutic targets in Alzheimer's disease? J Neurochem. 2012; 120 Suppl 1:167-85.

[28] Leissring MA, Farris W, Chang AY, Walsh DM, Wu X, Sun X, Frosch MP, Selkoe DJ. Enhanced proteolysis of beta-amyloid in APP transgenic mice prevents plaque formation, secondary pathology, and premature death. Neuron. 2003; 40: 1087-93.

[29] Qiu WQ, Folstein MF. Insulin, insulin-degrading enzyme and amyloid-beta peptide in Alzheimer's disease: review and hypothesis. Neurobiol Aging. 2006; 27: 190-8.

[30] Miners JS, Barua N, Kehoe PG, Gill S, Love S. Aβ-degrading enzymes: potential for treatment of Alzheimer disease. J Neuropathol Exp Neurol. 2011; 70: 944-59.

[31] Aisen PS, Gauthier S, Vellas B, Briand R, Saumier D, Laurin J, Garceau D. Alzhemed: a potential treatment for Alzheimer's disease. Curr Alzheimer Res. 2007; 4: 473-8.

[32] Aisen PS, Gauthier S, Ferris SH, Saumier D, Haine D, Garceau D, Duong A, Suhy J, Oh J, Lau WC, Sampalis J. Tramiprosate in mild-to-moderate Alzheimer's disease _ a randomized, double-blind, placebo-controlled, multi-centre study (The Alphase study). Arch Med Sci. 2011; 7: 102-11.

[33] Fenili D, Brown M, Rappaport R, McLaurin J. Properties of scyllo-inositol as a thera-peutic treatment of AD-like pathology. J Mol Med (Berl). 2007; 85: 603-11.

[34] Hawkes CA, Deng LH, Shaw JE, Nitz M, McLaurin J. Small molecule beta-amyloid inhibitors that stabilize protofibrillar structures in vitro improve cognition and pathology in a mouse model of Alzheimer's disease. Eur J Neurosci. 2010; 31: 203-13.

[35] Salloway S, Sperling R, Keren R, Porsteinsson AP, van Dyck CH, Tariot PN, Gilman S, Arnold D, Abushakra S, Hernandez C, Crans G, Liang E, Quinn G, Bairu M, Pastrak A, Cedarbaum JM; ELND005-AD201 Investigators. A phase 2 randomized trial of ELND005, scyllo-inositol, in mild to moderate Alzheimer disease. Neurology. 2011; 77: 1253-62.

[36] Adlard PA, Cherny RA, Finkelstein DI, Gautier E, Robb E, Cortes M, Volitakis I, Liu X, Smith JP, Perez K, Laughton K, Li QX, Charman SA, Nicolazzo JA, Wilkins S, Deleva K, Lynch T, Kok G, Ritchie CW, Tanzi RE, Cappai R, Masters CL, Barnham KJ, Bush AI. Rapid restoration of cognition in Alzheimer's transgenic mice with 8-hydroxy quinoline analogs is associated with decreased interstitial Abeta. Neuron. 2008 59: 43-55.

[37] Faux NG, Ritchie CW, Gunn A, Rembach A, Tsatsanis A, Bedo J, Harrison J, Lannfelt L, Blennow K, Zetterberg H, Ingelsson M, Masters CL, Tanzi RE, Cummings JL, Herd

CM, Bush AI. PBT2 rapidly improves cognition in Alzheimer's Disease: additional phase II analyses. J Alzheimers Dis. 2010; 20: 509-16.

[38]   Klajnert B, Cladera J, Bryszewska M. Molecular interactions of dendrimers with amyloid peptides: pH dependence. Biomacromolecules. 2006; 7: 2186-91.

[39]   Klajnert B, Cortijo-Arellano M, Cladera J, Bryszewska M. Influence of dendrimer's structure on its activity against amyloid fibril formation. Biochem Biophys Res Commun. 2006; 345: 21-8.

[40]   Klementieva O, Benseny-Cases N, Gella A, Appelhans D, Voit B, Cladera J. Dense shell glycodendrimers as potential nontoxic anti-amyloidogenic agents in Alzheimer's disease. Amyloid-dendrimer aggregates morphology and cell toxicity. Biomacromolecules. 2011; 12: 3903-9.

[41]   Schenk D, Barbour R, Dunn W, Gordon G, Grajeda H, Guido T, Hu K, Huang J, Johnson-Wood K, Khan K, Kholodenko D, Lee M, Liao Z, Lieberburg I, Motter R, Mutter L, Soriano F, Shopp G, Vasquez N, Vandevert C, Walker S, Wogulis M, Yednock T, Games D, Seubert P. Immunization with amyloid-beta attenuates Alzheimer-disease-like pathology in the PDAPP mouse. Nature. 1999; 400:173-7.

[42]   Janus C, Pearson J, McLaurin J, Mathews PM, Jiang Y, Schmidt SD, Chishti MA, Horne P, Heslin D, French J, Mount HT, Nixon RA, Mercken M, Bergeron C, Fraser PE, St George-Hyslop P, Westaway D. A beta peptide immunization reduces behavioural impairment and plaques in a model of Alzheimer's disease. Nature. 2000; 408: 979-82.

[43]   Morgan D, Diamond DM, Gottschall PE, Ugen KE, Dickey C, Hardy J, Duff K, Jantzen P, DiCarlo G, Wilcock D, Connor K, Hatcher J, Hope C, Gordon M, Arendash GW. A beta peptide vaccination prevents memory loss in an animal model of Alzheimer's disease. Nature. 2000; 408: 982-5.

[44]   Orgogozo JM, Gilman S, Dartigues JF, Laurent B, Puel M, Kirby LC, Jouanny P, Dubois B, Eisner L, Flitman S, Michel BF, Boada M, Frank A, Hock C. Subacute meningoence-phalitis in a subset of patients with AD after Abeta42 immunization. Neurology. 2003; 61: 46-54.

[45]   Nicoll JA, Wilkinson D, Holmes C, Steart P, Markham H, Weller RO. Neuropathology of human Alzheimer disease after immunization with amyloid-beta peptide: a case report. Nat Med. 2003; 9: 448-52.

[46]   Ferrer I, Boada Rovira M, Sánchez Guerra ML, Rey MJ, Costa-Jussá F. Neuropathology and pathogenesis of encephalitis following amyloid-beta immunization in Alzheimer's disease. Brain Pathol. 2004; 14: 11-20.

[47]   Meyer-Luehmann M, Mora JR, Mielke M, Spires-Jones TL, de Calignon A, von Andrian UH, Hyman BT. T cell mediated cerebral hemorrhages and microhemorrhages during passive Abeta immunization in APPPS1 transgenic mice. Mol Neurodegener. 2011; 6: 22.

[48] Patton RL, Kalback WM, Esh CL, Kokjohn TA, Van Vickle GD, Luehrs DC, Kuo YM, Lopez J, Brune D, Ferrer I, Masliah E, Newel AJ, Beach TG, Castaño EM, Roher AE. Amyloid-beta peptide remnants in AN-1792-immunized Alzheimer's disease patients: a biochemical analysis. Am J Pathol. 2006; 169: 1048-63.

[49] Nicoll JA, Barton E, Boche D, Neal JW, Ferrer I, Thompson P, Vlachouli C, Wilkinson D, Bayer A, Games D, Seubert P, Schenk D, Holmes C. Abeta species removal after abeta42 immunization. J Neuropathol Exp Neurol. 2006 ; 65: 1040-8.

[50] Serrano-Pozo A, William CM, Ferrer I, Uro-Coste E, Delisle MB, Maurage CA, Hock C, Nitsch RM, Masliah E, Growdon JH, Frosch MP, Hyman BT. Beneficial effect of human anti-amyloid-beta active immunization on neurite morphology and tau pathology. Brain. 2010; 133: 1312-27.

[51] Agadjanyan MG, Ghochikyan A, Petrushina I, Vasilevko V, Movsesyan N, Mkrtichyan M, Saing T, Cribbs DH. Prototype Alzheimer's disease vaccine using the immunodominant B cell epitope from beta-amyloid and promiscuous T cell epitope pan HLA DR-binding peptide. J Immunol. 2005; 174:1580-6.

[52] McLaurin J, Cecal R, Kierstead ME, Tian X, Phinney AL, Manea M, French JE, Lambermon MH, Darabie AA, Brown ME, Janus C, Chishti MA, Horne P, Westaway D, Fraser PE, Mount HT, Przybylski M, St George-Hyslop P. Therapeutically effective antibodies against amyloid-beta peptide target amyloid-beta residues 4-10 and inhibit cytotoxicity and fibrillogenesis. Nat Med. 2002; 8: 1263-9.

[53] Lemere CA, Maier M, Jiang L, Peng Y, Seabrook TJ. Amyloid-beta immunotherapy for the prevention and treatment of Alzheimer disease: lessons from mice, monkeys, and humans. Rejuvenation Res. 2006; 9: 77-84.

[54] Wilcock DM, Alamed J, Gottschall PE, Grimm J, Rosenthal A, Pons J, Ronan V, Symmonds K, Gordon MN, Morgan D. Deglycosylated anti-amyloid-beta antibodies eliminate cognitive deficits and reduce parenchymal amyloid with minimal vascular consequences in aged amyloid precursor protein transgenic mice. J Neurosci. 2006; 26: 5340-6.

[55] Solomon B, Frenkel D. Immunotherapy for Alzheimer's disease. Neuropharmacology. 2010; 59: 303-9.

[56] Delrieu J, Ousset PJ, Caillaud C, Vellas B. 'Clinical trials in Alzheimer's disease': immunotherapy approaches. J Neurochem. 2012; 120 Suppl 1:186-93.

[57] Golde TE, Schneider LS, Koo EH. Anti-aβ therapeutics in Alzheimer's disease: the need for a paradigm shift. Neuron. 2011; 69: 203-13.

[58] Morris M, Maeda S, Vossel K, Mucke L. The many faces of tau. Neuron. 2011; 70: 410-26.

[59] Huang Y, Mucke L. Alzheimer mechanisms and therapeuthic strategies. Cell 2012; 148: 1204-22.

[60] Wischik CM, Edwards PC, Lai RY, Roth M, Harrington CR. Selective inhibition of Alzheimer disease-like tau aggregation by phenothiazines. Proc Natl Acad Sci USA. 1996; 93:11213-8.

[61] O'Leary JC 3rd, Li Q, Marinec P, Blair LJ, Congdon EE, Johnson AG, Jinwal UK, Koren J 3rd, Jones JR, Kraft C, Peters M, Abisambra JF, Duff KE, Weeber EJ, Gestwicki JE, Dickey CA. Phenothiazine-mediated rescue of cognition in tau transgenic mice requires neuroprotection and reduced soluble tau burden. Mol Neurodegener. 2010; 5: 45.

[62] Gura T. Hope in Alzheimer's fight emerges from unexpected places. Nat Med. 2008; 14: 894.

[63] Yoshiyama Y, Higuchi M, Zhang B, Huang SM, Iwata N, Saido TC, Maeda J, Suhara T, Trojanowski JQ, Lee VM. Synapse loss and microglial activation precede tangles in a P301S tauopathy mouse model. Neuron. 2007; 53: 337-51.

[64] Chambraud B, Sardin E, Giustiniani J, Dounane O, Schumacher M, Goedert M, Baulieu EE. A role for FKBP52 in Tau protein function. Proc Natl Acad Sci U S A. 2010; 107: 2658-63.

[65] Taniguchi S, Suzuki N, Masuda M, Hisanaga S, Iwatsubo T, Goedert M, Hasegawa M. Inhibition of heparin-induced tau filament formation by phenothiazines, polyphenols, and porphyrins. J Biol Chem. 2005; 280: 7614-23.

[66] Gong CX, Iqbal K. Hyperphosphorylation of microtubule-associated protein tau: a promising therapeutic target for Alzheimer disease. Curr Med Chem. 2008; 15: 2321-8.

[67] Mi K, Johnson GV. The role of tau phosphorylation in the pathogenesis of Alzheimer's disease. Curr Alzheimer Res. 2006; 3: 449-63.

[68] Hernández F, de Barreda EG, Fuster-Matanzo A, Goñi-Oliver P, Lucas JJ, Avila J. The role of GSK3 in Alzheimer disease. Brain Res Bull. 2009; 80: 248-50.

[69] Mazanetz MP, Fischer PM. Untangling tau hyperphosphorylation in drug design for neurodegenerative diseases. Nat Rev Drug Discov. 2007; 6: 464-79.

[70] Noble W, Planel E, Zehr C, Olm V, Meyerson J, Suleman F, Gaynor K, Wang L, LaFrancois J, Feinstein B, Burns M, Krishnamurthy P, Wen Y, Bhat R, Lewis J, Dickson D, Duff K. Inhibition of glycogen synthase kinase-3 by lithium correlates with reduced tauopathy and degeneration in vivo. Proc Natl Acad Sci U S A. 2005; 102: 6990-5.

[71] Grandjean EM, Aubry JM. Lithium: updated human knowledge using an evidence-based approach. Part II: Clinical pharmacology and therapeutic monitoring. CNS Drugs. 2009; 23: 331-49.

[72] Alvarez A, Toro R, Cáceres A, Maccioni RB. Inhibition of tau phosphorylating protein kinase cdk5 prevents beta-amyloid-induced neuronal death. FEBS Lett. 1999; 459: 421-6

[73]   Zheng YL, Kesavapany S, Gravell M, Hamilton RS, Schubert M, Amin N, Albers W, Grant P, Pant HC. A Cdk5 inhibitory peptide reduces tau hyperphosphorylation and apoptosis in neurons. EMBO J. 2005; 24: 209-20.

[74]   Wen Y, Planel E, Herman M, Figueroa HY, Wang L, Liu L, Lau LF, Yu WH, Duff KE. Interplay between cyclin-dependent kinase 5 and glycogen synthase kinase 3 beta mediated by neuregulin signaling leads to differential effects on tau phosphorylation and amyloid precursor protein processing. J Neurosci. 2008; 28: 2624-32.

[75]   Cheung ZH, Ip NY. Cdk5: a multifaceted kinase in neurodegenerative diseases. Trends Cell Biol. 2012; 22: 169-75.

[76]   Li L, Sengupta A, Haque N, Grundke-Iqbal I, Iqbal K. Memantine inhibits and reverses the Alzheimer type abnormal hyperphosphorylation of tau and associated neurodegeneration. FEBS Lett. 2004; 566: 261-9.

[77]   Cheng Y, Feng Z, Zhang QZ, Zhang JT. Beneficial effects of melatonin in experimental models of Alzheimer disease. Acta Pharmacol Sin. 2006; 27: 129-39.

[78]   Torrent L, Ferrer I. PP2A and Alzheimer disease. Curr Alzheimer Res. 2012; 9: 248-56.

[79]   Ittner LM, Ke YD, Delerue F, Bi M, Gladbach A, van Eersel J, Wölfing H, Chieng BC, Christie MJ, Napier IA, Eckert A, Staufenbiel M, Hardeman E, Götz J. Dendritic function of tau mediates amyloid-beta toxicity in Alzheimer's disease mouse models. Cell. 2010; 142: 387-97.

[80]   Roberson ED, Scearce-Levie K, Palop JJ, Yan F, Cheng IH, Wu T, Gerstein H, Yu GQ, Mucke L. Reducing endogenous tau ameliorates amyloid beta-induced deficits in an Alzheimer's disease mouse model. Science. 2007; 316: 750-4.

[81]   Roberson ED, Halabisky B, Yoo JW, Yao J, Chin J, Yan F, Wu T, Hamto P, Devidze N, Yu GQ, Palop JJ, Noebels JL, Mucke L. Amyloid-β/Fyn-induced synaptic, network, and cognitive impairments depend on tau levels in multiple mouse models of Alzheimer's disease. J Neurosci. 2011; 31: 700-11.

[82]   Sahara N, Murayama M, Mizoroki T, Urushitani M, Imai Y, Takahashi R, Murata S, Tanaka K, Takashima A. In vivo evidence of CHIP up-regulation attenuating tau aggregation. J Neurochem. 2005; 94:1254-63.

[83]   Min SW, Cho SH, Zhou Y, Schroeder S, Haroutunian V, Seeley WW, Huang EJ, Shen Y, Masliah E, Mukherjee C, Meyers D, Cole PA, Ott M, Gan L. Acetylation of tau inhibits its degradation and contributes to tauopathy. Neuron. 2010; 67: 953-66.

[84]   Cohen TJ, Guo JL, Hurtado DE, Kwong LK, Mills IP, Trojanowski JQ, Lee VM. The acetylation of tau inhibits its function and promotes pathological tau aggregation. Nat Commun. 2011; 2: 252.

[85]   Asuni AA, Boutajangout A, Quartermain D, Sigurdsson EM. Immunotherapy targeting
       pathological tau conformers in atangle mouse model reduces brain pathology with
       associated functional improvements. J Neurosci. 2007; 27: 9115-29.

[86]   Boimel M, Grigoriades N, Lourbopoulos A, Haber E, Abramsky O, Rosennmann H.
       Efficacy and safety of immunization with phosphorylated tau against neurofibrillary
       tangles in mice. Exp Neurol 2010; 224: 472-85.

[87]   Chai X, Wu S, Murray TK, Kinley R, Cella CV, Sims H, Buckner N, Hanmer J, Davies
       P, O'Neill MJ, Hutton ML, Citron M. Passive immunization with anti-Tau antibodies
       in two transgenic models: reduction of Tau pathology and delay of disease progression.
       J Biol Chem. 2011; 286: 34457-67.

[88]   Brunden KR, Yao Y, Potuzak JS, Ferrer NI, Ballatore C, James MJ, Hogan AM, Troja-
       nowski JQ, Smith AB 3rd, Lee VM. The characterization of microtubule-stabilizing
       drugs as possible therapeutic agents for Alzheimer's disease and related tauopathies.
       Pharmacol Res. 2011; 63: 341-51.

[89]   Zempel H, Thies E, Mandelkow E, Mandelkow EM. Abeta oligomers cause localized
       Ca(2+) elevation, missorting of endogenous Tau into dendrites, Tau phosphorylation,
       and destruction of microtubules and spines. J Neurosci. 2010; 30: 11938-50.

[90]   Zhang B, Maiti A, Shively S, Lakhani F, McDonald-Jones G, Bruce J, Lee EB, Xie SX,
       Joyce S, Li C, Toleikis PM, Lee VM, Trojanowski JQ. Microtubule-binding drugs offset
       tau sequestration by stabilizing microtubules and reversing fast axonal transport
       deficits in a tauopathy model. Proc Natl Acad Sci USA. 2005; 102:: 227-31.

[91]   Brunden KR, Zhang B, Carroll J, Yao Y, Potuzak JS, Hogan AM, Iba M, James MJ, Xie
       SX, Ballatore C, Smith AB 3rd, Lee VM, Trojanowski JQ. Epothilone D improves
       microtubule density, axonal integrity, and cognition in a transgenic mouse model of
       tauopathy. J Neurosci. 2010; 30:13861-6.

[92]   Vulih-Shultzman I, Pinhasov A, Mandel S, Grigoriadis N, Touloumi O, Pittel Z, Gozes
       I. Activity-dependent neuroprotective protein snippet NAP reduces tau hyperphos-
       phorylation and enhances learning in a novel transgenic mouse model. J Pharmacol
       Exp Ther. 2007; 323: 438-49.

[93]   Gozes I, Stewart A, Morimoto B, Fox A, Sutherland K, Schmeche D. Addressing
       Alzheimer's disease tangles: from NAP to AL-108. Curr Alzheimer Res. 2009; 6: 455-60.

[94]   Nunomura A, Perry G, Aliev G, Hirai K, Takeda A, Balraj EK, Jones PK, Ghanbari H,
       Wataya T, Shimohama S, Chiba S, Atwood CS, Petersen RB, Smith MA. Oxidative
       damage is the earliest event in Alzheimer disease. J Neuropathol Exp Neurol. 2001;
       60:759-67.

[95]   Nunomura A, Perry G, Pappolla MA, Friedland RP, Hirai K, Chiba S, Smith MA.
       Neuronal oxidative stress precedes amyloid-beta deposition in Down syndrome. J
       Neuropathol Exp Neurol. 2000; 59: 1011-7

[96]   Perry G, Smith MA. Is oxidative damage central to the pathogenesis of Alzheimer disease? Acta Neurol Belg. 1998; 98:175-9.

[97]   Praticò D, Uryu K, Leight S, Trojanoswki JQ, Lee VM. Increased lipid peroxidation precedes amyloid plaque formation in an animal model of Alzheimer amyloidosis. J Neurosci. 2001; 21: 4183-7.

[98]   Praticò D, Clark CM, Liun F, Rokach J, Lee VY, Trojanowski JQ. Increase of brain oxidative stress in mild cognitive impairment: a possible predictor of Alzheimer disease. Arch Neurol. 2002 59(6):972-6. Erratum in: Arch Neurol 2002; 59:1475.

[99]   Martínez A, Portero-Otin M, Pamplona R, Ferrer I. Protein targets of oxidative damage in human neurodegenerative diseases with abnormal protein aggregates. Brain Pathol. 2010; 20: 281-97.

[100] Terni B, Boada J, Portero-Otin M, Pamplona R, Ferrer I. Mitochondrial ATP-synthase in the entorhinal cortex is a target of oxidative stress at stages I/II of Alzheimer's disease pathology. Brain Pathol. 2010; 20: 222-33.

[101] Praticò D. Evidence of oxidative stress in Alzheimer's disease brain and antioxidant therapy: lights and shadows. Ann N Y Acad Sci. 2008; 1147: 70-8.

[102] Bonda DJ, Wang X, Perry G, Nunomura A, Tabaton M, Zhu X, Smith MA. Oxidative stress in Alzheimer disease: a possibility for prevention. Neuropharmacology. 2010; 59: 290-4

[103] Richard T, Pawlus AD, Iglésias ML, Pedrot E, Waffo-Teguo P, Mérillon JM, Monti JP. Neuroprotective properties of resveratrol and derivatives. Ann N Y Acad Sci. 2011; 1215: 103-8.

[104] Li F, Gong Q, Dong H, Shi J. Resveratrol, a neuroprotective supplement for Alzheimer's disease. Curr Pharm Des. 2012; 18: 27-33.

[105] Mancuso C, Bates TE, Butterfield DA, Calafato S, Cornelius C, De Lorenzo A, Dinkova Kostova AT, Calabrese V. Natural antioxidants in Alzheimer's disease. Expert Opin Investig Drugs. 2007; 16:1921-31.

[106] Belkacemi A, Doggui S, Dao L, Ramassamy C. Challenges associated with curcumin therapy in Alzheimer disease. Expert Rev Mol Med. 2011; 13:e34.

[107] Hamaguchi T, Ono K, Yamada M. REVIEW: Curcumin and Alzheimer's disease. CNS Neurosci Ther. 2010; 16: 285-97.

[108] Mandel SA, Amit T, Weinreb O, Reznichenko L, Youdim MB. Simultaneous manipulation of multiple brain targets by green tea catechins: a potential neuroprotective strategy for Alzheimer and Parkinson diseases. CNS Neurosci Ther. 2008; 14: 352-65.

[109] Spagnoli A, Lucca U, Menasce G, Bandera L, Cizza G, Forloni G, Tettamanti M, Frattura L, Tiraboschi P, Comelli M, et al. Long-term acetyl-L-carnitine treatment in Alzheimer's disease. Neurology. 1991; 41: 1726-32.

[110] Montgomery SA, Thal LJ, Amrein R. Meta-analysis of double blind randomized controlled clinical trials of acetyl-L-carnitine versus placebo in the treatment of mild cognitive impairment and mild Alzheimer's disease. Int Clin Psychopharmacol. 2003; 18: 61-71.

[111] Nishida Y, Yokota T, Takahashi T, Uchihara T, Jishage K, Mizusawa H. Deletion of vitamin E enhances phenotype of Alzheimer disease model mouse. Biochem Biophys Res Commun. 2006; 350: 530-6.

[112] Viña J, LLoret A, Giraldo E, Badia MC, Alonso MD. Antioxidant pathways in Alzheimer's disease: possibilities of intervention. Curr Pharm Des 2011; 17: 3861-4.

[113] Harrison FE, Hosseini AH, McDonald MP, May JM. Vitamin C reduces spatial learning deficits in middle-aged and very old APP/PSEN1 transgenic and wild-type mice. Pharmacol Biochem Behav. 2009; 93: 443-50.

[114] Murakami K, Murata N, Ozawa Y, Kinoshita N, Irie K, Shirasawa T, Shimizu T. Vitamin C restores behavioral deficits and amyloid- oligomerization without affecting plaque formation in a mouse model of Alzheimer's disease. J Alzheimers Dis. 2011; 26: 7-18.

[115] Zandi PP, Anthony JC, Khachaturian AS, Stone SV, Gustafson D, Tschanz JT, Norton MC, Welsh-Bohmer KA, Breitner JC; Cache County Study Group. Reduced risk of Alzheimer disease in users of antioxidant vitamin supplements: the Cache County Study. Arch Neurol. 2004; 61: 82-8

[116] Boothby LA, Doering PL. Vitamin C and vitamin E for Alzheimer's disease. Ann Pharmacother. 2005; 39: 2073-80.

[117] Birks J, Grimley Evans J. Ginkgo biloba for cognitive impairment and dementia. Cochrane Database Syst Rev. 2009; (1):CD003120.

[118] Tchantchou F, Xu Y, Wu Y, Christen Y, Luo Y. EGb 761 enhances adult hippocampal neurogenesis and phosphorylation of CREB in transgenic mouse model of Alzheimer's disease. FASEB J. 2007; 21: 2400-8.

[119] Galasko DR, Peskind E, Clark CM, Quinn JF, Ringman JM, Jicha GA, Cotman C, Cottrell B, Montine TJ, Thomas RG, Aisen P; for the Alzheimer's Disease Cooperative Study. Antioxidants for Alzheimer disease: a randomized clinical trial with cerebrospinal fluid biomarker measures. Arch Neurol. 2012 Mar 19.

[120] Holmquist L, Stuchbury G, Berbaum K, Muscat S, Young S, Hager K, Engel J, Münch G. Lipoic acid as a novel treatment for Alzheimer's disease and related dementias. Pharmacol Ther. 2007; 113:154-64.

[121] Maczurek A, Hager K, Kenklies M, Sharman M, Martins R, Engel J, Carlson DA, Münch G. Lipoic acid as an anti-inflammatory and neuroprotective treatment for Alzheimer's disease. Adv Drug Deliv Rev. 2008; 60: 1463-70.

[122]   Pocernich CB, Butterfield DA. Elevation of glutathione as a therapeutic strategy in Alzheimer disease. Biochim Biophys Acta. 2012; 1822: 625-30.

[123]   Adair JC, Knoefel JE, Morgan N. Controlled trial of N-acetylcysteine for patients with probable Alzheimer's disease. Neurology. 2001; 578: 1515-7.

[124]   Orsucci D, Mancuso M, Ienco EC, LoGerfo A, Siciliano G. Targeting mitochondrial dysfunction and neurodegeneration by means of coenzyme Q10 and its analogues. Curr Med Chem. 2011; 18: 4053-64

[125]   Beal MF. Mitochondrial dysfunction and oxidative damage in Alzheimer's and Parkinson's diseases and coenzyme Q10 as a potential treatment. J Bioenerg Biomembr. 2004; 36: 381-6.

[126]   Dumont M, Kipiani K, Yu F, Wille E, Katz M, Calingasan NY, Gouras GK, Lin MT, Beal MF. Coenzyme Q10 decreases amyloid pathology and improves behavior in a transgenic mouse model of Alzheimer's disease. J Alzheimers Dis. 2011; 27: 211-23.

[127]   McManus MJ, Murphy MP, Franklin JL. The mitochondria-targeted antioxidant MitoQ prevents loss of spatial memory retention and early neuropathology in a transgenic mouse model of Alzheimer's disease. J Neurosci. 2011; 31:15703-15.

[128]   Hensley K. Neuroinflammation in Alzheimer's disease: mechanisms, pathologic consequences, and potential for therapeutic manipulation. J Alzheimers Dis. 2010; 21:1-14.

[129]   McGeer PL, McGeer E, Rogers J, Sibley J. Anti-inflammatory drugs and Alzheimer disease. Lancet. 1990; 335:1037.

[130]   Kaufmann WE, Andreasson KI, Isakson PC, Worley PF. Cyclooxygenases and the central nervous system. Prostaglandins. 1997; 54: 601-24.

[131]   Lim GP, Yang F, Chu T, Chen P, Beech W, Teter B, Tran T, Ubeda O, Ashe KH, Frautschy SA, Cole GM. Ibuprofen suppresses plaque pathology and inflammation in a mouse model for Alzheimer's disease. J Neurosci. 2000; 20: 5709-14.

[132]   Jantzen PT, Connor KE, DiCarlo G, Wenk GL, Wallace JL, Rojiani AM, Coppola D, Morgan D, Gordon MN. Microglial activation and beta -amyloid deposit reduction caused by a nitric oxide-releasing nonsteroidal anti-inflammatory drug in amyloid precursor protein plus presenilin-1 transgenic mice. J Neurosci. 2002; 22: 2246-54.

[133]   Yan Q, Zhang J, Liu H, Babu-Khan S, Vassar R, Biere AL, Citron M, Landreth G. Anti-inflammatory drug therapy alters beta-amyloid processing and deposition in an animal model of Alzheimer's disease. J Neurosci. 2003; 23: 7504-9.

[134]   Heneka MT, Sastre M, Dumitrescu-Ozimek L, Hanke A, Dewachter I, Kuiperi C, O'Banion K, Klockgether T, Van Leuven F, Landreth GE. Acute treatment with the PPARgamma agonist pioglitazone and ibuprofen reduces glial inflammation and Abeta1-42 levels in APPV717I transgenic mice. Brain. 2005; 128: 1442-53.

[135] Lim GP, Yang F, Chu T, Gahtan E, Ubeda O, Beech W, Overmier JB, Hsiao-Ashec K, Frautschy SA, Cole GM. Ibuprofen effects on Alzheimer pathology and open field activity in APPsw transgenic mice. Neurobiol Aging. 2001; 22: 983-91.

[136] Quinn J, Montine T, Morrow J, Woodward WR, Kulhanek D, Eckenstein F. Inflammation and cerebral amyloidosis are disconnected in an animal model of Alzheimer's disease. J Neuroimmunol. 2003; 137: 32-41.

[137] Sung S, Yang H, Uryu K, Lee EB, Zhao L, Shineman D, Trojanowski JQ, Lee VM, Praticò D. Modulation of nuclear factor-kappa B activity by indomethacin influences A beta levels but not A beta precursor protein metabolism in a model of Alzheimer's disease. Am J Pathol. 2004; 165: 2197-206.

[138] Kukar T, Murphy MP, Eriksen JL, Sagi SA, Weggen S, Smith TE, Ladd T, Khan MA, Kache R, Beard J, Dodson M, Merit S, Ozols VV, Anastasiadis PZ, Das P, Fauq A, Koo EH, Golde TE. Diverse compounds mimic Alzheimer disease-causing mutations by augmenting Abeta42 production. Nat Med. 2005; 11: 545-50.

[139] Jaturapatporn D, Isaac MG, McCleery J, Tabet N. Aspirin, steroidal and non-steroidal anti-inflammatory drugs for the treatment of Alzheimer's disease. Cochrane Database Syst Rev. 2012; CD006378.

[140] Coma M, Serenó L, Da Rocha-Souto B, Scotton TC, España J, Sánchez MB, Rodríguez M, Agulló J, Guardia-Laguarta C, Garcia-Alloza M, Borrelli LA, Clarimón J,Lleó A, Bacskai BJ, Saura CA, Hyman BT, Gómez-Isla T. Triflusal reduces dense-core plaque load, associated axonal alterations and inflammatory changes, and rescues cognition in a transgenic mouse model of Alzheimer's disease. Neurobiol Dis. 2010; 38: 482-91.

[141] Mosconi L, Pupi A, De Leon MJ. Brain glucose hypometabolism and oxidative stress in preclinical Alzheimer's disease. Ann NY Acad Sci 2008; 147: 180-95.

[142] Ferrer I. Altered mitochondria, energy metabolism, voltage-dependent anion channel, and lipid rafts converge to exhaust neurons in Alzheimer's disease. J Bioenerg Biomembr. 2009; 41: 425-31.

[143] Ferreira IL, Resende R, Ferreiro E, Rego AC, Pereira CF.Multiple defects in energy metabolism in Alzheimer's disease. Curr Drug Targets. 2010; 11: 1193-206.

[144] Ankarcrona M, Mangialasche F, Winblad B. Rethinking Alzheimer's disease therapy: are mitochondria the key? J Alzheimers Dis. 2010; 20 Suppl 2: S579-90

[145] Cunnane S, Nugent S, Roy M, Courchesne-Loyer A, Croteau E, Tremblay S, Castellano A, Pifferi F, Bocti C, Paquet N, Begdouri H, Bentourkia M, Turcotte E, Allard M, Barberger-Gateau P, Fulop T, Rapoport SI. Brain fuel metabolism, aging, and Alzheimer's disease. Nutrition. 2011; 27: 3-20.

[146] Kapogiannis D, Mattson MP. Disrupted energy metabolism and neuronal circuit dysfunction in cognitive impairment and Alzheimer's disease. Lancet Neurol. 2011; 10: 187-98.

[147] Jagust WJ, Seab JP, Huesman RH, Valk PE, Mathis CA, Reed BR, Coxson PG, Budinger TF. Diminished glucose transport in Alzheimer's disease: dynamic PET studies. J Cereb Blood Flow Metab. 1991; 11: 323-30.

[148] Pedersen WA, Flynn ER. Insulin resistance contributes to aberrant stress responses in the Tg2576 mouse model of Alzheimer's disease. Neurobiol Dis 2004; 17: 500-6.

[149] Landreth G, Jiang Q, Mandrekar S, Heneka M. PPARgamma agonists as therapeutics for the treatment of Alzheimer's disease. Neurotherapeutics. 2008; 5: 481-9.

[150] Bak AM, Egefjord L, Gejl M, Steffensen C, Stecher CW, Smidt K, Brock B, Rungby J. Targeting amyloid-beta by glucagon-like peptide -1 GLP-1) in Alzheimer's disease and diabetes. Expert Opin Ther Targets. 2011; 15: 1153-62.

[151] Bomfim TR, Forny-Germano L, Sathler LB, Brito-Moreira J, Houzel JC, Decker H, Silverman MA, Kazi H, Melo HM, McClean PL, Holscher C, Arnold SE, Talbot K, Klein WL, Munoz DP, Ferreira ST, De Felice FG. An anti-diabetes agent protects the mouse brain from defective insulin signaling caused by Alzheimer's disease-associated Aβ oligomers. J Clin Invest. 2012; 122: 1339-53.

[152] Miichi Y, Sakurai T, Akisaki T, Yokono K. Effects of insulin and amyloid β(1-42) oligomers on glucose incorporation and mitochondrial function in cultured rat hippocampal neurons. Geriatr Gerontol Int. 2011; 11: 517-24.

[153] Miller BW, Willett KC, Desilets AR. Rosiglitazone and pioglitazone for the treatment of Alzheimer's disease. Ann Pharmacother. 2011; 45: 1416-24.

[154] Van der Auwera I, Wera S, Van Leuven F, Henderson ST. A ketogenic diet reduces amyloid beta 40 and 42 in a mouse model of Alzheimer's disease. Nutr Metab. 2005; 2: 28.

[155] Yao J, Chen S, Mao Z, Cadenas E, Brinton RD. 2-Deoxy-D-glucose treatment induces ketogenesis, sustains mitochondrial function, and reduces pathology in female mouse model of Alzheimer's disease. PLoS One. 2011; 6:e21788.

[156] Henderson ST, Vogel JL, Barr LJ, Garvin F, Jones JJ, Costantini LC. Study of the ketogenic agent AC-1202 in mild to moderate Alzheimer's disease: a randomized, double-blind, placebo-controlled, multicenter trial. Nutr Metab. 2009; 6:31.

[157] Brewer GJ, Wallimann TW. Protective effect of the energy precursor creatine against toxicity of glutamate and beta-amyloid in rat hippocampal neurons. J Neurochem. 2000; 74: 1968-78.

[158] Sullivan PG, Geiger JD, Mattson MP, Scheff SW. Dietary supplement creatine protects against traumatic brain injury. Ann Neurol. 2000; 48: 723-9.

[159] Caspersen C, Wang N, Yao J, Sosunov A, Chen X, Lustbader JW, Xu HW, Stern D, McKhann G, Yan SD. Mitochondrial Abeta: a potential focal point for neuronal metabolic dysfunction in Alzheimer's disease. FASEB J. 2005; 19: 2040-1.

[160] Lustbader JW, Cirilli M, Lin C, Xu HW, Takuma K, Wang N, Caspersen C, Chen X, Pollak S, Chaney M, Trinchese F, Liu S, Gunn-Moore F, Lue LF, Walker DG, Kuppus-amy P, Zewier ZL, Arancio O, Stern D, Yan SS, Wu H. ABAD directly links Abeta to mitochondrial toxicity in Alzheimer's disease. Science. 2004; 304: 448-52.

[161] Lim YA, Grimm A, Giese M, Mensah-Nyagan AG, Villafranca JE, Ittner LM, Eckert A, Götz J. Inhibition of the mitochondrial enzyme ABAD restores the amyloid-β-mediated deregulation of estradiol. PLoS One. 2011; 6: e28887

[162] Yao J, Du H, Yan S, Fang F, Wang C, Lue LF, Guo L, Chen D, Stern DM, Gunn Moore FJ, Xi Chen J, Arancio O, Yan SS. Inhibition of amyloid-beta (Abeta)peptide-binding alcohol dehydrogenase-Abeta interaction reduces Abeta accumulation and improves mitochondrial function in a mouse model of Alzheimer's disease. J Neurosci. 2011; 31: 2313-20.

[163] Yamada K, Inagaki N. Neuroprotection by KATP channels. J Mol Cell Cardiol.2005 ; 38: 945-9.

[164] Liu D, Pitta M, Lee JH, Ray B, Lahiri DK, Furukawa K, Mughal M, Jiang H, Villarreal J, Cutler RG, Greig NH, Mattson MP. The KATP channel activator diazoxide amelio-rates amyloid-β and tau pathologies and improves memory in the 3xTgAD mouse model of Alzheimer's disease. J Alzheimers Dis. 2010; 22: 443-57.

[165] Sabbagh MN, Shill HA. Latrepirdine, a potential novel treatment for Alzheimer's disease and Huntington's chorea. Curr Opin Investig Drugs. 2010; 11: 80-91.

[166] Bachurin S, Lermontova N, Shevtzova E, Serkova T, Kireeva E. Comparative study of Tacrine and Dimebon action on mitochondrial permeability transition and β-amyloid-induced neurotoxicity. J Neurochem. 1999; 73(Suppl S): S185.

[167] Lermontova NN, Redkozubov AE, Shevtsova EF, Serkova TP, Kireeva EG, Bachurin SO.Dimebon and tacrine inhibit neurotoxic action of β-amyloid in culture and block L-type Ca2+ channels. Bull Exp Biol Med. 2001; 132:1079–83.

[168] Shevtsova EP, Grigoriev VV, Kireeva EG, Koroleva IV, Bachurin SO. Dimebon as mitoprotective and antiaging drug. Biochim Biophys Acta. 2006 (Suppl S) Abs P2.3.4.

[169] Doody RS, Gavrilova SI, Sano M, Thomas RG, Aisen PS, Bachurin SO, Seely L, Hung D; dimebon investigators. Effect of dimebon on cognition, activities of daily living, behaviour, and global function in patients with mild-to-moderate Alzheimer's disease: a randomised, double-blind, placebo-controlled study. Lancet. 2008; 372: 207-15.

[170] Francis PT, Ramírez MJ, Lai MK. Neurochemical basis for symptomatic treatment of Alzheimer's disease. Neuropharmacology. 2010; 59: 221-9.

[171] Geula C, Nagykery N, Nicholas A, Wu CK. Cholinergic neuronal and axonal abnor-malities are present early in aging and in Alzheimer disease. J Neuropathol Exp Neurol. 2008; 67: 309-18.

[172] Mufson EJ, Counts SE, Perez SE, Ginsberg SD. Cholinergic system during the progres-sion of Alzheimer's disease: therapeutic implications. Expert Rev Neurother. 2008; 8: 1703-18.

[173] Fisher A. Cholinergic treatments with emphasis on m1 muscarinic agonists as potential disease-modifying agents for Alzheimer's disease. Neurotherapeutics. 2008; 5: 433-42.

[174] Higgins JP, Flicker L. Lecithin for dementia and cognitive impairment. Cochrane Database Syst Rev. 2003; CD001015.

[175] Birks J. Cholinesterase inhibitors for Alzheimer's disease. Cochrane Database Syst Rev. 2006; (1):CD005593.

[176] Wilcock GK, Dawbarn D. Current pharmacological approaches to treating Alzheimer's disease. In: Neurobiology of Alzheimer's Disease. Third edition. Edited by David Dawbarn and Shelley J. Allen. Oxford University Press. 2007. Pp 359-390.

[177] Herrmann N, Chau SA, Kircanski I, Lanctôt KL. Current and emerging drug treatment options for Alzheimer's disease: a systematic review. Drugs. 2011; 71: 2031-65.

[178] Fischer W, Wictorin K, Björklund A, Williams LR, Varon S, Gage FH. Amelioration of cholinergic neuron atrophy and spatial memory impairment in aged rats by nerve growth factor. Nature. 1987; 329: 65-8.

[179] Caccamo A, Oddo S, Billings LM, Green KN, Martinez-Coria H, Fisher A, LaFerla FM. M1 receptors play a central role in modulating AD-like pathology in transgenic mice. Neuron. 2006; 49: 671-82.

[180] Nitsch RM, Slack BE, Wurtman RJ, Growdon JH. Release of Alzheimer amyloid precursor derivatives stimulated by activation of muscarinic acetylcholine receptors. Science. 1992; 258: 304-7.

[181] Wolf BA, Wertkin AM, Jolly YC, Yasuda RP, Wolfe BB, Konrad RJ, Manning D, Ravi S, Williamson JR, Lee VM. Muscarinic regulation of Alzheimer's disease amyloid precursor protein secretion and amyloid beta-protein production in human neuronal NT2N cells. J Biol Chem. 1995; 270: 4916-22.

[182] Woodruff-Pak DS, Gould TJ. Neuronal nicotinic acetylcholine receptors: involvement in Alzheimer's disease and schizophrenia. Behav Cogn Neurosci Rev. 2002; 1: 5-20.

[183] Parri RH, Dineley TK. Nicotinic acetylcholine receptor interaction with beta-amyloid: molecular, cellular, and physiological consequences. Curr Alzheimer Res. 2010; 7: 27-39.

[184] Nordberg A, Hellström-Lindahl E, Lee M, Johnson M, Mousavi M, Hall R, Perry E, Bednar I, Court J. Chronic nicotine treatment reduces beta-amyloidosis in the brain of a mouse model of Alzheimer's disease (APPsw). J Neurochem. 2002; 81:655-8.

[185] Oddo S, Caccamo A, Green KN, Liang K, Tran L, Chen Y, Leslie FM, LaFerla FM. Chronic nicotine administration exacerbates tau pathology in a transgenic model of Alzheimer's disease. Proc Natl Acad Sci U S A. 2005; 102: 3046-51.

[186] Haydar SN, Dunlop J. Neuronal nicotinic acetylcholine receptors - targets for the development of drugs to treat cognitive impairment associated with schizophrenia and Alzheimer's disease. Curr Top Med Chem. 2010; 10:144-52.

[187] Ren K, Thinschmidt J, Liu J, Ai L, Papke RL, King MA, Hughes JA, Meyer EM. alpha7 Nicotinic receptor gene delivery into mouse hippocampal neurons leads to functional receptor expression, improved spatial memory-related performance, and tau hyperphosphorylation. Neuroscience. 2007; 145: 314-22

[188] Kihara T, Shimohama S, Urushitani M, Sawada H, Kimura J, Kume T, Maeda T, Akaike A. Stimulation of alpha4beta2 nicotinic acetylcholine receptors inhibits beta-amyloid toxicity. Brain Res. 1998; 792: 331-4.

[189] Tam SW, Zaczek R. Linopirdine. A depolarization-activated releaser of transmitters for treatment of dementia. Adv Exp Med Biol. 1995; 363:47-56.

[190] Lachowicz JE, Duffy RA, Ruperto V, Kozlowski J, Zhou G, Clader J, Billard W, Binch H 3rd, Crosby G, Cohen-Williams M, Strader CD, Coffin V. Facilitation of acetylcholine release and improvement in cognition by a selective M2 muscarinic antagonist, SCH 72788. Life Sci. 2001; 68: 2585-92.

[191] Clader JW, Wang Y. Muscarinic receptor agonists and antagonists in the treatment of Alzheimer's disease. Curr Pharm Des. 2005; 11: 3353-61.

[192] Rockwood K, Beattie BL, Eastwood MR, Feldman H, Mohr E, Pryse-Phillips W, Gauthier S. A randomized, controlled trial of linopirdine in the treatment of Alzheimer's disease. Can J Neurol Sci. 1997; 24:140-5.

[193] Boyle CD, Lachowicz JE. Orally active and selective benzylidene ketal M2 muscarinic receptor antagonists for the treatment of Alzheimer's disease. Drug Dev Res 2002; 56: 310 –20.

[194] Palop JJ, Mucke L. Amyloid-beta-induced neuronal dysfunction in Alzheimer's disease: from synapses toward neural networks. Nat Neurosci. 2010; 13: 812-8.

[195] Hu NW, Ondrejcak T, Rowan MJ. Glutamate receptors in preclinical rserarch on Alzheimer's disease: update on recent advances. Pharmacol Biochem Behav 2012; 100: 855-62.

[196] Keller JN, Mark RJ, Bruce AJ, Blanc E, Rothstein JD, Uchida K, Waeg G, Mattson MP. 4-Hydroxynonenal, an aldehydic product of membrane lipid peroxidation, impairs glutamate transport and mitochondrial function in synaptosomes. Neuroscience. 1997; 80: 685-96.

[197] Li S, Hong S, Shepardson NE, Walsh DM, Shankar GM, Selkoe D. Soluble oligomers of amyloid Beta protein facilitate hippocampal long-term depression by disrupting neuronal glutamate uptake. Neuron. 2009; 62: 788-801.

[198] Cissé M, Halabisky B, Harris J, Devidze N, Dubal DB, Sun B, Orr A, Lotz G, Kim DH, Hamto P, Ho K, Yu GQ, Mucke L. Reversing EphB2 depletion rescues cognitive functions in Alzheimer model. Nature. 2011; 469: 47-52.

[199] Hoey SE, Williams RJ, Perkinton MS. Synaptic NMDA receptor activation stimulates alpha-secretase amyloid precursor protein processing and inhibits amyloid-beta production. J Neurosci. 2009; 29: 4442-60.

[200] Bordji K, Becerril-Ortega J, Nicole O, Buisson A. Activation of extrasynaptic, but not synaptic, NMDA receptors modifies amyloid precursor protein expression pattern and increases amyloid-ß production. J Neurosci. 2010; 30:15927-42.

[201] Francis PT. Glutamatergic approaches to the treatment of cognitive and behavioural symptoms of Alzheimer's disease. Neurodegener Dis. 2008; 5: 241-3.

[202] Lynch G, Gall CM. Glutamate-based therapeutic approaches: ampakines. Curr Opin Pharmacol. 2006; 6: 82-8.

[203] Granger R, Deadwyler S, Davis M, Moskovitz B, Kessler M, Rogers G, Lynch G. Facilitation of glutamate receptors reverses an age-associated memory impairment in rats. Synapse. 1996; 22: 332-7.

[204] Bartolini L, Casamenti F, Pepeu G. Aniracetam restores object recognition impaired by age, scopolamine, and nucleus basalis lesions. Pharmacol Biochem Behav. 1996; 53: 277-83.

[205] Johnson SA, Simmon VF. Randomized, double-blind, placebo-controlled international clinical trial of the Ampakine CX516 in elderly participants with mild cognitive impairment: a progress report. J Mol Neurosci. 2002; 19: 197-200.

[206] Myhrer T, Paulsen RE. Infusion of D-cycloserine into temporal-hippocampal areas and restoration of mnemonic function in rats with disrupted glutamatergic temporal systems. Eur J Pharmacol. 1997; 328: 1-7.

[207] Schwartz BL, Hashtroudi S, Herting RL, Schwartz P, Deutsch SI. d-Cycloserine enhances implicit memory in Alzheimer patients. Neurology. 1996; 46: 420-4.

[208] Parsons CG, Stöffler A, Danysz W. Memantine: a NMDA receptor antagonist that improves memory by restoration of homeostasis in the glutamatergic system—too little activation is bad, too much is even worse. Neuropharmacology. 2007; 53: 699-723.

[209] Reisberg B, Doody R, Stöffler A, Schmitt F, Ferris S, Möbius HJ; Memantine Study Group. Memantine in moderate-to-severe Alzheimer's disease. N Engl J Med. 2003; 348:1333-41.

[210] McKeage K. Memantine: a review of its use in moderate to severe Alzheimer's disease. CNS Drugs. 2009; 23: 881-97.

[211] Danysz W, Parsons CG. The NMDA receptor antagonist memantine as asymptomatological and neuroprotective treatment for Alzheimer's disease: preclinical evidence. Int J Geriatr Psychiatry. 2003; 18(Suppl 1): S23-32.

[212] Dong H, Yuede CM, Coughlan C, Lewis B, Csernansky JG. Effects of memantine on neuronal structure and conditioned fear in the Tg2576 mouse model of Alzheimer's disease. Neuropsychopharmacology. 2008; 33: 3226-36.

[213] Scholtzova H, Wadghiri YZ, Douadi M, Sigurdsson EM, Li YS, Quartermain D, Banerjee P, Wisniewski T. Memantine leads to behavioral improvement and amyloid reduction in Alzheimer's-disease-model transgenic mice shown as by micromagnetic resonance imaging. J Neurosci Res. 2008; 86: 2784-91.

[214] Martinez-Coria H, Green KN, Billings LM, Kitazawa M, Albrecht M, Rammes G, Parsons CG, Gupta S, Banerjee P, LaFerla FM. Memantine improves cognition and reduces Alzheimer's-like neuropathology in transgenic mice. Am J Pathol. 2010; 176: 870-80.

[215] Filali M, Lalonde R, Rivest S. Subchronic memantine administration on spatial learning, exploratory activity, and nest-building in an APP/PS1 mouse model of Alzheimer's disease. Neuropharmacology. 2011; 60: 930-6.

[216] Schneider LS, Dagerman KS, Higgins JP, McShane R. Lack of evidence for the efficacy of memantine in mild Alzheimer disease. Arch Neurol. 2011; 68: 991-8.

[217] Bowen DM, Allen SJ, Benton JS, Goodhardt MJ, Haan EA, Palmer AM, Sims NR, Smith CC, Spillane JA, Esiri MM, Neary D, Snowdon JS, Wilcock GK, Davison AN. Biochemical assessment of serotonergic and cholinergic dysfunction and cerebral atrophy in Alzheimer's disease. J Neurochem. 1983; 41: 266-72.

[218] Arai H, Ichimiya Y, Kosaka K, Moroji T, Iizuka R. Neurotransmitter changes in early- and late-onset Alzheimer-type dementia. Prog Neuropsychopharmacol Biol Psychiatry. 1992; 16: 883-90.

[219] Geldenhuys WJ, Van der Schyf CJ. Role of serotonin in Alzheimer's disease: a new therapeutic target? CNS Drugs. 2011; 25: 765-81.

[220] Nelson RL, Guo Z, Halagappa VM, Pearson M, Gray AJ, Matsuoka Y, Brown M, Martin B, Iyun T, Maudsley S, Clark RF, Mattson MP. Prophylactic treatment with paroxetine ameliorates behavioral deficits and retards the development of amyloid and tau pathologies in 3xTgAD mice. Exp Neurol. 2007; 205:166-76.

[221] Cirrito JR, Disabato BM, Restivo JL, Verges DK, Goebel WD, Sathyan A, Hayreh D, D'Angelo G, Benzinger T, Yoon H, Kim J, Morris JC, Mintun MA, Sheline YI. Serotonin signaling is associated with lower amyloid-β levels and plaques in transgenic mice and humans. Proc Natl Acad Sci U S A. 2011; 108: 14968-73.

[222] Schechter LE, Dawson LA, Harder JA. The potential utility of 5-HT1A receptor antagonists in the treatment of cognitive dysfunction associated with Alzheimer s disease. Curr Pharm Des. 2002; 8:139-45.

[223] Schechter LE, Smith DL, Rosenzweig-Lipson S, Sukoff SJ, Dawson LA, Marquis K, Jones D, Piesla M, Andree T, Nawoschik S, Harder JA, Womack MD, Buccafusco J, Terry AV, Hoebel B, Rada P, Kelly M, Abou-Gharbia M, Barrett JE, Childers W. Lecozotan (SRA-333): a selective serotonin 1A receptor antagonist that enhances the stimulated release of glutamate and acetylcholine in the hippocampus and possesses cognitive-enhancing properties. J Pharmacol Exp Ther. 2005; 314:1274-89.

[224] Patat A, Parks V, Raje S, Plotka A, Chassard D, Le Coz F. Safety, tolerability, pharmacokinetics and pharmacodynamics of ascending single and multiple doses of lecozotan in healthy young and elderly subjects. Br J Clin Pharmacol. 2009; 67: 299-308.

[225] Upton N, Chuang TT, Hunter AJ, Virley DJ. 5-HT6 receptor antagonists as novel cognitive enhancing agents for Alzheimer's disease. Neurotherapeutics 2008; 5: 458-69.

[226] Cho S, Hu Y. Activation of 5-HT4 receptors inhibits secretion of beta-amyloid peptides and increases neuronal survival. Exp Neurol. 2007; 203: 274-8.

[227] Russo O, Cachard-Chastel M, Rivière C, Giner M, Soulier JL, Berthouze M, Richard T, Monti JP, Sicsic S, Lezoualc'h F, Berque-Bestel I. Design, synthesis, and biological evaluation of new 5-HT4 receptor agonists: application as amyloid cascade modulators and potential therapeutic utility in Alzheimer's disease. J Med Chem. 2009; 52: 2214-25.

[228] Knafo S, Alonso-Nanclares L, Gonzalez-Soriano J, Merino-Serrais P, Fernaud-Espinosa I, Ferrer I, DeFelipe J. Widespread changes in dendritic spines in a model of Alzheimer's disease. Cereb Cortex. 2009; 19: 586-92.

[229] Smith DL, Pozueta J, Gong B, Arancio O, Shelanski M. Reversal of long-term dendritic spine alterations in Alzheimer disease models. PNAS 2009; 106: 16877-82.

[230] Albasanz JL, Dalfó E, Ferrer I, Martín M. Impaired metabotropic glutamate receptor/ phospholipase C signaling pathway in the cerebral cortex in Alzheimer's disease and dementia with Lewy bodies correlates with stage of Alzheimer's-disease-related changes. Neurobiol Dis. 2005; 20: 685-93.

[231] Albasanz JL, Perez S, Barrachina M, Ferrer I, Martín M. Up-regulation of adenosine receptors in the frontal cortex in Alzheimer's disease. Brain Pathol. 2008; 18: 211-9.

[232] Coleman P, Federoff H, Kurlan R. A focus on the synapse for neuroprotection in Alzheimer disease and other dementias. Neurology. 2004; 63:1155-62.

[233] Arendt T. Alzheimer's disease as a disorder of mechanisms underlying structural brain self-organization. Neuroscience. 2001; 102: 723-65.

[234] Palop JJ, Mucke L. Synaptic depression and aberrant excitatory network activity in Alzheimer's disease: two faces of the same coin? Neuromolecular Med. 2010; 12: 48-55.

[235] Martin V, Fabelo N, Santpere G, Puig B, Marín R, Ferrer I, Diaz M. Lipid alterations in lipid rafts from Alzheimer's disease human brain córtex. J Alzheimers Dis 2010; 19: 489-502.

[236] Darios F, Davletov B. Omega-3 and omega-6 fatty acids stimulate cell membrane expansion by acting on syntaxin 3. Nature. 2006; 440: 813-7.

[237] Florent-Béchard S, Desbène C, Garcia P, Allouche A, Youssef I, Escanyé MC, Koziel V, Hanse M, Malaplate-Armand C, Stenger C, Kriem B, Yen-Potin FT, Olivier JL, Pillot T, Oster T. The essential role of lipids in Alzheimer's disease. Biochimie. 2009; 91: 804-9.

[238] Oster T, Pillot T. Docosahexaenoic acid and synaptic protection in Alzheimer's disease mice. Biochim Biophys Acta. 2010; 1801: 791-8.

[239] Secades JJ, Lorenzo JL. Citicoline: pharmacological and clinical review, 2006 update. Methods Find Exp Clin Pharmacol. 2006; Suppl B:1-56.

[240] Proctor DT, Coulson EJ, Dodd PR. Post-synaptic scaffolding protein interactions with glutamate receptors in synaptic dysfunction and Alzheimer's disease. Prog Neurobiol. 2011; 93: 509-21.

[241] Kaplan DR, Miller FD. Neurotrophin signal transduction in the nervous system. Curr Opin Neurobiol. 2000; 10: 381-91.

[242] Montero CN, Hefti F. Rescue of lesioned septal cholinergic neurons by nerve growth factor: specificity and requirement for chronic treatment. J Neurosci. 1988; 8: 2986-99.

[243] Allard S, Leon WC, Pakavathkumar P, Bruno MA, Ribeiro-da-Silva A, Cuello AC. Impact of the NGF maturation and degradation pathway on the cortical cholinergic system phenotype. J Neurosci. 2012; 32: 2002-12.

[244] Cuello AC, Bruno MA, Allard S, Leon W, Iulita MF. Cholinergic involvement in Alzheimer's disease. A link with NGF maturation and degradation. J Mol Neurosci. 2010; 40: 230-5.

[245] Bruno MA, Leon WC, Fragoso G, Mushynski WE, Almazan G, Cuello AC. Amyloid beta-induced nerve growth factor dysmetabolism in Alzheimer disease. J Neuropathol Exp Neurol. 2009; 68: 857-69.

[246] Pedraza CE, Podlesniy P, Vidal N, Arévalo JC, Lee R, Hempstead B, Ferrer I, Iglesias M, Espinet C. Pro-NGF isolated from the human brain affected by Alzheimer's disease induces neuronal apoptosis mediated by p75NTR. Am J Pathol. 2005; 166: 533-43.

[247] Podlesniy P, Kichev A, Pedraza C, Saurat J, Encinas M, Perez B, Ferrer I, Espinet C. Pro-NGF from Alzheimer's disease and normal human brain displays distinctive abilities to induce processing and nuclear translocation of intracellular domain of p75NTR and apoptosis. Am J Pathol. 2006; 169:119-31.

[248] Kichev A, Ilieva EV, Piñol-Ripoll G, Podlesniy P, Ferrer I, Portero-Otín M, Pamplona R, Espinet C. Cell death and learning impairment in mice caused by in vitro modified

pro-NGF can be related to its increased oxidative modifications in Alzheimer disease. Am J Pathol. 2009; 175: 2574-85.

[249] Eriksdotter Jönhagen M, Nordberg A, Amberla K, Bäckman L, Ebendal T, Meyerson B, Olson L, Seiger, Shigeta M, Theodorsson E, Viitanen M, Winblad B, Wahlund LO. Intracerebroventricular infusion of nerve growth factor in three patients with Alzheimer's disease. Dement Geriatr Cogn Disord. 1998; 9: 246-57.

[250] Cattaneo A, Capsoni S, Paoletti F. Towards noninvasive nerve growth factor therapies for Alzheimer's disease. J Alzheimers Dis. 2008; 15:255-83.

[251] Ferrer I, Marín C, Rey MJ, Ribalta T, Goutan E, Blanco R, Tolosa E, Martí E. BDNF and full-length and truncated TrkB expression in Alzheimer disease. Implications in therapeutic strategies. J Neuropathol Exp Neurol. 1999; 58: 729-39.

[252] Connor B, Young D, Yan Q, Faull RL, Synek B, Dragunow M. Brain-derived neurotrophic factor is reduced in Alzheimer's disease. Brain Res Mol Brain Res. 1997; 49: 71-81.

[253] Holsinger RM, Schnarr J, Henry P, Castelo VT, Fahnestock M. Quantitation of BDNF mRNA in human parietal cortex by competitive reverse transcription-polymerase chain reaction: decreased levels in Alzheimer's disease. Brain Res Mol Brain Res. 2000; 76: 347-54.

[254] Hock C, Heese K, Hulette C, Rosenberg C, Otten U. Region-specific neurotrophin imbalances in Alzheimer disease: decreased levels of brain-derived neurotrophic factor and increased levels of nerve growth factor in hippocampus and cortical areas. Arch. Neurol 2000; 57: 846–51.

[255] Nagahara AH, Tuszynski MH. Potential therapeutic uses of BDNF in neurological and psychiatric disorders. Nat Rev Drug Discov. 2011; 10: 209-19.

[256] Nagahara AH, Merrill DA, Coppola G, Tsukada S, Schroeder BE, Shaked GM, Wang L, Blesch A, Kim A, Conner JM, Rockenstein E, Chao MV, Koo EH, Geschwind D, Masliah E, Chiba AA, Tuszynski MH. Neuroprotective effects of brain-derived neurotrophic factor in rodent and primate models of Alzheimer's disease. Nat Med. 2009; 15: 331-7.

[257] Blurton-Jones M, Kitazawa M, Martinez-Coria H, Castello NA, Müller FJ, Loring JF, Yamasaki TR, Poon WW, Green KN, LaFerla FM. Neural stem cells improve cognition via BDNF in a transgenic model of Alzheimer disease. Proc Natl Acad Sci U S A. 2009; 106: 13594-9.

[258] Finch CE, Laping NJ, Morgan TE, Nichols NR, Pasinetti GM. TGF-β1 is an organizer of response to neurodegeneration. J Cell Biochem. 1993; 53: 314–22.

[259] Brionne TC, Tesseur I, Masliah E, Wyss Coray T. Loss of TGF-β1 leads to increased neuronal cell death and microgliosis in mouse brain. Neuron. 2003; 40:1133–45.

[260] Caraci F, Spampinato S, Sortino MA, Bosco P, Battaglia G, Bruno V, Drago F, Nicoletti F, Copani A. Dysfunction of TGF-β1 signaling in Alzheimer's disease: perspectives for neuroprotection. Cell Tissue Res. 2012 347;: 291-301.

[261] Caraci F, Battaglia G, Busceti C, Biagioni F, Mastroiacovo F, Bosco P, Drago F, Nicoletti F, Sortino MA, Copani A. TGF-beta 1 protects against Abeta-neurotoxicity via the phosphatidylinositol-3-kinase pathway. Neurobiol Dis. 2008; 30: 234-42.

[262] Sortino MA, Chisari M, Merlo S, Vancheri C, Caruso M, Nicoletti F, Canonico PL, Copani A. Glia mediates the neuroprotective action of estradiol on beta-amyloid-induced neuronal death. Endocrinology. 2004; 145: 5080-6.

[263] Bruno V, Battaglia G, Casabona G, Copani A, Caciagli F, Nicoletti F. Neuroprotection by glial metabotropic glutamate receptors is mediated by transforming growth factor-beta. J Neurosci. 1998; 18: 9594-600.

[264] Caraci F, Battaglia G, Bruno V, Bosco P, Carbonaro V, Giuffrida ML, Drago F, Sortino MA, Nicoletti F, Copani A. TGF-beta1 pathway as a new target for neuroprotection in Alzheimer's disease. CNS Neurosci Ther. 2009; 17: 237-249.

[265] Vollmar P, Haghikia A, Dermietzel R, Faustmann PM. Venlafaxine exhibits an anti-inflammatory effect in an inflammatory co-culture model. Int J Neuropsychopharmacol. 2008; 11:111-7.

[266] Arnon R, Aharoni R. Mechanism of action of glatiramer acetate in multiple sclerosis and its potential for the development of new applications. Proc Natl Acad Sci USA. 2004; 101 (Suppl 2): 14593-8.

[267] Zhang H, Zou K, Tesseur I, Wyss-Coray T. Small molecule tgf-beta mimetics as potential neuroprotective factors. Curr Alzheimer Res. 2005; 2: 183-6.

[268] Scheibel AB, Tomiyasu U. Dendritic sprouting in Alzheimer's presenile dementia. Exp Neurol. 1978; 60:1-8.

[269] Ferrer I, Aymami A, Rovira A, Grau Veciana JM. Growth of abnormal neurites in atypical Alzheimer's disease. A study with the Golgi method. Acta Neuropathol. 1983; 59:167-70.

[270] Arendt T. Synaptic degeneration in Alzheimer's disease. Acta Neuropathol. 2009; 118: 167-79.

[271] Barnett A, Brewer GJ. Autophagy in aging and Alzheimer's disease: pathologic or protective? J Alzheimers Dis. 2011; 25: 385-94.

[272] Harris H, Rubinsztein DC. Control of autophagy as a therapy for neurodegenerative disease. Nat Rev Neurol. 2011; 8: 108-17.

[273] Nixon RA, Wegiel J, Kumar A, Yu WH, Peterhoff C, Cataldo A, Cuervo AM. Extensive involvement of autophagy in Alzheimer disease: an immuno-electron microscopy study. J Neuropathol Exp Neurol. 2005; 64: 113-22.

[274] Barrachina M, Maes T, Buesa C, Ferrer I. Lysosome-associated membrane protein 1 (LAMP-1) in Alzheimer's disease. Neuropathol Appl Neurobiol. 2006; 32: 505-16.

[275] Li L, Zhang X, Le W. Autophagy dysfunction in Alzheimer's disease. Neurodegener Dis. 2010; 7: 265-71.

[276] Moreira PI, Santos RX, Zhu X, Lee HG, Smith MA, Casadesus G, Perry G. Autophagy in Alzheimer's disease. Expert Rev Neurother. 2010; 10: 1209-18.

[277] Lee S, Sato Y, Nixon RA. Primary lysosomal dysfunction causes cargo-specific deficits of axonal transport leading to Alzheimer-like neuritic dystrophy. Autophagy. 2011; 7: 1562-3.

[278] Sanchez-Varo R, Trujillo-Estrada L, Sanchez-Mejias E, Torres M, Baglietto-Vargas D, Moreno-Gonzalez I, De Castro V, Jimenez S, Ruano D, Vizuete M, Davila JC, Garcia-Verdugo JM, Jimenez AJ, Vitorica J, Gutierrez A. Abnormal accumulation of autophagic vesicles correlates with axonal and synaptic pathology in young Alzheimer's mice hippocampus. Acta Neuropathol. 2012; 123: 53-70.

[279] Nixon RA, Yang DS. Autophagy failure in Alzheimer's disease--locating the primary defect. Neurobiol Dis. 2011; 43: 38-45.

[280] Caccamo A, Majumder S, Richardson A, Strong R, Oddo S. Molecular interplay between mammalian target of rapamycin (mTOR), amyloid-beta, and Tau: effects on cognitive impairments. J Biol Chem. 2010; 285: 13107-20.

[281] Spilman P, Podlutskaya N, Hart MJ, Debnath J, Gorostiza O, Bredesen D, Richardson A, Strong R, Galvan V. Inhibition of mTOR by rapamycin abolishes cognitive deficits and reduces amyloid-beta levels in a mouse model of Alzheimer's disease. PLoS One. 2010; 5: e9979.

[282] Majumder S, Richardson A, Strong R, Oddo S. Inducing autophagy by rapamycin before, but not after, the formation of plaques and tangles ameliorates cognitive deficits. PLoS One. 2011; 6: e25416.

[283] Yang DS, Stavrides P, Mohan PS, Kaushik S, Kumar A, Ohno M, Schmidt SD, Wesson D, Bandyopadhyay U, Jiang Y, Pawlik M, Peterhoff CM, Yang AJ, Wilson DA, St George-Hyslop P, Westaway D, Mathews PM, Levy E, Cuervo AM, Nixon RA. Reversal of autophagy dysfunction in the TgCRND mouse model of Alzheimer's disease ameliorates amyloid pathologies and memory deficits. Brain. 2011; 134: 258-77.

[284] Laplante M, Sabatini DM. mTOR signaling in growth control and disease. Cell. 2012; 149: 274-93.

[285] Sarkar S, Floto RA, Berger Z, Imarisio S, Cordenier A, Pasco M, Cook LJ, Rubinsztein DC. Lithium induces autophagy by inhibiting inositol monophosphatase. J Cell Biol. 2005; 170:1101-11.

[286] Williams A, Sarkar S, Cuddon P, Ttofi EK, Saiki S, Siddiqi FH, Jahreiss L, Fleming A, Pask D, Goldsmith P, O'Kane CJ, Floto RA, Rubinsztein DC. Novel targets for Hun-

tington's disease in an mTOR-independent autophagy pathway. Nat Chem Biol. 2008; 4: 295-305.

[287]   Frautschy SA, Cole GM. Why pleiotropic interventions are needed for Alzheimer's disease. Mol Neurobiol. 2010; 41: 392-409.

[288]   Bajda M, Guzior N, Ignasik M, Malawska B. Multi-target-directed ligands in Alzheimer's disease treatment. Curr Med Chem. 2011; 18: 4949-75.

[289]   Hashimoto M, Hossain S. Neuroprotective and ameliorative actions of polyunsaturated fatty acids against neuronal diseases: beneficial effect of docosahexaenoic acid on cognitive decline in Alzheimer's disease. J Pharmacol Sci. 2011; 116: 150-62.

[290]   Fredholm BB, Battig K, Holmen J, Nehlig A, Zvartau EE. Actions of caffeine in the brain with special reference to factors that contribute to its widespread use. Pharmacol Rev. 1999; 51: 83-133.

[291]   Marques S, Batalha VL, Vaqueiro Lops L, Fleming Outeiro T. Modulating Alzheimer's disease through caffeine: a putative link to epigenetics. J Alzheimers Dis 2011; 24: 161-71.

[292]   Arendash GW, Scleif W, Rezai-Zadech K, Jackson EK, Zacharia LC, Cracchiolo JR, Shippy D, Tan J. Caffeine protects Alzheimer's mice against cognitive impairmenmt and reduces brain beta-amyloid production. Neuroscience (2006) 142: 941-52.

[293]   Dall'Igna OP, Fett P, Gomes MW, Souza DO, Cunha RA, Lara DR. Caffeine and adenosine A (2a) receptor antagonists prevent beta-amyloid (25-30)-induced cognitive deficits in mice. Exp Neurol. 2007; 203: 241-5.

[294]   Ritchie K, Carriere I, de Mendonca A, Portet F, Dartigues JF, Rouaud O, Barberger-Gateau P, Ancelin ML. The neuroprotective effects of caffeine: a prospective population study. Neurology. 2007; 69: 536-45.

[295]   Santos C, Lunet N, Azevedo A, de Mendonca A, Richtie K, Barros H. Caffeine intake and dementia: systematic review and meta-analysis. J Alzheimers Dis. 2010; suppl 1: S187-204.

[296]   Eskelinen MH, Kivipelto M. Caffeine as a protective factor in dementia and Alzheimer's disease. J Alzheimers Dis 2010; 20 suppl 1: S167-74.

[297]   Singh M, Dykens JA, Simpkins JW. Novel mechanisms for estrogen-induced neuroprotection. Exp Biol Med. 2006; 231: 514-21.

[298]   Pike CJ, Carroll JC, Rosario ER, Barron AM. Protective actions of sex steroid hormones in Alzheimer's disease. Front Neuroendocrinol. 2009; 30: 239-58.

[299]   Correia SC, Santos RX, Cardoso S, Carvalho C, Santos MS, Oliveira CR, Moreira PI. Effects of estrogen in the brain: is it a neuroprotective agent in Alzheimer's disease? Curr Aging Sci. 2010; 3:113-26.

[300] Alonso A, Gonzalez C. Neuroprotective role of estrogens: relationship with insulin/ IGF-1 signaling. Front Biosci. 2012; 4: 607-19.

[301] Carroll JC, Rosario ER, Chang L, Stanczyk FZ, Oddo S, LaFerla FM, Pike CJ. Progesterone and estrogen regulate Alzheimer-like neuropathology in female 3xTg-AD mice. J Neurosci. 2007; 27:13357-65.

[302] Fillit H, Weinreb H, Cholst I, Luine V, McEwen B, Amador R, Zabriskie J. Observations in a preliminary open trial of estradiol therapy for senile dementia-Alzheimer's type. Psychoneuroendocrinology. 1986; 11: 337–45.

[303] Craig MC, Murphy DG. Estrogen therapy and Alzheimer's dementia. Ann N Y Acad Sci. 2010; 1205: 245-53.

[304] Campbell VA, Gowran A. Alzheimer's disease: taking the edge off with cannabinoids? Br J Pharmacol 2007; 152: 655-62.

[305] Van Der Stelt M, Mazzola C, Espositp G, Mathias I, Petrosino S, De Filippis D et al. Endocannabinoids and b-amyloid-induced neurotoxicity in vivo: effect of pharmacological elevation of endocannabinoid levels. Cell Mol Life Sci. 2006; 63: 1410–24.

[306] Aso E, Palomer E, Juvés S, Maldonado R, Muñoz FJ, Ferrer I. CB1 agonist ACEA protects neurons and reduces the cognitive impairment of AβPP/PS1 mice. J Alzheimers Dis. 2012; 30: 439-59.

[307] Ramírez BG, Blázquez C, Gómez del Pulgar T, Guzmán M, de Ceballos ML. Prevention of Alzheimer's disease pathology by cannabinoids: neuroprotection mediated by blockade of microglial activation. J Neurosci. 2005; 25:1904-13.

[308] Martín-Moreno AM, Brera B, Spuch C, Carro E, García-García L, Delgado M, Pozo MA, Innamorato NG, Cuadrado A, Ceballos ML. Prolonged oral cannabinoid administration prevents neuroinflammation, lowers β-amyloid levels and improves cognitive performance in Tg APP 2576 mice. J Neuroinflammation. 2012; 9:8.

[309] Esposito G, De Filippis D, Carnuccio R, Izzo AA, Iuvone T. The marijuana component cannabidiol inhibits beta-amyloid-induced tau protein hyperphosphorylation through Wnt/beta-catenin pathway rescue in PC12 cells. J Mol Med 2006; 84: 253.8.

[310] Galve-Roperh I, Aguada T, Palazuelos J, Guzman M. The endocannabinoid system and neurogenesis in health and disease. Neuroscientist 2007; 13: 109–14.

[311] Harvey BS, Ohlsson KS, Mååg JL, Musgrave IF, Smid SD. Contrasting protective effects of cannabinoids against oxidative stress and amyloid-β evoked neurotoxicity in vitro. Neurotoxicology. 2012; 33: 138-46.

[312] Noonan J, Tanveer R, Klompas A, Gowran A, McKiernan J, Campbell VA. Endocannabinoids prevent β-amyloid-mediated lysosomal destabilization in cultured neurons. J Biol Chem. 2010; 285: 38543-54.

[313] Eubanks LM, Rogers CJ, Beuscher AE 4th, Koob GF, Olson AJ, Dickerson TJ, Janda KD. A molecular link between the active component of marijuana and Alzheimer's disease pathology. Mol Pharm. 2006; 3: 773-7.

[314] Sirén AL, Fasshauer T, Bartels C, Ehrenreich H. Therapeutic potential of erythropoietin and its structural or functional variants in the nervous system. Neurotherapeutics. 2009; 6: 108-27.

[315] Sun ZK, Yang HQ, Pan J, Zhen H, Wang ZQ, Chen SD, Ding JQ. Protective effects of erythropoietin on tau phosphorylation induced by beta-amyloid. J Neurosci Res. 2008; 86: 3018-27.

[316] Li G, Ma R, Huang C, Tang Q, Fu Q, Liu H, Hu B, Xiang J. Protective effect of erythropoietin on beta-amyloid-induced PC12 cell death through antioxidant mechanisms. Neurosci Lett. 2008; 442:143-7.

[317] Adamcio B, Sargin D, Stradomska A, Medrihan L, Gertler C, Theis F, Zhang M, Müller M, Hassouna I, Hannke K, Sperling S, Radyushkin K, El-Kordi A, Schulze L, Ronnenberg A, Wolf F, Brose N, Rhee JS, Zhang W, Ehrenreich H. Erythropoietin enhances hippocampal long-term potentiation and memory. BMC Biol. 2008; 6:37.

[318] Ponce LL, Navarro JC, Ahmed O, Robertson CS. Erythropoietin neuroprotection with traumatic brain injury. Pathophysiology. 2012 Mar 13.

[319] Shepardson NE, Shankar GM, Selkoe DJ. Cholesterol level and statin use in Alzheimer disease: I. Review of epidemiological and preclinical studies. Arch Neurol. 2011; 68: 1239-44.

[320] Pac-Soo C, Lloyd DG, Vizcaychipi MP, Ma D. Statins: the role in the treatment and prevention of Alzheimer's neurodegeneration. J Alzheimers Dis. 2011; 27: 1-10.

[321] Chauhan NB, Siegel GJ, Feinstein DL. Effects of lovastatin and pravastatin on amyloid processing and inflammatory response in TgCRND8 brain. Neurochem Res. 2004; 29: 1897-911.

[322] Li L, Cao D, Kim H, Lester R, Fukuchi K. Simvastatin enhances learning and memory independent of amyloid load in mice. Ann Neurol. 2006; 60: 729-39.

[323] Weinreb O, Amit T, Bar-Am O, Youdim MB. Ladostigil: a novel multimodal neuroprotective drug with cholinesterase and brain-selective monoamine oxidase inhibitory activities for Alzheimer's disease treatment. Curr Drug Targets. 2012; 13: 483-94.

[324] Wang R, Yan H, Tang XC. Progress in studies of huperzine A, a natural cholinesterase inhibitor from Chinese herbal medicine. Acta Pharmacol Sin. 2006; 27:1-26.

[325] Peng Y, Lee DY, Jiang L, Ma Z, Schachter SC, Lemere CA. Huperzine A regulates amyloid precursor protein processing via protein kinase C and mitogen-activated protein kinase pathways in neuroblastoma SK-N-SH cells over-expressing wild type human amyloid precursor protein 695. Neuroscience. 2007; 150: 386-95.

[326] Ved HS, Koenig ML, Dave JR, Doctor BP. Huperzine A, a potential therapeutic agent for dementia, reduces neuronal cell death caused by glutamate. Neuroreport. 1997; 8: 963-8.

[327] Li J, Wu HM, Zhou RL, Liu GJ, Dong BR. Huperzine A for Alzheimer's disease. Cochrane Database Syst Rev. 2008; 16:CD005592.

[328] Huang TC, Lu KT, Wo YY, Wu YJ, Yang YL. Resveratrol protects rats from Aβ-induced neurotoxicity by the reduction of iNOS expression and lipid peroxidation. PLoS One. 2011; 6: e29102.

[329] Li F, Gong Q, Dong H, Shi J. Resveratrol, a neuroprotective supplement for Alzheimer's disease. Curr Pharm Des. 2012; 18: 27-33.

[330] Davinelli S, Sapere N, Zella D, Bracale R, Intrieri M, Scapagnini G. Pleiotropic protective effects of phytochemicals in Alzheimer's disease. Oxid Med Cell Longev. 2012; 2012:386527.

[331] Allison AC, Cacabelos R, Lombardi VR, Alvarez XA, Vigo C. Celastrol, a potent antioxidant and anti-inflammatory drug, as a possible treatment for Alzheimer'sdisease.

[332] Neuropsychopharmacol Biol Psychiatry. 2001; 25: 1341-1357.

[333] Paris D, Ganey NJ, Laporte V, Patel NS, Beaulieu-Abdelahad D, Bachmeier C, March A, Ait-Ghezala G, Mullan MJ. Reduction of beta-amyloid pathology by celastrol in a transgenic mouse model of Alzheimer'sdisease. J Neuroinflammation. 2010;7: 17.

[334] Murray ME, Graff-Radford NR, Ross OA, Petersen RC, Duara R, Dickson DW. Neuropathologically defined subtypes of Alzheimer's disease with distinct clinical characteristics: a retrospective study. Lancet Neurol. 2011; 10: 785-796.

[335] Reiman EM, Langbaum JB, Fleisher AS, Caselli RJ, Chen K, Ayutyanont N, Quiroz YT, Kosik KS, Lopera F, Tariot PN.Alzheimer's Prevention Initiative: a plan to accelerate the evaluation of presymptomatic treatments. J Alzheimers Dis. 2011; 26 Suppl 3:321-329.

[336] Henderson ST, Poirier J. Pharmacogenetic analysis of the effects of polymorphisms in APOE, IDE and IL1B on a ketone body based therapeutic on cognition in mild to moderate Alzheimer's disease; a randomized, double-blind, placebo-controlled study. BMC Med Genet. 2011; 12:137.

Epidemiology, Clinical Presentation and Prevention

Chapter 3

Epidemiology of Alzheimer's Disease

Weili Xu, Camilla Ferrari and Hui-Xin Wang

Additional information is available at the end of the chapter

1. Introduction

1.1. Global aging

The aging of populations has become a worldwide phenomenon [1]. In 1990, 26 nations had more than two million elderly citizens aged 65 years and older, and the projections indicate that an additional 34 countries will join the list by 2030. In 2000, the number of old people (65+ years) in the world was estimated to be 420 million and it was projected to be nearly one billion by 2030, with the proportion of old people increasing from 7 to 12%. The largest increase in absolute numbers of old people will occur in developing countries; it will almost triple from 249 million in 2000 to an estimated 690 million in 2030. The developing regions' sharing the worldwide aging population will increase from 59 to 71% [2]. Developed countries, which have already shown a dramatic increase in people over 65 years of age will experience a progressive aging of the elderly population. Underlying global population aging is a process known as the "demographic transition" in which mortality and then fertility decline [3]. Decreasing fertility and lengthening life expectancy have together reshaped the age structure of the population in most regions of the planet by shifting relative weight from younger to older groups.

Both developed and developing countries will face the challenge of coping with a high frequency of chronic conditions, such as dementia, which is a characteristic of aging societies. These conditions impair the ability of older persons to function optimally in the community and reduce well-being among affected individuals and their families. Further, these conditions are associated with significant health care costs that must be sustained by the society at large. Thus, the global trend in the phenomenon of population aging has a dramatic impact on public health, healthcare financing and delivery systems throughout the world [4]. Due to the aging of the population, dementia has become a major challenge to elderly care and public health.

1.2. Dementia and Alzheimer's disease

Dementia is defined as a clinical syndrome, and characterized by the development of multiple cognitive deficits that are severe enough to interfere with daily functioning, including social and professional functioning. The cognitive deficits include memory impairment and at least one of the other cognitive domains, such as aphasia, apraxia, agnosia or disturbances in executive functioning [5, 6]. Alzheimer's disease is the most common cause of dementia in the elderly, accounting for 60-70% of all demented cases [7]. Alzheimer's disease is strictly a neuropathological diagnosis determined by the presence of neurofibrillary tangles and senile plaques in the brain of patients with dementia. The disease frequently starts with memory impairment, but is invariably followed by a progressive global cognitive impairment [8]. Vascular dementia is the second most common cause of dementia in the elderly after Alzheimer's disease. Vascular dementia is defined as loss of cognitive function resulting from ischemic, hypoperfusive, or haemorrhagic brain lesions due to cerebrovascular disease or cardiovascular pathology. Diagnosis of vascular dementia requires cognitive impairment; vascular brain lesions, often predominantly subcortical, as demonstrated by brain imaging; a temporal link between stroke and dementia; and exclusion of other causes of dementia [9]. The combination of Alzheimer's disease and vascular dementia pathological changes in the brains of older people are extremely common, making mixed dementia probably the most common type of dementia [10].

Alzheimer's disease was first identified more than 100 years ago, but research into its symptoms, causes, risk factors and treatment has gained momentum only in the last 30 years. Although research has revealed a great deal about Alzheimer's, the precise physiologic changes that trigger the development of Alzheimer's disease largely remain unknown. The only exceptions are certain rare, inherited forms of the disease caused by known genetic mutations. Alzheimer's disease affects people in different ways, but the most common symptom pattern begins with gradually worsening ability to remember new information. This occurs because disruption of brain cell function usually begins in brain regions involved in forming new memories. As damage spreads, individuals experience other difficulties. The following are warning signs of Alzheimer's disease: memory loss that disrupts daily life; challenges in planning or solving problems; difficulty completing familiar tasks at home, at work or at leisure; confusion with time or place; trouble understanding visual images and spatial relationships; new problems with words in speaking or writing; misplacing things and losing the ability to retrace steps; decreased or poor judgment; withdrawal from work or social activities; and changes in mood and personality. As the disease progresses, the individual's cognitive and functional abilities decline. In advanced Alzheimer's disease, people need help with basic activities of daily living, such as bathing, dressing, eating and using the bathroom. Those in the final stages of the disease lose their ability to communicate, fail to recognize loved ones and become bed-bound and reliant on around-the-clock care. When an individual has difficulty moving because of Alzheimer's disease, they are more vulnerable to infections, including pneumonia (infection of the lungs).

2. Occurrence of Alzheimer's disease

The occurrence of a disease can be measured as proportion of people affected by the disease in a defined population at a specific time point (prevalence), or as number of new cases that occur during a specific time period in a population at risk for developing that disease (incidence). The prevalence reflects the public health burden of the disease, whereas the incidence indicates the risk of developing that disease. The prevalence is determined by both incidence and duration of the disease, and in certain circumstances, the prevalence may be estimated as incidence × average disease duration.

2.1. Prevalence

Based on the available epidemiological data, a group of experts estimated that 24.3 million people have dementia today, with 4.6 million new cases of dementia every year (one new case every 7 seconds). The number of people affected will double every 20 years to 81.1 million by 2040 [11]. Similar estimates have been reported previously [12]. Most people with dementia live in developing countries. China and its western Pacific neighbours have the highest number of people with dementia (6 million), followed by the European Union (5.0 million), USA (2.9 million), and India (1.5 million). The rates of increase in the number of dementia cases are not uniform across the world; numbers in developed countries are forecasted to increase by 100% between 2001 and 2040, but to increase by more than 300% in India, China, and other south Asian and western Pacific countries [11]. About 70% of these cases were attributed to Alzheimer's disease [11, 13]. The pooled data of population-based studies in Europe suggests that the age-standardized prevalence in people 65+ years old was 6.4 % for dementia and 4.4 % for Alzheimer's disease [14]. In the US, a study of a national representative sample of people aged >70 years yielded a prevalence for Alzheimer's disease of 9.7 % [15].

Worldwide, the global prevalence of dementia was estimated to be 3.9 % in people aged 60+ years, with the regional prevalence being 1.6 % in Africa, 4.0 % in China and Western Pacific regions, 4.6 % in Latin America, 5.4 % in Western Europe, and 6.4 % in North America [11]. A meta-analysis including 18 studies from China during 1990-2010 showed prevalence of Alzheimer's disease of 1.9% [16]. More than 25 million people in the world are currently affected by dementia, most suffering from Alzheimer's disease, with around 5 million new cases occurring every year [11]. The number of people with dementia is anticipated to double every 20 years. Despite different inclusion criteria, several meta-analyses and nationwide surveys have yielded roughly similar age-specific prevalence of AD across regions (Figure 1) [17]. The age-specific prevalence of Alzheimer's disease almost doubles every 5 years after aged 65. Among developed nations, approximately 1 in 10 older people aged ≥ 65 is affected by some degree of dementia, whereas more than one third of very old people aged ≥85 years may have dementia-related symptoms and signs [18, 19]. There is a similar pattern of dementia subtypes across the world, with Alzheimer's disease and vascular dementia, the two most common forms of dementia, accounting for 50 % to 70 % and 15 % to 25 %, respectively, of all dementia cases.

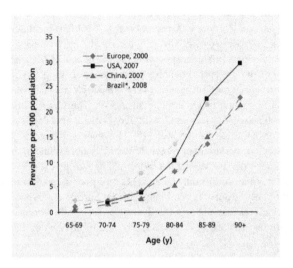

Figure 1. Age-specific prevalence of Alzheimer's disease (per 100 population) across continents and countries. *prevalence of all types of dementia [17].

Epidemiological research of dementia and AD in low- and middle-income countries has drawn much attention in recent years. A systematic review estimated that the overall prevalence of Alzheimer's disease in developing countries was 3.4 % (95 % CI,1.6 % - 5.0 %) [20]. The prevalence of dementia (DSM-IV criteria) in people aged 65+ years in seven developing nations varied widely from less than 0.5 % to more than 6 %, which is substantially lower than in developed countries [21]. Indeed, the prevalence rates of dementia in India and rural Latin America were approximately a quarter of the rates in European countries. However, the prevalence of AD in persons 65+ years in urban areas of China was 3.5 %, and even higher (4.8 %) after post-hoc correction for negative screening errors [22], which is generally comparable with those from Western nations. Similar prevalence rates of dementia were also reported from the urban populations of Latin American nations such as Havana in Cuba (6.4 %) and São Paulo in Brazil (5.1 %) [20, 23, 24].

2.2. Incidence

The global annual incidence of dementia is around 7.5 per 1,000 persons [11]. The incidence rate of dementia increases exponentially with age, from approximately one per 1,000 person-year in people aged 60-64 years to more than 70 per 1,000 person-year in 90+ year-olds. The incidence rates of dementia across regions are quite similar in the younger-old (<75 years), but greater variations are seen among the older ages [25]. Slightly lower rates have been detected in the USA in comparison with Europe and Asia, and this is possibly due to differences in the study designs and the case ascertainment procedures. The pooled incidence rate of Alzheimer's disease among people 65+ years of age in Europe was 19.4 per 1000 person-year [26]. The pooled data from two large-scale community-based studies of people aged ≥65 years in the US Seattle and Baltimore areas yielded an incidence rate for Alzheimer's disease of 15.0 (male, 13.0; female, 16.9) per 1000 person-year [27, 28]. The incidence rate of Alzheimer's disease increases almost exponentially with increasing age until 85 years of age (Figure 2) [17]. A consistently exponential increase, with advancing age in Alzheimer incidence suggests that Alzheimer's disease is an inevitable consequence of aging, whereas a convergence to or a decline at certain age may suggest that very old people may have reduced vulnerability, owing perhaps to genetic or environmental factors. The Cache County Study further found that the incidence of AD increased with age, peaked, and then started to decline at extreme old ages for both men and women [29]. However, some meta-analyses and large-scale studies in Europe provided no evidence for the potential decline in the incidence of dementia and Alzheimer's disease among the oldest-old age groups [26, 30, 31]. The apparent decline suggested in some studies may be an artifact of poor response rate and survival effect in these very old age groups. Several studies from Europe observed a higher incidence rate of Alzheimer's disease among women than men, especially among the oldest-old age groups, whereas studies in North America found no significant gender difference [17].

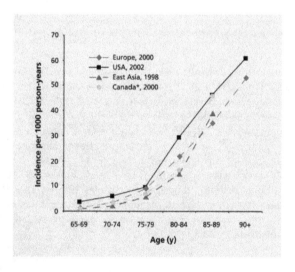

Figure 2. Age-specific incidence of Alzheimer's disease (per 1 000 person years) across continents and countries. *incidence of all types of dementia [17].

There appears to be some geographic variations in the incidence of Alzheimer's disease. The pooled data of eight European studies suggested a geographical dissociation across Europe, with higher incidence rates being found among the oldest-old people of north-western countries than among southern countries [26]. The incidence rates of Alzheimer's disease were reported to be slightly lower in North America than in Europe. Differences in methodology (e.g., differences in study design and procedure of case ascertainment), rather than real different regional distributions of the disease, may be partly responsible for the geographic variations. The study using identical methods in UK found no evidence of variation in dementia incidence among five areas in England and Wales [30]. Studies have confirmed that AD incidence in developing countries is generally lower than in North America and Europe. For example, the incidence rate of AD among people aged 65+ years was 7.7 per 1 000 person-year in Brazil and 3.2 per 1 000 person-year in India [20, 32].

3. Prognosis and impact

Dementia is one of the leading causes of death in older people. However, death certificates grossly underreport its cause, even when multiple underlying causes of death are taken into account. The community-based follow-up studies could provide reliable data on mortality. In the Swedish Kungsholmen Project of people aged 75 years or over, the mortality rate of dementia was 2.4 per 100 person-year; 70% of incident dementia cases died within five years following the diagnosis. In three years, more than 50% of the dementia cases reached the severe stage. In the Kungsholmen Project, the proportion of severe dementia among prevalent cases increased from 19% at baseline to 48% after three years, and to 78% after seven years. This progression is due to both cognitive and functional decline [33]. Dementia is strongly associated with disability as it has been found to be the major determinant of developing dependence and functional decline over three years. Approximately half of the persons who developed functional dependence in a three year period can attribute to dementia [34]. In industrialised countries, mental disease and cognitive impairment are the most prevalent disorders among older adults living in nursing homes or other institutions. However, institutionalisation of demented patients varies depending on age structure, urban or rural residence, and other cultural aspects. In a 75+ year old population, 70% of incident dementia cases died in the five years following the diagnosis, accounting for a mortality rate specific for dementia of 2.4 per 100 person-years. Dementia triples the risk of death [35]. The demands of healthcare and social service of the huge and rapidly growing numbers of dementia patients have a major economic impact at the societal level [36]. The worldwide direct costs for dementia in 2003 were estimated at 156 billion USD in the main scenario of a worldwide prevalence of 27.7 million demented persons. It is obvious that due to these costs and the expected increase in the number of elderly people in developing countries, the dementing conditions will present a great challenge [37,38].

4. Risk and protective factors

Alzheimer's disease is multifactorial disorder that is determined by genetic and environmental factors as well as their interactions. Population-based prospective study is the major epidemiological approach to identifying influential factors for chronic multifactorial diseases such as dementia, in which the life-course approach should be taken into consideration. Age is the most powerful determinant of Alzheimer's disease, and gene mutations contribute to a small proportion of all cases. The strong association of Alzheimer's disease with increasing age may partially reflect the cumulative effect of different risk and protective factors over the lifespan, including the effect of complex interactions of genetic susceptibility, psychosocial factors, biological factors, and environmental exposures experienced over the lifespan. Evidence from epidemiological, neuroimaging, and neuropathological research, supports the role of genetic, vascular, and psychosocial factors in the development of Alzheimer's disease, whereas evidence for the etiologic role of dietary or nutritional factors, occupational exposures, and inflammation is less clear [39].

4.1. Genetic factors

Mutations in amyloid precursor protein, presenilin-1, and presenilin-2 genes can cause early-onset familial Alzheimer's disease that account for no more than 5% of all cases. The majority of AD cases are sporadic, with considerable heterogeneity in their risk profiles and neuropathological features.

4.1.1. Apolipoprotein E ε4 (APOE ε4)

The *APOE* ε4 allele is the only established susceptibility gene for both early- and late-onset Alzheimer's disease, and is a susceptibility gene, being neither necessary nor sufficient for the development of Alzheimer's disease. *APOE* ε4 is one of three common forms (ε2, ε3 and ε4) of the *APOE* gene, which provides the blue print for a protein that carries cholesterol in the bloodstream. Everyone inherits one form of the *APOE* gene from each parent. Those who inherit one *APOE* ε4 gene have increased risk of developing Alzheimer's disease and of developing it at an earlier age than those who inherit the ε2 or ε3 forms of the *APOE* gene [40]. Those who inherit two *APOE*-ε4 genes have an even higher risk. Unlike inheriting a known genetic mutation for Alzheimer's disease, inheriting one or two copies of this form of the *APOE* gene does not guarantee that an individual will develop Alzheimer's disease. The risk effect of the *APOE* ε4 allele decreases with increasing age, and after age 75, 15–20% of Alzheimer's cases are attributable to *APOE* genotype [41]. Several other genes have been examined as possible candidates, but the reports are sporadic, and the results are inconsistent [42].

However, not all (4-carriers develop dementia. Studies have demonstrated that high education, active leisure activities, or maintaining vascular health seems to reduce the risk of dementia related to APOE ε4 [40, 41]. The ε4-carriers with these characteristics appear to have similar dementia-free survival time to non ε4-carriers. Further, the obese related FTO gene may interact with *APOE* ε4 to increase the risk of Alzheimer's disease [44].

4.1.2. Family history

Individuals who have a parent, brother or sister with Alzheimer's are more likely to develop the disease than those who do not have a first-degree relative with Alzheimer's [45-47]. Those who have more than one first-degree relative with Alzheimer's disease are at even higher risk of developing the disease [48]. When diseases run in families, heredity (genetics), shared environmental and /or lifestyle factors or both may play a role.

4.2. Biological risk factors

Increasing age is a well-established risk factor for Alzheimer's disease. The incidence of Alzheimer's disease almost doubles with every 5 years of age [49, 50]. Female sex is often associated with an increased risk of AD, especially at the oldest-old age [25]. Men seem to be at greater risk for vascular dementia than women [51].

4.3. Vascular disorders and risk factors

A number of vascular risk factors and disorders have been linked to Alzheimer's disease, but some factors may have a differential association with the risk of Alzheimer's disease depending on the age when the exposure is assessed.

4.3.1. Blood pressure

Several studies have consistently reported an association between midlife high blood pressure and increased risk of dementia and Alzheimer's disease [52, 53]. Hypertension has been linked to neurodegenerative markers in the brain, suggesting that long-term high blood pressure may play a causal role in the neurodegenerative process itself or by causing brain atrophy. In very old people, the deleterious effect of high blood pressure is less evident, whereas low blood pressure seems to be predictive of dementia and Alzheimer's disease. As dementia has a long latent period, low blood pressure may be a sign of impending illness [54], which was confirmed by the longitudinal data from the Kungsholmen Project, suggesting the involvement of late life low blood pressure and cerebral hypo-perfusion in the development of dementia and Alzheimer's disease [55]. All these findings suggest that the relation of blood pressure to dementia may be age-dependent [25].

Recent follow-up studies have suggested that the protective effect of antihypertensive therapy on dementia and AD may depend on the duration of treatment and the age when people take the medications; the more evident efficacy was seen among young-old people (i.e., <75 years) and those with long-term treatment [56, 57]. Evidence from clinical trials of antihypertensive therapy and dementia is summarized in the section on intervention trials towards primary prevention. Antihypertensive treatment may protect against dementia and AD by postponing atherosclerotic process, reducing the number of cerebrovascular lesions, and improving cerebral perfusion [52]. It has also been suggested that some antihypertensive agents (e.g., calcium-channel antagonists) may have neuroprotective effects. The recent neuropathological study found substantially less Alzheimer neuropathological changes (i.e., neuritic plaque and neurofibrillary tangle densities) in the medicated hypertension group than non-hypertensive group, which may reflect a salutary effect of antihypertensive therapy against Alzheimer's disease-associated neuropathology [57].

4.3.2. Cardiovascular disease

A healthy heart helps ensure that enough blood is pumped through blood vessels to the brain. The follow-up data of the Cardiovascular Health Study showed that cardiovascular disease was associated with an increased risk of Alzheimer's disease, especially in people with peripheral arterial disease [58], suggesting that extensive peripheral atherosclerosis is a risk factor for Alzheimer's disease. Other cardiovascular diseases, such as heart failure and atrial fibrillation, have been independently related to increased risk of dementia. In the Kungsholmen Project, heart failure was associated with a more than 80% increased risk of dementia and Alzheimer's disease [59].

4.3.3. Cerebrovascular disease

Cerebrovascular changes such as haemorrhagic infarcts, small and large ischemic cortical infarcts, vasculo-pathie, and white matter changes all increase the risk of dementia [13]. Systematic reviews of population-based studies reveal an approximately two- to four-fold increased risk of incident dementia associated with clinical stroke (post-stroke dementia). Multiple cerebral infarcts, recurrent and strategic strokes are main risk factors for post-stroke dementia. Silent stroke and white matter lesions detected on neuroimaging are associated with increased risk of dementia and cognitive decline. Spontaneous cerebral emboli were related to both AD and VaD. Some studies reported an association of stroke with Alzheimer's disease and cognitive decline [60]. Cerebral vascular lesions may interact with neurodegenerative lesions to produce a dementia syndrome in individuals not having sufficient neurodegenerative damages to express dementia [25]. Neuropathological studies suggested that cerebrovascular lesions, atherosclerosis, and neurodegenerative changes in the brain often coexist, and may be coincident processes converging to cause additive damage to the aging brain and to promote clinical expression of the dementia syndrome [61].

4.3.4. Diabetes mellitus

A potential link between diabetes and cognitive impairment was first reported more than 80 years ago. The association of diabetes with these cognitive changes is now well established [62]. There is substantial evidence suggesting that type 2 diabetes is associated with cognitive impairment involving both memory and executive function [63-65]. Several large longitudinal population-based studies have also shown that the rate of cognitive decline is accelerated in elderly people with type 2 diabetes [66]. An increased risk of not only vascular dementia but also neurodegenerative type dementia among persons with diabetes has been reported in several longitudinal studies [67-70], and the risk effect was confirmed by a systematic review [71]. Midlife diabetes or a longer duration of diabetes may play a crucial role in dementia and Alzheimer's disease [68, 72]. Overall, diabetes leads to a 20-70% greater decline in cognitive performance, and a 60% higher risk of dementia [73]. In addition, borderline or prediabetes or impaired glucose tolerance, is also linked to an increased risk of dementia and Alzheimer's disease in very old people [74].

4.3.5. Overweight and obesity

Similar to hypertension, recent studies suggested a lifespan-dependent relation of obesity with dementia [75, 76]. A higher body mass index (BMI) at middle age was related to an increased risk of dementia in late life [77, 78]. A greater decline in BMI approximately 10 years prior to dementia onset was detected, which is in line with the other studies suggesting an association of accelerated BMI decline with Alzheimer's disease [79, 80]. Low BMI in late life and weight loss may be related to high risk of dementia and Alzheimer's disease [81], but low BMI and weight loss can be interpreted as markers of preclinical Alzheimer's disease, especially when measured less than 10 years prior to clinical diagnosis [25]. In line with these findings, several follow-up studies of older people suggested that accelerated decline in BMI was associated with future development of Alzheimer's disease [79, 82, 83]. Low BMI in late life was related to a higher risk for Alzheimer's disease over a subsequent 5- to 6-year period [81]. Thus, late-life low BMI and weight loss can be interpreted as markers for preclinical Alzheimer's disease, particularly when measured just a few years prior to clinical diagnosis of the disease [17].

4.3.6. Hyperlipidaemia

An association of elevated cholesterol at middle life with increased risk of late-life Alzheimer's disease was reported in some studies [53]. Controversial findings have also been reported on the relation of cholesterol in late life to dementia risk. Some cohort studies found no association or even an inverse association of total cholesterol with dementia risk [84]. A study showed a decline in total cholesterol at least 15 years before dementia onset [85]. Recently, a bidirectional cholesterol-cognition relationship has been reported. High midlife cholesterol was associated with poorer late-life cognition, but decreasing cholesterol after midlife may reflect poorer cognitive status [86].

4.3.7. The metabolic syndrome

Instead of exploring the effect of its subcomponents, several studies have assessed the relationship between metabolic syndrome as a whole and the risk of Alzheimer's disease or cognitive decline. A clustering of interrelated metabolic risk factors such as diabetes, obesity, hypertension and dyslipidaemia has received increasing attention in the past few years. Several components of the metabolic syndrome have been individually related to cognitive outcomes. A prospective study found that the metabolic syndrome contributed to cognitive decline [87]. But this finding was not confirmed in a population of the oldest old. The concept of the metabolic syndrome may be less valid in this age group [88]. Finally, two studies showed that metabolic syndrome was associated with an increased risk of Alzheimer's disease [89, 90].

4.3.8. Alcohol consumption

Excessive alcohol intake can cause alcoholic dementia and may increase the risk of vascular dementia. Heavier alcohol intake at middle age was associated with increased risk of late-life dementia [91]. By contrast, increasing evidence suggests that light to moderate alcohol consumption may be associated with a reduced risk of dementia and cognitive decline [92], a similar effect as observed for cardiovascular disease [25]. In a meta-analysis of 15 prospective studies on the effect of alcohol on dementia risk, light to moderate alcohol consumption was associated with a reduction in the risk of Alzheimer's disease and dementia [93]. However, the role of moderate alcohol consumption in dementia still remains controversial because the inverse association may be due to information bias, the confounding of healthy lifestyles and high socioeconomic status, different approaches in assessments of alcohol consumption, or outcome misclassification.

4.3.9. Cigarette smoking

The relationship between smoking and cognitive decline remains uncertain. Case-control studies have largely suggested that smoking lowers the risk of Alzheimer's disease [13]. Some prospective studies have found an increased risk of Alzheimer's disease associated with smoking [94]. A meta-analysis that examined the association between smoking and Alzheimer's disease while accounting for tobacco-industry affiliation found that the combined results of 18 cross-sectional studies without industry affiliations yielded no association [95]. Analysis of 14 cohort studies without tobacco-industry affiliations yielded a significant increase in the risk of Alzheimer's disease [13]. In the Kungsholmen Project, smoking affected survival in Alzheimer's disease cases more than in non-demented subjects, and the protective effect of smoking on the Alzheimer's disease was no longer present when incident Alzheimer's cases were studied [7] suggesting that previously reported association of cigarette smoking with low prevalence of dementia was probably due to survival bias.

4.3.10. Diet and nutrients

Diets high in fish, fruits and vegetables are high in anti-oxidants and polyunsaturated fatty acids (PUFAs). In some observational studies, high or supplementary intake of vitamins C, E, B6, B12, and folate has been related to a decreased risk of Alzheimer's disease [96, 97]. Indeed, low levels of B12 and folate were found to be related to an increased risk of Alzheimer's disease in a study from the Kungsholmen Project [98]. Investigations on the effect of dietary PUFAs on the risk of cognitive dysfunction proved inconclusive. Several studies showed that the consumption of PUFAs led to reduction in the risk of Alzheimer's disease and dementia, mild cognitive impairment [99]. Population-based studies suggested that moderate to high intake of unsaturated fats at midlife is protective, whereas a moderate intake of saturated fats may increase the risk of dementia and Alzheimer's disease [100, 101], especially among *APOE* ε4 carriers [102, 103]. Fatty acids may affect dementia through various mechanisms such as atherosclerosis and inflammation. Adherence to 'Mediterranean diet' (higher intake of fish, fruits, and vegetables rich in antioxidants) was associated with a reduced risk of Alzheimer's disease independent of vascular pathways [104].

4.4. Psychosocial factors

Psychological factors include social economic status, education attainment in early life, and work complexity in adult-life and leisure activities. Evidence from epidemiological research has been accumulating that some psychosocial factors and healthy lifestyle may postpone the onset of dementia, possibly by enhancing cognitive reserve.

4.4.1. Social economic status

A number of studies have found that higher socioeconomic status (SES) is associated with a reduced risk of developing Alzheimer's disease [105-107]. In most of these studies, SES was assessed based on occupational attainment, current income to reflect socioeconomic level in adulthood, or educational attainment. Findings from a prospective study, however, suggested that early life socioeconomic status assessed at the household or community level was related to level of cognition in late life but not to rate of cognitive decline or risk of Alzheimer's disease [47].

4.4.2. High education

Numerous longitudinal studies have consistently shown that a higher educational achievement in early life is associated with a decreased incidence of dementia, and of Alzheimer's disease in particular. Low dementia prevalence among highly educated persons has been reported by numerous surveys. Educational attainment and lifespan mental activity associated with childhood education may reduce the risk of dementia [25]. The cognitive reserve hypothesis has been proposed to interpret this association such that education could enhance neural and cognitive reserve that may provide compensatory mechanisms to cope with degenerative pathological changes in the brain, and therefore delay onset of the dementia syndrome [17]. Alternatively, educational achievement may be a surrogate or an indicator of intelligent quotient, early life living environments, and occupational toxic exposure experienced over adulthood [108].

4.4.3. Physical activity

Basic science and observational evidence on humans strongly supports the hypothesis that increased physical activity prevents the onset of dementia. Regular exercise, even low-intensity activity such as walking, has been associated with reduced risk of dementia and cognitive decline [109-111]. In the Kungsholmen Project, the component of physical activity presenting in various leisure activities, rather than sports and any specific physical exercise, was related to a decreased dementia risk [110]. A strong protective effect of regular physical activity in middle age against the development of dementia and Alzheimer's disease in late life was reported, especially for persons with the *APOE* ε4 allele [112]. As it may take years to achieve high levels of physical fitness, brief periods of exercise training may not have substantial benefits on cognitive processes, but could still be detectable in the subsets of cognitive domains that are more sensitive to the age related decrements. Physical activity is important not only in promoting general and vascular health, but also in promoting brain plasticity, and it may also affect several gene transcripts and neurotropic factors that are relevant for the maintenance of cognitive functions. There is now increasing amounts of trial evidence to support this hypothesis in terms of cognitive benefits in healthy older adults as well as in people at risk for dementia. However, to date there are no RCTs confirm that increased physical activity prevents dementia.

4.4.4. Mentally stimulating activity

Various types of mentally demanding activities have been examined in relation to dementia and AD, including knitting, gardening, dancing, playing board games and musical instruments, reading, social and cultural activities, and watching specific television programs, which often showed a protective effect [113]. Due to the cultural and individual differences in choosing specific activities, some researchers summarize mentally stimulating activities into a composite score, which showed that a cognitive activity score involving participation in seven common activities with information processing as a central component was associated with a reduced risk of AD, even after controlling for APOE ε4 allele, medical conditions, and depressive symptoms [114, 115]. The Swedish Twin Study showed that greater complexity of work, and particularly complex work with people, may reduce the risk of Alzheimer's disease [116]. The Canadian Study of Health and Aging found that high complexity of work appeared to be associated with a reduced risk of dementia, but mostly for vascular dementia [117]. In supporting of these findings, the recent neuroimaging study suggested that a high level of complex mental activity across the lifespan was correlated with a reduced rate of hippocampal atrophy [118].

4.4.5. Social network and social engagement

A poor social network or social disengagement in late life was associated with an elevated risk of dementia. Evidence from longitudinal observational studies suggests that a poor social network or social disengagement is associated with cognitive decline and dementia [119, 120]. The risk for dementia and AD was also increased in older people with increasing social isolation and less frequent and unsatisfactory contacts with relatives and friends. Furthermore, low social engagement in late life and a decline in social engagement from middle age to late life were associated with a doubly increased risk of developing dementia and AD in late life. Rich social networks and high social engagement imply better social support, leading to better access to resources and material goods [123]. Rich and large social networks also provide affective and intellectual stimulation that could influence cognitive function and different health outcomes through behavioural, psychological, and physiological pathways [122]. Finally, a recent study suggested that low neuroticism in combination with high extraversion was the personality trait associated with the lowest dementia risk, and among socially isolated individuals even low neuroticism alone seemed to decrease the risk of dementia [121].

4.4.6. Depression

Recent evidence suggests a strong relationship between depression and Alzheimer's disease. A lifetime history of major depression has been considered as a risk factor for later development of Alzheimer's disease [124, 125]. The presence of depressive symptoms can affect the conversion of mild cognitive impairment to Alzheimer's disease. Neuronal plaques and neurofibrillary tangles, the two major hallmarks of Alzheimer's disease brain, are more pronounced in the brains of Alzheimer's disease patients with comorbid depression as compared with Alzheimer's disease patients without depression. On the other hand, neurodegenerative phenomena have been observed in different brain regions of patients with a history of depression. Recent evidence suggests that molecular mechanisms and cascades that underlie the pathogenesis of major depression, such as chronic inflammation and hyper-activation of hypothalamic–pituitary–adrenal (HPA) axis, are also involved in the pathogenesis of Alzheimer's disease [125]. A recent study has shown that depression increased the risk of dementia among patients with diabetes [126].

4.5. Other factors

4.5.1. Inflammation

Inflammation is known to be involved in the atherosclerotic process. Thus, serum inflammatory makers may be associated with dementia. Some cohort studies found such an association, and C-reactive protein may be the most promising in predicting dementia risk [127]. In addition, long-term use of non-steroidal anti-inflammatory drugs was suggested to be associated with a lower risk of AD [25].

4.5.2. Hormone replacement therapy

Hormone replacement therapy in postmenopausal women has been frequently reported to be associated with a lower risk of AD. An association between hormone replacement therapy and a reduced risk of dementia and Alzheimer's disease among postmenopausal women had been frequently reported in numerous observational studies until 2004 when, instead of a protective effect, a significantly increased risk of dementia associated with estrogenic therapy was found in the Women's Health Study [128].

4.5.3. Occupational exposures

Manual work involving goods production has been associated with an increased risk of AD and dementia. Occupation and occupational exposures (e.g., electromagnetic fields and heavy metals) may play a role in dementia and Alzheimer's disease [129, 130]. Data from the Kungsholmen Project showed that manual work involving goods production was associated with an increased risk of dementia and Alzheimer's disease [130], and specifically a risk effect was detected with electromagnetic exposure [129]. Occupational exposure to extremely-low-frequency electromagnetic fields (ELF-EMF) has been related to an increased risk of dementia and AD in a number of follow-up studies [129, 131]. The meta-analysis of epidemiological evidence suggests an association between occupational exposure to ELF-EMF and AD [132].

4.5.4. Head trauma and traumatic brain injury

For many years, head trauma has been suggested as a possible risk factor for Alzheimer's disease, and it has been extensively investigated in several studies, but this possible association still remains controversial. Moderate head injuries are associated with twice the risk of developing Alzheimer's compared with no head injuries, and severe head injuries are associated with 4.5 times the risk [133, 134]. Moderate head injury is defined as a head injury resulting in loss of consciousness or post-traumatic amnesia lasting more than 30 minutes; if either of these lasts more than 24 hours, the injury is considered severe. These increased risks have not been shown for individuals experiencing mild head injury or any number of common mishaps, such as bumping one's head while exiting a car. Groups that experienced repeated head injuries, such as boxers, football players and combat veterans, may be at increased risk of dementia, late-life cognitive impairment and evidence of tau tangles (a hallmark of Alzheimer's) at autopsy [135-138]. Additional research is needed to better understand the association between brain injury and increased risk of Alzheimer's disease.

5. Summary of evidence from systematic review

Meta-analyses and systematic reviews have provided robust evidence that cognitive reserve (a concept combining the benefits of education, occupation, and mental activities) [139], physical activity and exercise [140, 141], midlife obesity [142], alcohol intake [93], and smoking [142] are the most important modifiable risk factors for Alzheimer's disease. There is insufficient overall evidence from epidemiological studies to support any association between dietary or supplementary antioxidant or B vitamins and altered risk of incident dementia [143, 144]. Data from several independent time points from a large Swedish epidemiological study suggest that better social networks and social activities might be associated with reduced incidence of Alzheimer's disease [119], but this has not been examined systematically in other large epidemiological cohorts [61].

Many treatable medical conditions have also been associated with an increased risk of Alzheimer's disease, including stroke [145], diabetes [146], midlife hypertension [52], and midlife hypercholesterolemia [147, 148]. Blood pressure and cholesterol both seem to be reduced in late life and in the prodromal to Alzheimer's disease; thus, the difference between midlife and late life is an important distinction. There is probably an important relation between some of these conditions and the lifestyle factors mentioned previously, and interventions to promote healthy living will probably reduce the incidence of diabetes and stroke as well as having other, more direct, effects on dementia. There is limited evidence about the potential effect of management of diabetes or stroke on the risk of subsequent dementia, more intervention trials on this topic are needed (Table 1) [61,149].

Less than two decades have passed since the first incidence data for Alzheimer's disease and other dementias were reported, during which there have been many achievements in the understanding of risk and protective factors of Alzheimer's disease. Accumulated evidence from epidemiological research strongly supports a role for lifestyle and cardiovascular risk factors in the pathogenesis and development of dementia. However, none of these factors has been proven to have a causal relation specifically with Alzheimer's disease. Indeed, this topic is further complicated by the fact that the traditional diagnosis of dementia subtypes has been challenged by population-based neuropathological and neuroimaging studies. Research has shown a range of dementia-associated brain abnormalities from pure vascular lesions at one end to pure Alzheimer's pathologies at the other, with most dementia cases

being attributable to both vascular disease and neurodegeneration.

Factors	Systematic review	Results
Overweight and obesity	Meta-analysis of ten studies. Sixteen articles on 15 prospective studies with 3.2-36 years follow-up	Overweight: Dementia RR 1.26 (95% CI 1.10–1.44); Alzheimer's disease 1.35 (95% CI 1·19–1.54) Obesity: Dementia RR 1.64 (95% CI 1.34-2.00); Alzheimer's disease RR 2.04 (95% CI 1.59-2.62)
Smoking	Meta-analysis of four prospective studies with 2–25 years follow-up in over 17 000 people. In the four studies the dementia ORs were 3·17 (95% CI 1.37–7.35), 1.42 (1.07–1.89), 1.60 (1.00–2.57), and 1.63 (1.00–2.67)	Dementia RR 2.2 (95% CI 1.3–3.6)
Physical activity	13 prospective studies focusing on Alzheimer's disease, dementia, or both, with at least 150 000 participants	Dementia RR 0.72 (95% CI 0.60–0.86); Alzheimer's disease 0.55 (95% CI 0.36–0.84)
Cognitive reserve (intelligence, occupation, and education)	22 prospective studies with at least 29 000 participants followed up for a median of 7.1 years	Dementia OR 0.54 (95% CI 0.49–0.59)
Alcohol	15 longitudinal studies with 2–8 years follow-up and at least 14 000 participants	Dementia RR 0.74 (95% CI 0.61–0.91); Alzheimer's disease 0.72 (0.61–0.86)
Medical conditions		
Midlife hypertension	At least 15 years follow-up in most studies, with at least 16 000 participants	Four of five longitudinal studies focusing on midlife hypertension suggested that it is a significant risk factor for incident dementia (RR 1.24–2.8 in different studies) The biggest differences were reported in studies using 160/95 mm Hg as the threshold for hypertension
Stroke	16 studies with at least 25 000 participants, mainly included patients aged 65 years and over	12 of 16 studies showed significant association between stroke and incident dementia, with overall doubling of incidence
Diabetes	15 prospective cohort studies	Dementia RR 1.47 (95% CI 1.25–1.73); Alzheimer's disease RR 1.39 (95% CI 1.16–1.66)

Factors	Systematic review	Results
Midlife hypercholes-terolemia	18 studies, but only five assessed high cholesterol specifically in midlife. All five midlife studies had over 15 years follow-up and a total of over 15 000 participants	Four of five longitudinal studies in midlife suggested a significant positive association between high total cholesterol and incident dementia. For overall difference the RR was 1·4–3·1
Intervention studies		
Hypertension	12 091 participants between the three trials (SHEP, SYST-EUR, and SCOPE) with mean follow-up of 3·3 years. Only SYST-EUR reported significant benefit	OR 0.89 (95% CI 0.69–1.16) for incident dementia
Statins for prevention of dementia	26 340 participants between the two trials (PROSPER and HPS), with follow-up of 3·2 and 5 years. Cognition was measured with different instruments at different timepoints	Neither of the two trials reported significant benefit of statin therapy
Vitamins B12 or fo-late	Four trials in older people without existing cognitive impairment	Three trials showed no benefit. One trial (the only that selected participants based on increased homocysteine) reported benefit with respect to global function

RR=relative risk. OR=odds ratio. SHEP=Systolic Hypertension in the Elderly Program. SYST-EUR=Systolic Hypertension in Europe. SCOPE=Study on Cognition and Prognosis in the Elderly. PROSPER=PROspective Study of Pravastatin in the Elderly at Risk. HPS=Heart Protection Study.

Table 1. Meta-analyses or systematic reviews of risk factors for dementia and Alzheimer's disease [61,149]

Population studies have identified many factors that could be important in reducing the risk of dementia, including factors that identify people at risk for dementia (vascular risk factors, depressive symptoms) and factors that may reduce the risk of dementia (cognitive, physical, and social activity, a diet rich in antioxidants and polyunsaturated fatty acids, vascular risk factor control). While early interventional studies have been less conclusive, future trials should continue to examine the effect of risk factor modification on cognitive outcomes. In particular, interventions that combine a number of factors, such as healthy nutrition along with cognitive, social, and physical activity, should be investigated. In the most optimistic view, dementia could be delayed or even prevented by these interventions. At worst, people will improve their overall health, especially their cardiovascular health, and enjoy a more cognitively and socially engaging life.

5.1. Intervention strategies against Alzheimer's disease

Despite the specific challenges posed by neurological disorders, such as Alzheimer's disease and other dementias, interventions need to be implemented to verify findings from the many population-based observational studies, which suggest that preventive and therapeutic interventions have great potential [150].

5.1.1. Vascular factors and related disorders

Most vascular risk factors and related disorders are modifiable or treatable that can serve as targets in the development of primary preventative strategies against dementia. For example, antihypertensive therapy has been shown to reduce the risk of dementia in observational studies, and this finding was partly confirmed by clinical trials. Furthermore, studies have confirmed that obesity and diabetes can be prevented by changing dietary habits and lifestyles, and that health education may help quit smoking. Finally, preventing recurrent cerebrovascular disease and maintaining sufficient cerebral blood perfusion seems to be critical for postponing expression of the dementia syndrome in older people. Thus, controlling high blood pressure and obesity, especially from middle age, and preventing diabetes and recurrent stroke could be the primary preventive measures against late-life dementia.

5.1.2. Intervention towards psychosocial factors and lifestyles

High educational achievements in early life can provide cognitive reserve that benefits the whole life in terms of cognitive health and delaying the onset of late-life dementia. Extensive social networks and active engagements in intellectually stimulating activities such as reading, doing crosswords, and playing board games may significantly lower the risk of dementia by providing cognitive reserve or by reducing psychosocial stress. It is likely that mentally and socially integrated lifestyles could postpone the onset of dementia [119]. Regular physical exercise may reduce the risk of the dementias resulting from cerebral atherosclerosis. Leisure activities with all three components of physical, mental, and social activities may have the most beneficial effect on dementia prevention. Many of the risk factors for dementia, such as hypertension, diabetes, and obesity, may be modified by diet. In addition, a diet high in antioxidants may reduce inflammation, which is associated with the risk of dementia. Thus, it is reasonable to suggest that the risk of dementia itself could be modified by diet. The treatment of depression also seems to improve cognitive function in people who are depressed. Taking together, the most promising strategy for the primary prevention of dementia may be to encourage people implementing multiple preventative measures throughout the life course, including high educational attainment in childhood and early adulthood, an active control of vascular factors (e.g., smoking) and disorders (e.g., hypertension and diabetes) in adulthood, and maintenance of mentally, physically, and socially active lifestyles during middle age and later in life.

6. Conclusions

Alzheimer's disease is a major cause of functional dependence, institutionalisation, and mortality among elderly people. Population-based studies have made a great contribution to our knowledge of Alzheimer's disease. Although many aspects of Alzheimer's disease are still unclear, we are now able to make more accurate diagnoses than before, and the pattern of dementia distribution has been sufficiently described to guide the planning of medical and social services. Epidemiological studies have shown that vascular risk factors in middle age and later in life significantly contribute to the development and progression of the dementia syndrome, whereas extensive social network and active engagement in social, physical, and mental activities may delay the onset of the dementing disorders. Hence, one of the promising strategies to deal with the tremendous challenge from the epidemic of dementia is to implement appropriate intervention measures from a life-course perspective. Achieving high education in early life and engaging mentally stimulating activity over adulthood to enhance cognitive reserve, and maintaining vascular health by adopting healthy lifestyles and optimally controlling vascular diseases to reduce the burden of vascular lesions in the brain. These preventive measures will enable people to maintain cognitive ability in late life, even though they may have developed a high load of Alzheimer pathologies in their brain.

Acknowledgements

Research grants were received from the Swedish council for working life and social research, the Swedish Research Council in Medicine and the Swedish Brain Power. This study was also supported in part by funds from the Loo and Hans Ostermans Foundation and the Foundation for Geriatric Diseases at Karolinska Institutet, the Gamla Tjänarinnor Foundation, Demensfonden and the Bertil Stohnes Foundation.

Author details

Weili Xu[1,2*], Camilla Ferrari[2,3] and Hui-Xin Wang[2]

*Address all correspondence to: weili.xu@ki.se

1 Department of Epidemiology, Tianjin Medical University, Tianjin, P.R., China

2 Aging Research Center, Karolinska Institutet-Stockholm University, Stockholm, Sweden

3 Department of Neurological and Psychiatric Sciences, University of Florence, Italy

References

[1] From the Centers for Disease Control and Prevention. Public health and aging: trends in aging--United States and worldwide. JAMA 2003;289(11):1371-1373.

[2] Kinsella K, Velkoff VA. The demographics of aging. Aging Clin Exp Res 2002;14(3): 159-169.

[3] Lunenfeld B. An Aging World - demographics and challenges. Gynecol Endocrinol 2008;24(1):1-3.

[4] Bennett DA. Editorial comment on 'Prevalence of dementia in the United States: the aging, demographics, and memory study' by Plassman et al. Neuroepidemiology 2007;29(1-2):133-135.

[5] American Psychiatric Association: Diagnostic and Statistical Manual of Mental Disorders, Third Edition-Revised (DSM-III-R). Washington, DC: American Psychiatric Association; 1987.

[6] American Psychiatric Association: Diagnostic and Statistical Manual of Mental Disorders, Fourth Edition (DSM-IV). Washington, DC: American Psychiatric Association; 1994.

[7] Fratiglioni L, Winblad B, von Strauss E. Prevention of Alzheimer's disease and dementia. Major findings from the Kungsholmen Project. Physiol Behav 2007;92(1-2): 98-104.

[8] Harvey R, Fox N, Rossor M. Dementia Handbook. London: Martin Dunitz; 1999.

[9] Roman GC. Vascular dementia: distinguishing characteristics, treatment, and prevention. J Am Geriatr Soc 2003;51(5 Suppl Dementia):S296-304.

[10] Korczyn AD, Vakhapova V. The prevention of the dementia epidemic. J Neurol Sci 2007;257(1-2):2-4.

[11] Ferri CP, Prince M, Brayne C, Brodaty H, Fratiglioni L, Ganguli M, et al. Global prevalence of dementia: a Delphi consensus study. Lancet 2005;366(9503):2112-2117.

[12] Wimo A, Winblad B, Aguero-Torres H, von Strauss E. The magnitude of dementia occurrence in the world. Alzheimer Dis Assoc Disord 2003;17(2):63-67.

[13] Reitz C, Brayne C, Mayeux R. Epidemiology of Alzheimer disease. Nat Rev Neurol 2011;7(3):137-152.

[14] Lobo A, Launer LJ, Fratiglioni L, Andersen K, Di Carlo A, Breteler MM, et al. Prevalence of dementia and major subtypes in Europe: A collaborative study of population-based cohorts. Neurologic Diseases in the Elderly Research Group. Neurology 2000;54(11 Suppl 5):S4-9.

[15] Plassman BL, Langa KM, Fisher GG, Heeringa SG, Weir DR, Ofstedal MB, et al. Prevalence of dementia in the United States: the aging, demographics, and memory study. Neuroepidemiology 2007;29(1-2):125-132.

[16] Zhang Y, Xu Y, Nie H, Lei T, Wu Y, Zhang L, et al. Prevalence of dementia and major dementia subtypes in the Chinese populations: A meta-analysis of dementia prevalence surveys, 1980-2010. J Clin Neurosci 2012;19(10):1333-1337.

[17] Qiu C, Kivipelto M, von Strauss E. Epidemiology of Alzheimer's disease: occurrence, determinants, and strategies toward intervention. Dialogues Clin Neurosci 2009;11(2):111-128.

[18] Corrada MM, Brookmeyer R, Berlau D, Paganini-Hill A, Kawas CH. Prevalence of dementia after age 90: results from the 90+ study. Neurology 2008;71(5):337-343.

[19] von Strauss E, Viitanen M, De Ronchi D, Winblad B, Fratiglioni L. Aging and the occurrence of dementia: findings from a population-based cohort with a large sample of nonagenarians. Arch Neurology 1999;56(5):587-592.

[20] Kalaria RN, Maestre GE, Arizaga R, Friedland RP, Galasko D, Hall K, et al. Alzheimer's disease and vascular dementia in developing countries: prevalence, management, and risk factors. Lancet Neurol 2008;7(9):812-826.

[21] Llibre Rodriguez JJ, Ferri CP, Acosta D, Guerra M, Huang Y, Jacob KS, et al. Prevalence of dementia in Latin America, India, and China: a population-based cross-sectional survey. Lancet 2008;372(9637):464-474.

[22] Zhang ZX, Zahner GE, Roman GC, Liu J, Hong Z, Qu QM, et al. Dementia subtypes in China: prevalence in Beijing, Xian, Shanghai, and Chengdu. Archives of neurology 2005;62(3):447-453.

[23] Llibre Rodriguez J, Valhuerdi A, Sanchez, II, Reyna C, Guerra MA, Copeland JR, et al. The prevalence, correlates and impact of dementia in Cuba. A 10/66 group population-based survey. Neuroepidemiology 2008;31(4):243-251.

[24] Scazufca M, Menezes PR, Vallada HP, Crepaldi AL, Pastor-Valero M, Coutinho LM, et al. High prevalence of dementia among older adults from poor socioeconomic backgrounds in Sao Paulo, Brazil. Int Psychogeriatr 2008;20(2):394-405.

[25] Qiu C, De Ronchi D, Fratiglioni L. The epidemiology of the dementias: an update. Curr Opin Psychiatry 2007;20(4):380-385.

[26] Fratiglioni L, Launer LJ, Andersen K, Breteler MM, Copeland JR, Dartigues JF, et al. Incidence of dementia and major subtypes in Europe: A collaborative study of population-based cohorts. Neurologic Diseases in the Elderly Research Group. Neurology 2000;54(11 Suppl 5):S10-15.

[27] Kawas C, Gray S, Brookmeyer R, Fozard J, Zonderman A. Age-specific incidence rates of Alzheimer's disease: the Baltimore Longitudinal Study of Aging. Neurology 2000;54(11):2072-2077.

[28] Kukull WA, Higdon R, Bowen JD, McCormick WC, Teri L, Schellenberg GD, et al. Dementia and Alzheimer disease incidence: a prospective cohort study. Arch Neurol 2002;59(11):1737-1746.

[29] Miech RA, Breitner JC, Zandi PP, Khachaturian AS, Anthony JC, Mayer L. Incidence of AD may decline in the early 90s for men, later for women: The Cache County study. Neurology 2002;58(2):209-218.

[30] Matthews F, Brayne C. The incidence of dementia in England and Wales: findings from the five identical sites of the MRC CFA Study. PLoS Med 2005;2(8):e193.

[31] Ravaglia G, Forti P, Maioli F, Martelli M, Servadei L, Brunetti N, et al. Incidence and etiology of dementia in a large elderly Italian population. Neurology 2005;64(9): 1525-1530.

[32] Chandra V, Pandav R, Dodge HH, Johnston JM, Belle SH, DeKosky ST, et al. Incidence of Alzheimer's disease in a rural community in India: the Indo-US study. Neurology 2001;57(6):985-989.

[33] Aguero-Torres H, Qiu C, Winblad B, Fratiglioni L. Dementing disorders in the elderly: evolution of disease severity over 7 years. Alzheimer Dis Assoc Disord 2002;16(4): 221-227.

[34] Aguero-Torres H, Fratiglioni L, Guo Z, Viitanen M, von Strauss E, Winblad B. Dementia is the major cause of functional dependence in the elderly: 3-year follow-up data from a population-based study. Am J Public Health 1998;88(10):1452-1456.

[35] Aguero-Torres H, Fratiglioni L, Guo Z, Viitanen M, Winblad B. Mortality from dementia in advanced age: a 5-year follow-up study of incident dementia cases. J Clin Epidemiol 1999;52(8):737-743.

[36] Cotter VT. The burden of dementia. Am J Manag Care 2007;13 Suppl 8:S193-197.

[37] Wimo A, Jonsson L, Winblad B. An estimate of the worldwide prevalence and direct costs of dementia in 2003. Dement Geriatr Cogn Disord 2006;21(3):175-181.

[38] Qiu C. Epidemiological findings of vascular risk factors in Alzheimer's disease: implications for therapeutic and preventive intervention. Expert Rev Neurother 2011;11(11):1593-1607.

[39] Qiu C, Kivipelto M, Fratiglioni L. Preventing Alzheimer disease and cognitive decline. Ann Inter Med 2011;154(3):211; author reply 212-213.

[40] Ferrari C, Xu WL, Wang HX, Winblad B, Sorbi S, Qiu C, et al. How can elderly apolipoprotein E epsilon4 carriers remain free from dementia? Neurobiol Aging 2012.

[41] Qiu C, Kivipelto M, Aguero-Torres H, Winblad B, Fratiglioni L. Risk and protective effects of the APOE gene towards Alzheimer's disease in the Kungsholmen project: variation by age and sex. J Neurol Neurosurg Psychiatry 2004;75(6):828-833.

[42] D'Introno A, Solfrizzi V, Colacicco AM, Capurso C, Amodio M, Todarello O, et al. Current knowledge of chromosome 12 susceptibility genes for late-onset Alzheimer's disease. Neurobiol Aging 2006;27(11):1537-1553.

[43] Wang HX, Gustafson DR, Kivipelto M, Pedersen NL, Skoog I, Windblad B, et al. Education halves the risk of dementia due to apolipoprotein epsilon4 allele: a collaborative study from the Swedish Brain Power initiative. Neurobiol Aging 2012;33(5):1007 e1001-1007.

[44] Keller L, Xu W, Wang HX, Winblad B, Fratiglioni L, Graff C. The obesity related gene, FTO, interacts with APOE, and is associated with Alzheimer's disease risk: a prospective cohort study. J Alzheimers Dis 2011;23(3):461-469.

[45] Green RC, Cupples LA, Go R, Benke KS, Edeki T, Griffith PA, et al. Risk of dementia among white and African American relatives of patients with Alzheimer disease. JAMA 2002;287(3):329-336.

[46] Fratiglioni L, Ahlbom A, Viitanen M, Winblad B. Risk factors for late-onset Alzheimer's disease: a population-based, case-control study. Ann Neurol 1993;33(3):258-266.

[47] Wilson RS, Scherr PA, Hoganson G, Bienias JL, Evans DA, Bennett DA. Early life socioeconomic status and late life risk of Alzheimer's disease. Neuroepidemiology 2005;25(1):8-14.

[48] Lautenschlager NT, Cupples LA, Rao VS, Auerbach SA, Becker R, Burke J, et al. Risk of dementia among relatives of Alzheimer's disease patients in the MIRAGE study: What is in store for the oldest old? Neurology 1996;46(3):641-650.

[49] Fratiglioni L, Rocca W. Epidemiology of dementia. In: Handbook of Neuropsychology (2nd Edition), Boller F and Cappa SF, eds Elsevier Science B.V.; 2001.

[50] McVeigh C, Passmore P. Vascular dementia: prevention and treatment. Clin Interv Aging 2006;1(3):229-235.

[51] Nelson NW. Differential diagnosis of Alzheimer's dementia and vascular dementia. Dis Mon 2007;53(3):148-151.

[52] Qiu C, Winblad B, Fratiglioni L. The age-dependent relation of blood pressure to cognitive function and dementia. Lancet Neurol 2005;4(8):487-499.

[53] Whitmer RA, Sidney S, Selby J, Johnston SC, Yaffe K. Midlife cardiovascular risk factors and risk of dementia in late life. Neurology 2005;64(2):277-281.

[54] Ruitenberg A, den Heijer T, Bakker SL, van Swieten JC, Koudstaal PJ, Hofman A, et al. Cerebral hypoperfusion and clinical onset of dementia: the Rotterdam Study. Ann Neurol 2005;57(6):789-794.

[55] Qiu C, von Strauss E, Fastbom J, Winblad B, Fratiglioni L. Low blood pressure and risk of dementia in the Kungsholmen project: a 6-year follow-up study. Arch Neurol 2003;60(2):223-228.

[56] Peila R, White LR, Masaki K, Petrovitch H, Launer LJ. Reducing the risk of dementia: efficacy of long-term treatment of hypertension. Stroke 2006;37(5):1165-1170.

[57] Haag MD, Hofman A, Koudstaal PJ, Breteler MM, Stricker BH. Duration of antihypertensive drug use and risk of dementia: A prospective cohort study. Neurology 2009;72(20):1727-1734.

[58] Newman AB, Fitzpatrick AL, Lopez O, Jackson S, Lyketsos C, Jagust W, et al. De-
      mentia and Alzheimer's disease incidence in relationship to cardiovascular disease in
      the Cardiovascular Health Study cohort. J Am Geriatr Soc 2005;53(7):1101-1107.

[59] Qiu CX, Winblad, B, Marengoni A, Klarin I, Fastbom J, Fratiglioni L. Heart failure
      and risk of dementia and Alzheimer disease: a population-based cohort study. Arch
      Intern Med 2006;166:1003-1008.

[60] Purandare N, Burns A, Daly KJ, Hardicre J, Morris J, Macfarlane G, et al. Cerebral
      emboli as a potential cause of Alzheimer's disease and vascular dementia: case-con-
      trol study. BMJ 2006;332(7550):1119-1124.

[61] Ballard C, Gauthier S, Corbett A, Brayne C, Aarsland D, Jones E. Alzheimer's disease.
      Lancet 2011;377(9770):1019-1031.

[62] Arvanitakis Z, Wilson RS, Bennett DA. Diabetes mellitus, dementia, and cognitive
      function in older persons. J Nutr Health Aging 2006;10(4):287-291.

[63] Cukierman T, Gerstein HC, Williamson JD. Cognitive decline and dementia in diabe-
      tes--systematic overview of prospective observational studies. Diabetologia
      2005;48(12):2460-2469.

[64] Luchsinger JA, Reitz C, Patel B, Tang MX, Manly JJ, Mayeux R. Relation of diabetes
      to mild cognitive impairment. Arch Neurol 2007;64(4):570-575.

[65] Arvanitakis Z, Wilson RS, Li Y, Aggarwal NT, Bennett DA. Diabetes and function in
      different cognitive systems in older individuals without dementia. Diabetes Care
      2006;29(3):560-565.

[66] Allen KV, Frier BM, Strachan MW. The relationship between type 2 diabetes and
      cognitive dysfunction: longitudinal studies and their methodological limitations. Eur
      J Pharmacol 2004;490(1-3):169-175.

[67] Xu W, Caracciolo B, Wang HX, Winblad B, Backman L, Qiu C, et al. Accelerated Pro-
      gression from Mild Cognitive Impairment to Dementia in People with Diabetes. Dia-
      betes 2010;59(11):2928-35

[68] Xu W, Qiu C, Gatz M, Pedersen NL, Johansson B, Fratiglioni L. Mid- and late-life dia-
      betes in relation to the risk of dementia: a population-based twin study. Diabetes
      2009;58(1):71-77.

[69] Xu WL, Qiu CX, Wahlin A, Winblad B, Fratiglioni L. Diabetes mellitus and risk of
      dementia in the Kungsholmen project: a 6-year follow-up study. Neurology
      2004;63(7):1181-1186.

[70] Xu WL, von Strauss E, Qiu CX, Winblad B, Fratiglioni L. Uncontrolled diabetes in-
      creases the risk of Alzheimer's disease: a population-based cohort study. Diabetolo-
      gia 2009;52(6):1031-1039.

[71] Biessels GJ, Staekenborg S, Brunner E, Brayne C, Scheltens P. Risk of dementia in dia-
      betes mellitus: a systematic review. Lancet Neurol 2006;5(1):64-74.

[72] Roberts RO, Geda YE, Knopman DS, Christianson TJ, Pankratz VS, Boeve BF, et al. Association of duration and severity of diabetes mellitus with mild cognitive impairment. Arch Neurol 2008;65(8):1066-1073.

[73] Strachan MW, Price JF, Frier BM. Diabetes, cognitive impairment, and dementia. Bmj 2008;336(7634):6.

[74] Xu W, Qiu C, Winblad B, Fratiglioni L. The effect of borderline diabetes on the risk of dementia and Alzheimer's disease. Diabetes 2007;56(1):211-216.

[75] Gustafson D. Adiposity indices and dementia. Lancet Neurol 2006;5(8):713-720.

[76] Whitmer RA. The epidemiology of adiposity and dementia. Curr Alzheimer Res 2007;4(2):117-122.

[77] Kivipelto M, Ngandu T, Fratiglioni L, Viitanen M, Kareholt I, Winblad B, et al. Obesity and vascular risk factors at midlife and the risk of dementia and Alzheimer disease. Arch Neurol 2005;62(10):1556-1560.

[78] Xu W, Atti A, Gatz M, Pedersen NL, Johansson B, Fratiglioni L. Midlife overweight and obesity increase dementia risk in old age: a population-based twin study. Neurology 2011;76(18):1568-74.

[79] Buchman AS, Wilson RS, Bienias JL, Shah RC, Evans DA, Bennett DA. Change in body mass index and risk of incident Alzheimer disease. Neurology 2005;65(6): 892-897.

[80] Johnson DK, Wilkins CH, Morris JC. Accelerated weight loss may precede diagnosis in Alzheimer disease. Arch Neurol 2006;63(9):1312-1317.

[81] Atti AR, Palmer K, Volpato S, Winblad B, De Ronchi D, Fratiglioni L. Late-life body mass index and dementia incidence: nine-year follow-up data from the Kungsholmen Project. J Am Geriatr Soc 2008;56(1):111-116.

[82] Johnson DK, Wilkins CH, Morris JC. Accelerated weight loss may precede diagnosis in Alzheimer disease. Arch Neurol 2006;63(9):1312-1317.

[83] Dahl AK, Lopponen M, Isoaho R, Berg S, Kivela SL. Overweight and obesity in old age are not associated with greater dementia risk. J Am Geriatr Soc 2008;56(12): 2261-2266.

[84] Mielke MM, Zandi PP, Sjogren M, Gustafson D, Ostling S, Steen B, et al. High total cholesterol levels in late life associated with a reduced risk of dementia. Neurology 2005;64(10):1689-1695.

[85] Stewart R, White LR, Xue QL, Launer LJ. Twenty-six-year change in total cholesterol levels and incident dementia: the Honolulu-Asia Aging Study. Arch Neurol 2007;64(1):103-107.

[86] Solomon A, Kareholt I, Ngandu T, Wolozin B, Macdonald SW, Winblad B, et al. Serum total cholesterol, statins and cognition in non-demented elderly. Neurobiol Aging 2007.

[87] Yaffe K, Kanaya A, Lindquist K, Simonsick EM, Harris T, Shorr RI, et al. The metabolic syndrome, inflammation, and risk of cognitive decline. JAMA 2004;292(18): 2237-2242.

[88] van den Berg E, Biessels GJ, de Craen AJ, Gussekloo J, Westendorp RG. The metabolic syndrome is associated with decelerated cognitive decline in the oldest old. Neurology 2007;69(10):979-985.

[89] Vanhanen M, Koivisto K, Moilanen L, Helkala EL, Hanninen T, Soininen H, et al. Association of metabolic syndrome with Alzheimer disease: a population-based study. Neurology 2006;67(5):843-847.

[90] Raffaitin C, Gin H, Empana JP, Helmer C, Berr C, Tzourio C, et al. Metabolic syndrome and risk for incident Alzheimer's disease or vascular dementia: the Three-City Study. Diabetes Care 2009;32(1):169-174.

[91] Anttila T, Helkala EL, Viitanen M, Kareholt I, Fratiglioni L, Winblad B, et al. Alcohol drinking in middle age and subsequent risk of mild cognitive impairment and dementia in old age: a prospective population based study. BMJ 2004;329(7465):539.

[92] Stampfer MJ, Kang JH, Chen J, Cherry R, Grodstein F. Effects of moderate alcohol consumption on cognitive function in women. N Engl J Med 2005;352(3):245-253.

[93] Anstey KJ, Mack HA, Cherbuin N. Alcohol consumption as a risk factor for dementia and cognitive decline: meta-analysis of prospective studies. Am J Geriatr Psychiatry 2009;17(7):542-555.

[94] Aggarwal NT, Bienias JL, Bennett DA, Wilson RS, Morris MC, Schneider JA, et al. The relation of cigarette smoking to incident Alzheimer's disease in a biracial urban community population. Neuroepidemiology 2006;26(3):140-146.

[95] Cataldo JK, Prochaska JJ, Glantz SA. Cigarette smoking is a risk factor for Alzheimer's Disease: an analysis controlling for tobacco industry affiliation. J Alzheimers Dis 2010;19(2):465-480.

[96] Luchsinger JA, Mayeux R. Dietary factors and Alzheimer's disease. Lancet Neurol 2004;3(10):579-587.

[97] Morris MC, Evans DA, Bienias JL, Tangney CC, Bennett DA, Aggarwal N, et al. Dietary intake of antioxidant nutrients and the risk of incident Alzheimer disease in a biracial community study. JAMA 2002;287(24):3230-3237.

[98] Wang HX, Wahlin A, Basun H, Fastbom J, Winblad B, Fratiglioni L. Vitamin B(12) and folate in relation to the development of Alzheimer's disease. Neurology 2001;56(9):1188-1194.

[99]   Kalmijn S, Launer LJ, Ott A, Witteman JC, Hofman A, Breteler MM. Dietary fat in-
       take and the risk of incident dementia in the Rotterdam Study. Ann Neu-
       rol1997;42(5):776-782.

[100] Morris MC, Evans DA, Bienias JL, Tangney CC, Bennett DA, Aggarwal N, et al. Diet-
       ary fats and the risk of incident Alzheimer disease. Arch Neurol 2003;60(2):194-200.

[101] Kalmijn S, Launer LJ, Ott A, Witteman JC, Hofman A, Breteler MM. Dietary fat in-
       take and the risk of incident dementia in the Rotterdam Study. Ann Neurol
       1997;42(5):776-782.

[102] Laitinen MH, Ngandu T, Rovio S, Helkala EL, Uusitalo U, Viitanen M, et al. Fat in-
       take at midlife and risk of dementia and Alzheimer's disease: a population-based
       study. Dement Geriatr Cogn Disord 2006;22(1):99-107.

[103] Kivipelto M, Rovio S, Ngandu T, Kareholt I, Eskelinen M, Winblad B, et al. Apolipo-
       protein E epsilon4 Magnifies Lifestyle Risks for Dementia: A Population Based
       Study. J Cell Mol Med 2008.

[104] Scarmeas N, Stern Y, Mayeux R, Luchsinger JA. Mediterranean diet, Alzheimer dis-
       ease, and vascular mediation. Arch Neurol 2006;63(12):1709-1717.

[105] Qiu C, Backman L, Winblad B, Aguero-Torres H, Fratiglioni L. The influence of edu-
       cation on clinically diagnosed dementia incidence and mortality data from the Kung-
       sholmen Project. Arch Neurol 2001;58(12):2034-2039.

[106] Evans DA, Hebert LE, Beckett LA, Scherr PA, Albert MS, Chown MJ, et al. Education
       and other measures of socioeconomic status and risk of incident Alzheimer disease
       in a defined population of older persons. Arch Neurol 1997;54(11):1399-1405.

[107] Borenstein AR, Wu Y, Mortimer JA, Schellenberg GD, McCormick WC, Bowen JD, et
       al. Developmental and vascular risk factors for Alzheimer's disease. Neurobiol Aging
       2005;26(3):325-334.

[108] Ngandu T, von Strauss E, Helkala EL, Winblad B, Nissinen A, Tuomilehto J, et al. Ed-
       ucation and dementia: what lies behind the association? Neurology 2007;69(14):
       1442-1450.

[109] Larson EB, Wang L, Bowen JD, McCormick WC, Teri L, Crane P, et al. Exercise is as-
       sociated with reduced risk for incident dementia among persons 65 years of age and
       older. Ann Intern Med 2006;144(2):73-81.

[110] Karp A, Paillard-Borg S, Wang HX, Silverstein M, Winblad B, Fratiglioni L. Mental,
       physical and social components in leisure activities equally contribute to decrease de-
       mentia risk. Dement Geriatr Cogn Disord 2006;21(2):65-73.

[111] Abbott RD, White LR, Ross GW, Masaki KH, Curb JD, Petrovitch H. Walking and de-
       mentia in physically capable elderly men. JAMA 2004;292(12):1447-1453.

[112] Rovio S, Kareholt I, Helkala EL, Viitanen M, Winblad B, Tuomilehto J, et al. Leisure-time physical activity at midlife and the risk of dementia and Alzheimer's disease. Lancet Neurol 2005;4(11):705-711.

[113] Crowe M, Andel R, Pedersen NL, Johansson B, Gatz M. Does participation in leisure activities lead to reduced risk of Alzheimer's disease? A prospective study of Swedish twins. J Gerontol B Psychol Sci Soc Sci 2003;58(5):P249-255.

[114] Wilson RS, Bennett DA, Bienias JL, Mendes de Leon CF, Morris MC, Evans DA. Cognitive activity and cognitive decline in a biracial community population. Neurology 2003;61(6):812-816.

[115] Wilson RS, Mendes De Leon CF, Barnes LL, Schneider JA, Bienias JL, Evans DA, et al. Participation in cognitively stimulating activities and risk of incident Alzheimer disease. JAMA 2002;287(6):742-748.

[116] Andel R, Crowe M, Pedersen NL, Mortimer J, Crimmins E, Johansson B, et al. Complexity of work and risk of Alzheimer's disease: a population-based study of Swedish twins. J Gerontol B Psychol Sci Soc Sci 2005;60(5):P251-258.

[117] Kroger E, Andel R, Lindsay J, Benounissa Z, Verreault R, Laurin D. Is complexity of work associated with risk of dementia? The Canadian Study of Health And Aging. American journal of epidemiology 2008;167(7):820-830.

[118] Valenzuela MJ, Sachdev P, Wen W, Chen X, Brodaty H. Lifespan mental activity predicts diminished rate of hippocampal atrophy. PLoS One 2008;3(7):e2598.

[119] Paillard-Borg S, Fratiglioni L, Xu W, Winblad B, Wang HX. An active lifestyle postpones dementia onset by more than one year in very old adults. J Alzheimers Dis Journal 2012;31(4):835-842.

[120] Fratiglioni L, Wang HX, Ericsson K, Maytan M, Winblad B. Influence of social network on occurrence of dementia: a community-based longitudinal study. Lancet 2000;355(9212):1315-1319.

[121] Wang HX, Karp A, Herlitz A, Crowe M, Kareholt I, Winblad B, et al. Personality and lifestyle in relation to dementia incidence. Neurology 2009;72(3):253-259.

[122] Saczynski JS, Pfeifer LA, Masaki K, Korf ES, Laurin D, White L, et al. The effect of social engagement on incident dementia: the Honolulu-Asia Aging Study. Am J Epidemiol 2006;163(5):433-440.

[123] Bennett DA, Schneider JA, Tang Y, Arnold SE, Wilson RS. The effect of social networks on the relation between Alzheimer's disease pathology and level of cognitive function in old people: a longitudinal cohort study. Lancet Neurol 2006;5(5):406-412.

[124] Wilson RS, Schneider JA, Bienias JL, Arnold SE, Evans DA, Bennett DA. Depressive symptoms, clinical AD, and cortical plaques and tangles in older persons. Neurology 2003;61(8):1102-1107.

[125] Caraci F, Copani A, Nicoletti F, Drago F. Depression and Alzheimer's disease: neuro-
        biological links and common pharmacological targets. Eur J Pharmacol 2010;626(1):
        64-71.

[126] Katon W, Lyles CR, Parker MM, Karter AJ, Huang ES, Whitmer RA. Association of
        depression with increased risk of dementia in patients with type 2 diabetes: the Dia-
        betes and Aging Study. Arch Gen Psychiatry 2012;69(4):410-417.

[127] DeLegge MH, Smoke A. Neurodegeneration and inflammation. Nutr Clin Pract
        2008;23(1):35-41.

[128] Whitmer RA, Quesenberry CP, Zhou J, Yaffe K. Timing of hormone therapy and de-
        mentia: the critical window theory revisited. Annal Neurology 2011;69(1):163-169.

[129] Qiu C, Fratiglioni L, Karp A, Winblad B, Bellander T. Occupational exposure to elec-
        tromagnetic fields and risk of Alzheimer's disease. Epidemiology 2004;15(6):687-694.

[130] Qiu C, Karp A, von Strauss E, Winblad B, Fratiglioni L, Bellander T. Lifetime princi-
        pal occupation and risk of Alzheimer's disease in the Kungsholmen project. Am J Ind
        Med 2003;43(2):204-211.

[131] Feychting M, Jonsson F, Pedersen NL, Ahlbom A. Occupational magnetic field expo-
        sure and neurodegenerative disease. Epidemiology 2003;14(4):413-419; discussion
        427-418.

[132] Garcia AM, Sisternas A, Hoyos SP. Occupational exposure to extremely low frequen-
        cy electric and magnetic fields and Alzheimer disease: a meta-analysis. Int J Epide-
        miol 2008;37(2):329-340.

[133] Plassman BL, Havlik RJ, Steffens DC, Helms MJ, Newman TN, Drosdick D, et al.
        Documented head injury in early adulthood and risk of Alzheimer's disease and oth-
        er dementias. Neurology 2000;55(8):1158-1166.

[134] Lye TC, Shores EA. Traumatic brain injury as a risk factor for Alzheimer's disease: a
        review. Neuropsychol Rev 2000;10(2):115-129.

[135] Roberts GW, Allsop D, Bruton C. The occult aftermath of boxing. J Neurol Neuro-
        surg Psychiatry 1990;53(5):373-378.

[136] Guskiewicz KM, Marshall SW, Bailes J, McCrea M, Cantu RC, Randolph C, et al. As-
        sociation between recurrent concussion and late-life cognitive impairment in retired
        professional football players. Neurosurgery 2005;57(4):719-726; discussion 719-726.

[137] Crawford FC, Vanderploeg RD, Freeman MJ, Singh S, Waisman M, Michaels L, et al.
        APOE genotype influences acquisition and recall following traumatic brain injury.
        Neurology 2002;58(7):1115-1118.

[138] Groswasser Z, Reider G, II, Schwab K, Ommaya AK, Pridgen A, Brown HR, et al.
        Quantitative imaging in late TBI. Part II: cognition and work after closed and pene-
        trating head injury: a report of the Vietnam head injury study. Brain Inj 2002;16(8):
        681-690.

[139] Valenzuela MJ, Sachdev P. Brain reserve and dementia: a systematic review. Psychol Med 2006;36(4):441-454.

[140] Hamer M, Chida Y. Physical activity and risk of neurodegenerative disease: a systematic review of prospective evidence. Psychol Med 2009;39(1):3-11.

[141] Wang HX, Xu W, Pei JJ. Leisure activities, cognition and dementia. Biochimica et biophysica acta 2012;1822(3):482-491.

[142] Lee Y, Back JH, Kim J, Kim SH, Na DL, Cheong HK, et al. Systematic review of health behavioral risks and cognitive health in older adults. Int Psychogeriatr 2010;22(2):174-187.

[143] Laurin D, Masaki KH, Foley DJ, White LR, Launer LJ. Midlife dietary intake of antioxidants and risk of late-life incident dementia: the Honolulu-Asia Aging Study. Am J Epidemiol 2004;159(10):959-967.

[144] Gray SL, Anderson ML, Crane PK, Breitner JC, McCormick W, Bowen JD, et al. Antioxidant vitamin supplement use and risk of dementia or Alzheimer's disease in older adults. J Am Geriatr Soc 2008;56(2):291-295.

[145] Savva GM, Stephan BC. Epidemiological studies of the effect of stroke on incident dementia: a systematic review. Stroke 2010;41(1):e41-46.

[146] Lu FP, Lin KP, Kuo HK. Diabetes and the risk of multi-system aging phenotypes: a systematic review and meta-analysis. PLoS One 2009;4(1):e4144.

[147] Anstey KJ, Lipnicki DM, Low LF. Cholesterol as a risk factor for dementia and cognitive decline: a systematic review of prospective studies with meta-analysis. Am J Geriatr Psychiatry 2008;16(5):343-354.

[148] Kivipelto M, Solomon A. Cholesterol as a risk factor for Alzheimer's disease - epidemiological evidence. Acta Neurol Scand Suppl 2006;185:50-57.

[149] Anstey KJ, Cherbuin N, Budge M, Young J. Body mass index in midlife and late-life as a risk factor for dementia: a meta-analysis of prospective studies. Obes Rev 2011;12(5):e426-37.

[150] Fratiglionia L, Qiu C. Prevention of cognitive decline in ageing: dementia as the target, delayed onset as the goal. Lancet Neurol 2011;10(9): 819-828.

Chapter 4

Alzheimer's Disease and Diabetes

Brent D. Aulston, Gary L. Odero, Zaid Aboud and
Gordon W. Glazner

Additional information is available at the end of the chapter

1. Introduction

"I have lost myself"

- Auguste Deter, the first patient diagnosed with Alzheimer's Disease, 1906

Identification of Alzheimer's Disease Alois Alzheimer was a German neuropathologist and among the first to identify and describe the hallmarks of what is known today as Alzheimer's disease (AD). In November of 1901, Dr. Alzheimer was presented with 51 year-old Auguste Deter who was suffering from mental incompetence, aphasia, disorientation, paranoia, and unprovoked bursts of anger. Deter's emotional and mental devastation became evident when she confided to Dr. Alzheimer "I have lost myself."

Symptoms similar to Deter's had been observed in patients for years and were considered a natural part of aging. However, it was unusual for such a pointed disease state to occur in someone so young. Over the next four and half years, Deter became increasingly demented, until her death at the age of 55. Upon examination of Deter's brain, Dr. Alzheimer found microscopic strands of protein which he described as "tangled bundles of fibrils" (neurofibrillary tangles) in addition to "miliary foci" (amyloid plaques). In 1906, at the 37th Conference of South-West German Psychiatrists in Tübingen, Alois Alzheimer presented Deter's case as, "a peculiar disease of the cerebral cortex."

To this day both the cause of and treatment for AD remain a mystery. AD is a multifaceted disease of great complexity, however, over 100 years of research has provided clues to its mechanisms. Of particular recent interest is the emerging realization that another rapidly growing disease, type 2 diabetes mellitus (T2DM), is linked to development of AD [1].

This chapter examines the current state of knowledge regarding the association of T2DM to vascular changes in the brain and the implications these changes have in AD development.

Other factors that contribute to AD such as insulin resistance and accumulation of the neurotoxic peptide amyloid beta (Aβ) are also examined. It's likely that no central cause of AD exists but rather, the disease represents a breakdown of several critical components involved in the general health and function of the brain.

Epidemiology of AD and T2DM AD is the most common form of dementia [2] and remains incurable. While the cause of AD remains unknown, several risk factors have been identified that may provide insight into the fundamentals of AD pathogenesis.

T2DM is a known risk factor for AD [1] suggesting that insulin signaling abnormalities play a central role in AD pathology. Moreover, AD brains show decreased insulin levels, decreased activity of insulin receptors and signs of compensatory mechanisms such as increased insulin receptor density [3] indicating AD as "type 3 diabetes" [4, 5].

Loss of insulin signaling in diabetes can occur by either type 1 or type 2 processes. Type 1 diabetes mellitus (T1DM) is characterized as an autoimmune disease that results in the destruction of insulin producing β cells found in the pancreas. In contrast, T2DM is a state of insulin resistance in which insulin levels are normal or elevated but tissues are unresponsive to its effects. While both T1DM and T2DM can lead to cognitive deficits, T2DM poses a greater risk for AD development [6, 7] and as a result the parallels between T2DM and AD are studied more vigorously than T1DM associations. Therefore, the majority of information presented here pertains to type 2 diabetic pathologies.

In addition to insulin resistance, T2DM is associated with the development of vascular dysfunction in the brain [8, 9]. T2DM is a risk factor for microvascular complications as well as macrovascular defects [10] such as stroke [11]. Vascular abnormalities are strongly associated with AD [12-16] implying further involvement of T2DM in disease onset.

2. Type 2 diabetes, vascular changes and Alzheimer's disease

Insulin signaling in the vasculature Activation of the insulin receptor (IR) leads to phosphorylation of insulin receptor substrate (IRS) which serve as docking proteins for phosphatidylinositol 3-kinase (PI3K). PI3K generates phosphatidyl-3,4,5-triphosphate (PIP$_3$) which then phosphorylates 3-phosphoinositide-dependent protein kinase-1 (PDK-1). Finally, PDK-1 phosphorylates Akt and stimulates endothelial nitric oxide synthase (eNOS) resulting in the production of nitric oxide (NO) and vascular relaxation [17, 18]. Interestingly, insulin receptor activation can also mediate vasoconstriction. Activation of IR can also lead to phosphorylation of Shc which then binds Grb-2 resulting in activation of Sos. This complex then activates Ras leading to phosphorylation Raf which results in activation of MAPK. Activation of MAPK stimulates release of endothelin-1 (ET-1), a vasoconstrictor [19-21]. By mediating vascular properties, insulin signaling plays a significant role in glucose and oxygen availability to the brain. Conversely, dysfunction in insulin signaling, as observed in T2DM, has profound detrimental effects on hemodynamics and, thus, maintenance of normative brain function.

Vascular complications associated with type 2 diabetes It is estimated that approximately 200 million people worldwide have diabetes and by 2025 the number is expected to increase to 333 million [22]. Epidemiological studies have indicated that patients with T2DM have a greater incidence of cardiovascular disease, cerebrovascular disease (CVD), hypertension and renal disease relative to the general population [8, 9]. In addition, a large number of population-based studies have identified diabetes as a risk factor for dementia [23-25], primarily as a result of CVD [26, 27]. At only 3% of body weight, the brain uses ~20% of the body's oxygen and ~25% of the body's blood glucose [28, 29], demonstrating that it is by far the most metabolically active organ. This oxygen and glucose consumption is constantly required, since brain neurons are obligate aerobic cells and have no other source of energy. The majority of this energy is used to maintain cellular ionic homeostasis, and thus when cerebral blood flow (CBF) ceases, brain function ends within seconds and damage to neurons occurs within minutes [30].

The vascular complications associated with diabetes can be divided into two classes based on the vascular etiology of their pathology: macrovascular (hypertension, coronary artery disease, atherosclerosis, stroke) and microvascular (neuropathy, retinopathy, nephropathy). Macrovascular complications are those that affect the larger (non-capillary) blood vessels. Statistics show that diabetes increases the risk of stroke and atherosclerosis [31]. Atherosclerosis accounts for 70% of morbidity associated with T2DM [32], while other studies have shown an association between the degree of hyperglycemia and increased risk of myocardial infarction and stroke [33-36]. While macrovascular complications themselves represent important pathological consequences of T2DM, they have also been shown to provide the etiological link between T2DM and the development of Alzheimer's disease.

Link between type 2 diabetes and Alzheimer's disease AD is an age-related disorder characterized by progressive cognitive decline and dementia. An estimated 5.3 million people in the United States are currently affected and represents the sixth-leading cause of death. Significant evidence has been provided that links T2DM to AD. For example, a comprehensive meta-analysis showed that the aggregate relative risk of AD for people with diabetes was 1.5 (95%-CI 1.2 to 1.8) [37]. Studies have shown that T2DM, impaired fasting glucose and increased islet amyloid deposition are more common in patients with Alzheimer's disease than in control subjects [38, 39]. Unsurprisingly, insulin signaling provides an important mechanistic link between T2DM and AD.

Ischemic CVD caused by T2DM is positively associated with AD through shared pathological mechanisms such as hyperinsulinemia, impaired insulin signaling, oxidative stress, inflammatory mechanisms and advanced glycation end-products (AGEs) [40]. Defective insulin signaling is associated with decreased cognitive ability and development of dementa, including AD [41], rendering signaling neurons more vulnerable to metabolic stress and accelerating neuronal dysfunction [42]. In vitro insulin-stimulated Akt phosphorylation is decreased in hyperinsulinemic conditions in cortical neurons [43]. Finally, all forms of amyloid beta (Aβ) (monomers, oligomers and Aβ-derived diffusible ligands (ADDLs)) can inhibit insulin signaling by directly binding to the insulin receptor and inhibit insulin signaling [44].

Mechanisms of macrovascular complications of diabetes A central pathological mechanism in diabetic-related macrovascular disease is atherosclerosis, which leads to the hardening of arterial walls throughout the body resulting in impaired blood flow. Although the mechanism for the susceptibility of diabetic patients to ischemic heart disease remains unclear, accumulating lines of evidence implicate hyperglycemia, hyperlipidemia and inflammation as playing key roles in the development of this disorder [45]. This link between obesity and both T2DM and atherosclerosis implicates elevated amounts of glucose oxidized LDL and free fatty acids (FFAs) in disease pathogenesis, potentially as triggers for the production of pro-inflammatory cytokines by macrophages [32].

In the insulin resistant state, there is a specific impairment in the vasodilatory PI3K pathway, whereas the Ras/MAPK-dependent pathway is unaffected [46, 47]. This results in decreased production of NO and an increased secretion of ET-1 in humans [48] leading to increased vasoconstriction. The decrease in NO production is significant in that NO protects blood vessels from endogenous injury by mediating molecular signals that prevent platelet and leukocyte interaction with the vascular wall and inhibit vascular smooth muscle cell proliferation and migration [49, 50]. Decreased production of NO allows for increased expression of proinflammatory transcription factor NF-κB, and subsequent expression of leukocyte adhesion molecules and production of chemokines and cytokines [51]. Activation of these proteins promote monocyte and vascular smooth muscle cell migration into the intima and formation of macrophage foam cells, initiating the morphological changes associated with the onset of atherosclerosis [52, 53].

High levels of FFAs are found in insulin-resistant individuals. FFAs generated by increased activity of hormone-sensitive lipase that contribute to and result in insulin resistance [54-56]. In vitro vascular endothelial cell culture treated with FFA resulted in decreased insulin-stimulated eNOS activity and NO production [57]. It is believed that FFA increases cellular levels of diacylglycerols, ceramide, and long-chain fatty acyl coenzyme A (CoA), all of which have been shown to activate protein kinase C (PKCβ1). Activation of PKCβ1 results in increased phosphorylation of IRS-1 that leads to reduced Akt and eNOS resulting in decreased vasodilatory capacity [58, 59]. Increase in FFAs result in an increase in reactive oxygen species (ROS) from NADPH and the mitochondrial electron transport chain [60]. The increase in ROS results in increased PKC which activates the hexosamine biosynthetic pathway leading to increased AGEs and subsequent decrease in endothelial-derived NO [60]. Hyperglycemia has been found to decrease activation of Akt and eNOS via O-GlcNAC of eNOS at the Akt phosphorylation sites [61, 62]. Hyperglycemia increases activation of PKCα, PKCβ, PKCδ resulting in decreased eNOS and concomitant increase in endothelial ET-1 [60]. T2DM is associated with vascular dysfunction as a result of increased atherosclerosis and decreased cerebral blood flow. The combination of both processes is decreased glucose and oxygen supply to vital organs such as the brain. The biochemical events leading to the macrovascular impairment has particular significance to brain health as the risk of stroke is a major complication of T2DM.

Type 2 diabetes and cardiovascular disease T2DM has been shown to be associated with an increased risk of coronary heart disease and stroke [63-66]. Insulin resistance, the mechanism underlying T2DM, has also been linked to a higher incidence and recurrence of stroke [67]. Two key pathological mediators of stroke observed in T2DM are intracranial stenosis [68] and

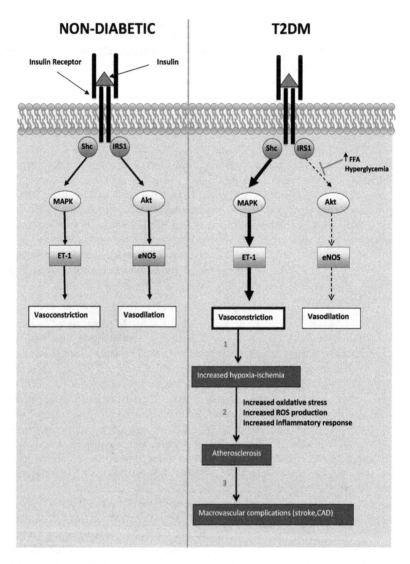

Figure 1. Pathways leading to macrovascular complications of type 2 diabetes mellitus (T2DM). In non-diabetic individuals (*left*), activation of the insulin receptor can result in activation of both vasodilatation and vasoconstriction. Under normative conditions, there is a balance of both processes to regulate the immediate metabolic requirements of various tissues. In type 2 diabetic patients (*right*), factors such as an increase in free fatty acids and hyperglycemia have been shown to specifically inhibit the Akt pathway while the MAPK pathway remains unaffected. This leads to an imbalance in homeostatic regulation of vascular function and hemodynamics (*1*). The resultant decrease in nutrient availability to affected tissues results in an increase in oxidative stress and ROS production and an increased inflammatory response (*2*). Released pro-inflammatory cytokines and macrophage recruitment instigates the onset of atherosclerosis, ultimately leading to macrovascular complications (*3*).

carotid atherosclerosis [69]. Insulin resistance has been associated with elevated expression of the fibrinolytic inhibitor plasminogen activator inhibitor 1 [70] resulting in decreased fibrinoyltic capacity and concurrent increased thrombosis due, in part, to an increase in platelet activation [71]. Insulin resistance has also been shown to induce endothelial dysfunction and inflammation [71], adversely affecting vascular function and initiating atherosclerosis, respectively. Collectively, these data implicate insulin resistance to the impairment of normative cerebrovascular function resulting in the activation of pathways that encourage the onset of stroke. Stroke could, in turn, exacerbate and/or initiate the onset of another disorder such as AD.

Pre-existing CVD has been identified as a significant risk factor for AD. The vascular hypothesis of AD posits that vascular dysfunction, such as stroke, is a pre-requisite for the development of this disorder. It has been reported that the risk of AD is three times greater after the occurrence of stroke [72]. Stroke may result in neurodegeneration [73, 74], resulting in the rapid cognitive decline observed in AD patients [75]. It has even been proposed that stroke may be the underlying cause of 50% of AD cases [74]. Conversely, individuals presenting with severe cognitive impairments, and possibly AD, may be at a greater risk for the development of stroke or CVD [76, 77].

The amyloid hypothesis of AD was long held as the prevailing theory explaining the etiology of AD. However, emerging evidence compiled from the last 20 years has suggested that the pathology associated with AD is vascular in origin. The vascular hypothesis of AD states that pre-existing cardiovascular dysfunction such as stroke, hypertension and atherosclerosis results in chronic cerebral hypoperfusion that could encourage the onset of AD. Several lines of evidence have been provided in support of this hypothesis. For example, it has been shown that cerebrovascular dysfunction precedes cognitive decline and the onset of neurodegenerative changes in AD and AD animal models [12, 13]. In rhesus monkeys, dystrophic axons labeled with amyloidogenic enzyme, BACE1, were found in close proximity or in direct contact with cortical blood vessels [78], asserting a tight association with AD pathology and vascular dysfunction. Clinical and epidemiological evidence provides further support of the vascular hypothesis.

AD patients show a greater degree of vascular narrowing of carotid arteries [65] and cerebral arteries of the Circle of Willis [79, 80]. In addition, large artery CVD was positively correlated to the frequency of neuritic plaques [81]. Several vascular risk factors such stroke (silent infarcts, transient ischemic attacks), atherosclerosis, hypertension, heart disease (coronary artery disease, atrial fibrillation) and diabetes mellitus have been associated with an increased risk AD-type dementia [82]. Between 60 to 90% of AD patients exhibit various cerebrovascular pathologies including White matter lesions, cerebral amyloid angiopathy (CAA), microinfarcts, small infarcts, hemorrhages and microvascular degeneration [12-16]. It believed that cardiovascular dysfunctions act as a nidus for accelerated Aβ deposition resulting in the onset of AD [83].

Aberrant blood brain barrier (BBB) function exposes neurons to neurotoxic substances. Chronic cerebral hypoperfusion is believed to render the brain more vulnerable to various insults, resulting in AD and associated cognitive loss [84]. Clinical observations in AD patients have revealed extensive degeneration of endothelium [85] and features indicative of BBB breakdown [86]. At the cellular level, AD is known to cause abnormal structural changes to arterioles and capillaries, swelling and increased number of pinocytotic vesciles in endothelial cells, decreased mitochondrial content, increased deposition of proteins of the basement membrane, reduced microvascular density and occasional swelling of astrocyte endfeet [87-92]. Aβ trafficking across the BBB deposition is also dependent on mechanisms of influx and efflux. Increased expression of receptor for advanced glycation endproducts (RAGE) may be responsible for Aβ influx from the blood to the brain has been reported in addition to a decrease in LRP1 receptors that are responsible for clearing Aβ from the brain to the blood [12, 93].

A functional consequence associated with BBB dysfunction is the resultant impairment in cerebral hemodynamics. AD impairs autoregulation, the mechanism that is responsible for the stabilization of blood flow to the brain in response to changes in cerebral perfusion pressure [94]. In an APP x PS1 mouse model neurovascular coupling, the process in which activation of a brain region evokes a local increase in blood flow, was impaired [95]. Finally, AD has shown to adversely affect vasomotor/vascular reactivity, the process that mediates vasodilatory or vasoconstrictor responses of cerebral blood vessels to hypercapnic or hypocapnic stimuli (ie. global or regional brain blood flow response to systemic changes in arterial CO_2) [96-98]. Cumulatively, the impairment of these processes adversely affects cerebral blood regulation that, in turn, would negatively affect nutrient availability to neurons. This would result in cerebral hypoperfusion, a process that is widely believed to initiate the onset of AD pathology.

There are a number of known direct links between biochemical pathways central to AD and hypoxia/ischemia. A rat model for vascular cognitive impairment has been developed referred to as the two-vessel occlusion model of cerebral ischemia. Studies found decreased cerebral blood flow up to 4 weeks, cognitive deficits, APP proteolysis to form Aβ-sized fragments [99-101]. Other studies have observed an overexpression of Aβ persisting for up to 3 months after surgery [102] and cognitive impairment [103], strongly suggesting that decreased CBF is a key mediator in the pathophysiology of AD. Several studies have been able to identify some of the molecular mechanisms as to how hypoxia/ischemia exerts its effects on AD-related genes.

APP expression increases following chronic cerebral hypoperfusion and ischemia [104, 105], and a greater proportion of APP is proteolytically cleaved by increased activity of amyloidogenic enzyme, BACE1, which is concurrently increased in AD following ischemic events [106]. Hypoxia inducible factor-1α (HIF-1α) plays an essential role in cellular and systemic responses to low oxygen and has been found to increase BACE1 mRNA expression [107]. Furthermore, BACE1 stabilization is enhanced in AD in addition to a decrease in its trafficking [108, 109]. Increased BACE results in greater γ-secretase-mediated production of Aβ [110]. In an APP overexpressing mouse model, chronic cerebral hypoperfusion as the result of cerebral amyloid angiopathy (pathological deposition of $Aβ_{1-40}$ in brain blood vessels) was followed by an increased rate of leptomeningeal Aβ precipitating the risk of microinfarcts [111]. Hypoxia/

ischemia not only causes increased amyloidogenic cleavage of APP and greater Aβ production, but also impairs Aβ degradation and trafficking [12, 112].

Decreased Aβ-degrading enzymes in response to hypoxic conditions increase the likelihood of developing pathological levels of Aβ in the brain [113-115]. Aβ serves not only as the end result of a pathological cascade, but Aβ itself has been found to contribute to dysfunction in components of the neurovascular unit. In endothelial cells Aβ was observed to decrease endothelial cell proliferation and accelerate senescence of endothelial cells in vivo and in vitro, inhibit VEGF-induced activation of Akt and eNOS in endothelial cells [116, 117]. Aβ has been found to decrease eNOS (via PKC-dependent pathway) resulting in decreased vascular tonus and decreased substance P-induced vasodilation of the basilar artery[118, 119]. In vascular smooth muscle cells (VSMCs), Aβ affects cellular morphological changes [120] and increases expression of transcription factors, serum response factor and myocardin, resulting in decreased Aβ clearance by downregulating LRP expression [12]. Finally, Aβ has been shown to cause retraction and swelling of astrocyte endfeet in an AD mouse model with CAA [121] as well as increase cholinergic denervation of cortical microvessels which, taken together, results in impaired functional hyperemia [122].

Type 2 diabetes and vascular dementia A significant number of population-based studies have indicated an increased risk for the development of dementia attributed to T2DM [23-25]. Due to the importance of insulin in the regulation of several cardiovascular functions, it is unsurprising that insulin resistance plays a role in the cerebrovascular mechanisms of T2DM-induced dementia. The presence of brain infarcts in demented diabetics who did not have AD has been reported 123. Interestingly, the association between T2DM and the development of AD and VaD has been found to be independent of hypertension and hypercholesterolemia [23] indicating that is CVD alone is not sufficient to initiate dementia. Non-cerebrovascular mechanisms such as peripheral hyperinsulinemia and generation of advanced glycation end-products also play in the etiology of T2DM-related dementia [124]. Studies have shown that the increased risk of developing vascular dementia was greater than developing AD in type 2 diabetics [7, 125, 126], indicating that although symptomatically similar and frequently confused [127], their etiologies are distinct.

Vascular dementia versus Alzheimer's dementia The leading cause of dementia is Alzheimer's disease accounting for 70-90% of all cases [127], while vascular dementia (VaD) accounts for the majority of the remaining incidents of dementia [128]. They share common risk factors including hypertension, diabetes mellitus, and hyperlipidemia. [129], highlighting the tight association between these two forms of dementia. In fact, it is now widely believed that AD and VaD are frequently present in the same brain. So-called "mixed dementia" has been observed in elderly people with cardiovascular risk factors in addition to slow progressive cognitive decline [130].

Differing clinical manifestations separate VaD from AD dementia. For example, VaD progression appears more varied than AD in relation to symptoms, its rate of progression and the disease outcome [131]. Increased damage to the ganglia-thalamo-cortical circuits specific to VaD results in problems with attention and the planning and speed of mental processing whereas the primary impairments characteristic of AD are memory and language-related

[132]. It has been suggested that differences in the clinical observations in AD and VaD patients may be due to the type, severity and location of vascular damage [133-135]. Furthermore, perturbations in vascular hemodynamics have been observed in VaD and AD [136, 137], however, AD patients had comparatively less impairment in cerebral perfusion than those with VaD [138] suggesting that hemodynamic disturbances may underlie different types of dementia [138]. While the precise mechanism that vascular risk factors initiate cognitive decline remains elusive [139], T2DM have been identified as an important contributing factor to the development of VaD.

Associations between vascular dementia and Alzheimer's dementia While regarded as two separate conditions, AD and VaD share common cerebrovascular pathologies such as CAA, endothelial cell and vascular smooth muscle cell degeneration, macro- and microinfarcts, hemorrhage and white matter changes [140-142]. These shared pathologies have been shown epidemiologically with almost 35% of AD patients showing evidence of cerebral infarction at autopsy [143, 144], and, conversely, VaD patients display AD-like pathology in the absence of pre-existing AD [145]. It has been postulated that CVD, thought to be the etiology of both disorders, not only result in dementia but also increase the likelihood of individuals with AD-related lesions for developing dementia [146, 147].

3. Insulin signaling in the brain

Insulin/IGF-1 pathway activation. The brain is a major metabolic organ that accounts for ~25% of the body's total glucose use [28, 29]. While glucose uptake in peripheral tissues requires insulin, in the brain this is considered to be an insulin-independent process. Insulin, however, along with Insulin-like Growth Factor-1 (IGF-1), are required for proper brain function as they provide critical neurotrophic support for neurons. IGF-1 and insulin share similar amino acid sequences/ tertiary structures [148] and are known to bind to and activate one anothers' receptors [149]. Both insulin and IGF-1 receptors are tyrosine kinases [150-152] that, when activated, phosphorylate substrate proteins such as IRS. IRS phosphorylation leads to down-stream activation of PI3K and Akt, a serine/threonine kinase and key mediator of insulin/ IFG-1's neurotrophic effects. Neuronal processes known to be, at least in part, under the control of insulin/IGF-1 include regulation of apoptotic proteins, transcription of both survival and pro-death genes, neurite outgrowth, and activity of metabolic proteins.

The source of brain insulin remains controversial. While preproinsulin mRNA has been reported in the neurons [153-155], very little insulin is synthesized in the brain [156]. Additionally, glial cells have been found not to be involved in insulin production [157], therefore, it is recognized that the majority of insulin in the brain is produced by pancreatic β cells [158-161]. In contrast, IGF-1 is produced locally in the brain and does not depend on growth hormone influence as is the case of liver and other tissues [148].

Neuronal insulin receptors are different than those found in the periphery [162]. Insulin receptors are present in one of two isoforms; the IR-A isoform that lacks exon 11 that the other isoform, IR-B, expresses [163, 164]. A major functional difference between the two isoforms is that IR-A has a higher affinity for the neurotrophic factor Insulin-like Growth Factor – 2 (IGF-II) [165] and a slightly higher affinity for insulin [166] and has also been shown to associate/dissociate with insulin quicker than IR-B [149]. Brain specific insulin receptors are mainly the IR-A isoform and as result of differential glycosylation have a lower molecular weight than their peripheral counterparts [162].

Structurally, the insulin receptor is a homodimer composed 2α chains and 2β chains held together with disulphide bonds [167-169]. Insulin receptor binding of insulin/IGF-1 results in a conformational change that activates the catalytic tyrosine kinase activity of the β subunits [170]. This activation of the insulin receptor results in autophosphorylation at multiple tyrosine residues [171, 172] including tyrosine 960 in the juxtamembrane region of the β subunit [173, 174]. Phosphorylation at this site is a vital component of the insulin signaling cascade because it provides a binding motif for the phospho-tyrosine binding (PTB) domain of IRS [173, 174]. Once docked to the insulin receptor, IRS is phosphorylated on tyrosine residues [170].

Tyrosine phosphorylation of IRS proteins creates binding sites for Src homology 2 (SH2) domain containing proteins such as PI3K [175]. PI3K catalyzes the production of 3'phosphoinositide secondary messengers which are critical to the insulin signaling cascade. PI3K is composed of a catalytic p110 subunit and a regulatory p85 subunit that contains SH2 domains that interact with activated IRS [176]. Formation of the IRS/PI3K complex increases the catalytic activity of the p110 subunit [177].

3'phosphoinositides produced by PI3K are important signal conductors that bind to PH (pleckstrin homology) domains on proteins such as IRS [177] and Akt [178]. This interaction is needed to bring IRS and AKT proteins towards the inner layer of the plasma membrane near the juxtamembrane region of the insulin receptor [179] and in close proximity to activating kinases, respectively [180-185]. Furthermore, binding of 3'phosphoinositides is required for Akt to be competent for phosphorylation [184, 186-188].

Akt has two phosphorylation sites, Thr 308 and Ser 473, capable of inducing catalytic activity [189]. PDK1, which also depends on 3'phosphoinosites for its function, phosphorylates Akt at Thr 308 [189, 190].While overexpression of PDK1 has been shown to activate Akt [186], optimal activation of Akt requires additional phosphorylation at Ser 473 by mTORC2 [191] which stabilizes the conformation state of Akt [192].

Akt mediates the neurotrophic effects of insulin/IGF-1, in part, by inhibiting pro-apoptotic machinery [193] and concomitantly activating anti-apoptotic proteins [194-198]. Akt's role in neurotrophic support also involves the regulation of survival transcription factors such as NF-κB [199] and CREB [198] as well as those involved in pro-death gene expression such as the FoxO family [200-202]. Moreover, Akt is involved in production of the neurotrophin BDNF [198], activation of proteins involved in neurite outgrowth (for review see: [203]) and regulation of the metabolic protein GSK-3β [204].

Akt and Bcl-2 family members The Bcl-2 family is a structurally related group of proteins that regulate cell death through effects on the mitochondria [205] (for review see [206, 207]). Bcl-2 members include the pro-apoptotic proteins BID, BIM, PUMA, BAD, NOXA, BAX, and BAK [205] along with anti-apoptotic mediators such as Bcl-2 and Bcl-xL [205]. Because Bcl-2 proteins possess the ability to form heterodimers with one another [208-210], their regulation of apoptosis can be described as a balancing act in which an increase of anti-apoptotic members leads to survival while increased pro-death proteins result in apoptosis.

Mitochondrial stress incurred by ROS can lead to elevated Ca^{2+} levels in the mitochondrial matrix [211, 212] resulting in increased mitochondrial membrane permeability and release of pro-apoptotic factors such as Cytochrome c, and AIF (apoptosis inducing factor) [213]. Bcl-xL is an anti-apoptotic Bcl-2 family member that prevents Ca^{2+} induced mitochondrial permeability [214]. In the absence of insulin/IGF-1 stimulation, the survival effects of Bcl-xL are blocked as Bcl-xL is complexed with the pro-death Bcl-2 family member Bad [215-217]. Akt liberates Bcl-xL by phosphorylating Bad [195-197, 218] allowing for mitochondrial stabilization.

Mitochondrial permeability marks a critical event in the cell death cascade. Akt promotes cell survival prior to Cytochrome c release through Bcl-xL activity but has also been found to act post apoptotic factor release. When Cytochrome c is released from the mitochondria, it will associate with Apaf-1, dATP and Caspase-9 forming a structure known as the apoptosome (For review see [219]). Formation of the apoptosome activates the proteolytic activity of caspase-9 which cleaves and activates other caspases critical to the apoptotic process [220, 221]. Akt blocks apoptosome formation by phosphorylating Caspase 9 [193].

Bcl-2 is another anti-apoptotic protein under the control of Akt [222]. Bcl-2's role in cell survival is similar to that of Bcl-xL in that in maintains mitochondrial membrane integrity [223]. Mitochondrial permeability has been linked to an oxidized shift in the mitochondria [224] while Bcl-2 has been shown to promote a more reduced state [225]. Upregulation of Bcl-2 may lead to higher cell reductive capacity [224] which is supported by the observation that Bcl-2 overexpressing cells show increased amounts of NADPH and are resistant to ROS generation [226].

The Bcl-2 promoter contains a cAMP response element site (CRE) that can enhance Bcl-2 expression by binding the transcription factor CREB. Akt is known to phosphorylate CREB which results in increased CREB binding to CBP and increased transcriptional activity [198]. Therefore, the ability of Akt to promote cell survival is mediated, in part, by influence over gene expression such as the up-regulation of Bcl-2 [227-230] and through direct protein interactions such as Bad phosphorylation resulting in Bcl-xL liberation [194-197].

Akt and transcription factor regulation Also under CREB transcriptional control is the neurotrophic factor BDNF [231, 232] which is essential for neuronal development, differentiation, synaptic plasticity, neuroprotection and restoration against a broad range of cellular insults [233]. BDNF has been a focus of AD research for its ability to stimulate non-amyloidogenic APP processing pathways [234, 235] in addition to protecting neuronal cultures against the cytotoxic effects of Aβ [236]. This indicates that decreased insulin signaling resulting in reduced BDNF production may be a contributing factor in AD development. In accordance, AD patients have decreased serum BDNF concentrations compared to healthy, elderly subjects [237-241] while reduced BDNF levels were associated with decreased cognitive performance in healthy individuals [242].

The transcription factor NF-κB is also under Akt control [199]. Like CREB, NF-κB plays critical roles in neuron survival [201, 243, 244] and is also involved in neurite outgrowth, myelin formation and axonal regeneration [245]. Genes for antioxidant proteins such as MnSOD [246] and Cu/ZnSOD [247] and anti-apoptotic proteins Bcl-2 and Bcl-xL are targets of NF-κB [248].

In its inactive form, NF-κB is bound to IκB proteins that sequester it to the cytosol (for review see [249, 250]). NF-κB is activated when IκB proteins are phosphorylated by IκB Kinase (IKK) complexes and targeted for degradation which allows NF-κB to translocate to the nucleus where it binds to regulatory DNA sequences [251]. The IKK complex consists of catalytic IKKα and IKKβ subunits and a regulatory IKKγ subunit [251]. Akt facilitates NF-κB activation by phosphorylating IKKα at a critical regulatory site that promotes IKK activation [252] and subsequent IκB degradation.

Akt influence is not limited to only survival transcription factors but extends to pro-death modulators as well [253, 254].The forkhead box class O (FoxO) family of transcription factors contribute to apoptosis through the induction of pro-death genes such as Fas L [201, 255, 256] and the Bcl-2 member BIM-1 [257]. Fas L facilitates apoptosis by activation of caspases [258] while BIM-1 activates the pro-apoptotic Bcl-2 family memeber BAX [259]. In the absence of Akt, FoxO transcription factors are transcriptionally active in the nucleus [200-202]. Akt phosphorylates FoxO family members at a conserved c-terminal sequence [253] which leads to nuclear exclusion and inhibition of transcriptional activity.

p53,another pro-death transcription factor known to be inactivated by Akt, [260] induces the expression of the pro-apoptotic Bcl-2 family member BAX. BAX proteins form oligomers that insert into the outer mitochondrial membrane which provide a passageway for Cytochrome c and other pro-apoptotic proteins to escape through [261]. Increased p53 activity leading to BAX expression has been linked to neuronal deprivation of neurotrophic factors [262].

Akt and neurite outgrowth Akt effects extend beyond apoptosis regulation as Akt also contributes to neurite outgrowth (for review see [203]). In hippocampal neurons Akt enhances characteristics such as dendritic length/complexity, caliber, and branching [263-267] with similar effects, excluding dendritic length, observed in dorsal root ganglia neurons [268-271]. Akt substrates implicated in neurite outgrowth include GSK-3β [272, 273], CREB [198], mTOR [274], peripherin [275], and β-catenin [276]. Akt may also work in conjunction with other pathways involved in neurite outgrowth. For example, Akt has been found to be complexed with Hsp-27 (heat shock protein) in spinal motor neurons following nerve injury [277] as well as in areas of regeneration following sciatic nerve axotomy [278].

Akt and GSK-3β Activity of the metabolic protein GSK-3β is also influenced by Akt. GSK-3β was originally identified for decreasing glycogen production through inhibition of glycogen synthase [272, 279-281]. However, GSK-3β is also involved in protein synthesis, cell proliferation/differentiation, microtubule dynamics, cell motility and apoptosis. Of particular interest, GSK-3β has also been shown to phosphorylate cytoskeletal associated tau proteins [282] which, in a diseased state, result in protein aggregates known as neurofibrillary tangles [283]. Neurofibrillary tangles have been linked to increased oxidative stress, mitochondrial dysfunction and apoptosis [284, 285] and are the most significant structural correlates of dementia in AD [286, 287]. IGF-1 protects neurons from ischemic damage by reducing GSK-3β activity [288] which implies a critical role of Akt in GSK- 3β regulation. Indeed, Akt has been shown to inhibit GSK-3β [204] thus demonstrating a direct role of insulin/IGF-1 signaling in the prevention of AD pathology.

Loss of insulin signaling While not a cause of death on its own, loss of insulin signaling in the brain leaves neurons vulnerable to a myriad of insults. Insulin signaling is known to protect against oxidative stress, mitochondrial collapse, over-activity of GSK-3β leading to hyperphosphorylation of tau, activation of death promoting transcription factors and forma-tion of apoptotic structures. Insulin also results in increased BDNF neurotrophic support as well as increased neurite outgrowth.

The mitochondrial permeability transition mediates apoptosis through the release of pro apoptotic factors. Insulin signaling maintains mitochondrial membrane integrity by increas-ing levels and activity of anti-apoptotic Bcl-2 family members [194-197, 227-230]. In the ab-sence of insulin signaling, the balance of Bcl-2 proteins tips in favor of pro-apoptotic members resulting in cell death. Post mitochondrial collapse, normal insulin signaling can still prevent apoptosis by blocking formation of apoptotic complexes [193, 229] while a state of insulin resistance allows this process to continue unimpeded.

Even under normal circumstances, ROS are produced in respiratory chain reactions in the mitochondria [289]. However, if not properly managed, ROS can cause oxidative damage to proteins, lipids, and nucleic acids. Insulin supplies cells with antioxidant proteins capable of diffusing the oxidative effects of ROS by activating protective transcription factors such as NF-κB [246, 247, 263]. Insulin resistance not only results in reduced antioxidants but also leaves cells susceptible to ROS mediated mitochondrial collapse because of the before men-tioned lack of anti-apoptotic Bcl-2 members.

The FoxO family of transcription factors is known to play a role in the cell's response to oxi-dative stress, however, their prolonged activation results in apoptosis [290]. Insulin signal-ing inactivates FoxO transcription factors through phosphorylation by Akt. Absence of insulin signaling allows FoxO members to remain in the nucleus and sustain transcription of pro-death genes [201, 255-257].

Insulin resistance is linked to structural changes in AD by overactive GSK-3β. Neurofibril-lary tangles are a pathological hallmark of AD [283] and produced by hyperphosphorylation of tau by GSK-3β. Under normal insulin signaling, GSK-3β is inactivated by Akt. Neurofi-brillary tangles are one of two significant pathological characteristics of AD the other being accumulation of Aβ [291]. Aβ toxicity and aggregation into plaques has devastating conse-quences in the brain such as synaptic disruption [292] and inhibition of LTP [293], interfer-ence of detoxifying enzymes [294], increased ROS and oxidative stress [295], increased vulnerability to calcium overload [296] and the before mentioned effects on brain vascula-ture. Aβ also depresses insulin signaling [297] which results in further loss of neurotrophic support. Insulin signaling, on the other, hand is involved in Aβ clearance [298] introducing a convoluted relationship between insulin and Aβ.

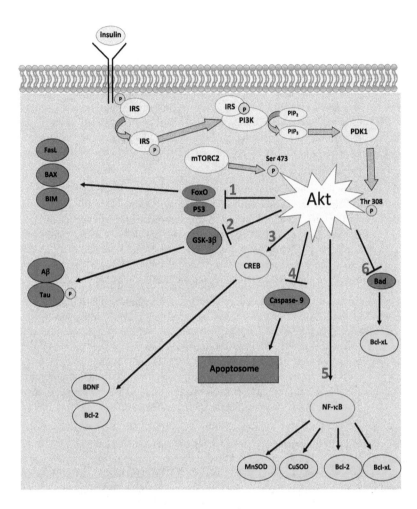

Figure 2. Insulin receptor binding of insulin triggers a complex signaling cascade (in blue) leading to activation of the serine/threonine kinase Akt. Upon binding of insulin, insulin receptors are autophophorylated and subsequently bind IRS proteins. IRS proteins are then phsophorylated by activated insulin receptors and complex with PI3K resulting in PI3K activation. Activated PI3K produces phospholipid secondary messengers by catalyzing the conversion of phosphatidylinositol 4,5-bisphosphate (PIP$_2$) to phosphatidylinositol 3,4,5-trisphosphate (PIP$_3$). PIP$_3$ messengers activate PDK1 which phosphorylates Akt at Threonine 308. Akt is further activated by phosphorylation at Ser 473 by mammalian target of rapamyicin 2 (mTORC2). Targets of activated Akt include pro-apoptotic mediators (in red) as well as pro-survival machinery (in green). Loss of insulin signaling (at sites labeled with numbers 1-6 in purple) allows FoxO and p53 transcription factors to remain active and (1) transcribe genes for pro-apoptotic proteins such as BIM, BAX and FasL. Akt inhibits the activity of GSK-3β that, when active, (2) causes increased amyloidogenic processing and hyperphosphorylation of tau. Other pro-apoptotic proteins inhibited by Akt include (3) caspase-9, which forms an apoptotic structure known as the apoptosome, and (6) Bad, which blocks activity of the ant-apoptotic protein Bcl-xL. Pro-survival modulators regulated by Akt include CREB and NF-κB. Reduction of CREB transcriptional activity as a result of a loss of insulin signaling leads to (4) decreased BDNF and Bcl-2 expression while inhibition of NF-κB leads to (5) reduced expression of anti-oxidants such as MnSOD and CuSOD as well as anti-apoptotic Bcl-2 family members.

4. Generation of Aβ

Background Aβ is a small peptide 38-43 amino acids in size long believed to have a major role in neurodegeneration and pathology of AD (for review see [299]). In sporadic AD (sAD), which accounts for over 90% of AD cases, Aβ's role in pathogensis is still under heavy investigation. The cause of familial AD (fAD), however, has been linked to 3 mutations involved in Aβ processing; presinilins 1 and 2 (PS1/PS2), which are part of Aβ producing complexes, and amyloid precursor protein (APP) from which Aβ is derived [300]. Successive cleavages of APP by β- and γ-secretases produce toxic Aβ peptides (for review see [301]) while cleavage by α-secretase produces the neuroprotective product Secreted APP alpha (sAPPα) [302].

While the physiological role of APP remains unknown, it has been suggested that APP plays a part in neurite outgrowth, synaptogenesis, neuronal trafficking along the axon, transmembrane signal transduction, cell adhesion and calcium metabolism, all of which still require in vivo evidence (for review see [303]). APP concentrations are elevated in the brain during the prenatal period in mice which implies a role of APP in brain development [304]. In the adult brain, APP is expressed in regions of synaptic modification [304] and has been shown to increase hippocampal neuronal response to glutamate [305].

APP belongs to a family of transmembrane proteins that includes APP-like protein 1 and 2 (APPLP1/APPLP2). All APP family members are processed in a similar fashion by α, β, and γ secretases [306-308], however the Aβ domain is unique to APP. Three isoforms of APP have been identified consisting of 695, 751, or 770 amino acids which arise from alternative splicing of the same gene located on chromosome 21 [309]. APP 751 and APP 770 are expressed in most tissues and contain a 56 amino acid Kunitz Protease inhibitor (KPI) domain not found in the neuron specific 695 isoform [310, 311]. mRNA levels of the 2 KPI containing isoforms are elevated in AD brains and are associated with Aβ deposition [312].

Synthesis of APP occurs in the endoplasmic reticulum where it is then transported through the golgi apparatus to the trans golgi network where the highest concentrations of APP are found in neurons [313-315]. From there, APP can be transported in secretory vesicles to the cell surface where α-secretases are located, however, Aβ production occurs within the trans golgi network where γ-secretase complexes are thought to reside [315-318].

APP cleavage Aβ generation requires cleavage of APP by β-secretase which has been indentified to be BACE1 [319-322]. Several studies have found that regions of the brain affected by AD have elevated BACE1 activity and levels [319, 320]. Once identified, BACE1 became a popular therapeutic target for AD treatment. However, BACE1 knockout mice have shown reduced survivability after birth and were smaller than wild-type littermates [323]. BACE1 knockouts also present with hyperactive behavior [323] and other abnormalities such as hypomyelination of peripheral nerves, reduced grip strength and elevated pain sensitivity [324].

APP cleavage by BACE1 results in two fragments: sAPPβ and Beta Carboxyl Terminal Fragment (βCTF) [301, 325]. sAPPβ has been identified as a ligand for Death Receptor 6 which mediates axonal pruning and neuronal death [326]. The remaining βCTF can be cleaved by γ secretase to produce Aβ [301]. γ-secretase is a complex composed of at least 4 components: PS1 or PS2, nicastrin, anterior pharynx defective-1 (APH-1) and presenilin enhancer-2 (PEN-2) [327, 328]. βCTF cleavage by γ secretase produces either $A\beta_{40}$ or $A\beta_{42}$ peptides [301]. $A\beta_{42}$ is the more hydrophic and amyloidogenic of the 2 species and makes up about 10% of Aβ produced [329]. An increased $A\beta_{42}/A\beta_{40}$ ratio has consistently been shown in fAD patients suggesting that $A\beta_{42}$ is critical to AD pathogensis [330, 331].

5. Aβ and insulin resistance

Aβ depresses insulin signaling Insulin resistance is recognized as a contributing factor in development of AD to the point that AD has been referred to as "type 3 diabetes" [4, 5]. This coincides with Aβ being a pathological hallmark of AD as Aβ contributes to insulin resistance [297]. Aβ oligomers are known impair insulin signaling in neurons [332] by competing with insulin for receptor binding sites [297] and studies have linked Aβ oligomers to decreased insulin receptor numbers [332].

Development of insulin resistance provides neurons with a dangerous dilemma as neurons rely on insulin signaling for Aβ clearance and inhibition of amyloidogenic processing. Insulin increases Aβ trafficking from the trans golgi-network leading to secretion [333]. Secretion of Aβ may be important in preventing neurodegeneration as intraneural Aβ accumulations have been found in brain regions prone to early AD in patients with mild cognitive impairment [334] and studies done with transgenic mice indicate that intracellular Aβ accumulation is an early event of the neuropathological phenotype [335-337]. Insulin signalling protects against Aβ toxicity [298] and inhibits GSK-3β activity [204] which, in addition to hyperphosphorylating tau, promotes amyloidogenic APP cleavage [160, 338].

Insulin signaling pathways in the brain are complex and depend on a delicate balance of cell activity to function properly. Accumulation of Aβ perturbs this balance resulting in insulin resistance and formation of a vicious cycle as insulin signaling is no longer able to clear and regulate Aβ. As Aβ oligomers increase, insulin resistance worsens. This cycle is perpetuated by competition between insulin and Aβ as substrates for IDE.

Insulin, Aβ and insulin degrading enzyme IDE is responsible for insulin degradation but has also been shown to degrade Aβ peptides [339-341], a process known to be decreased in AD brains [318]. Studies have shown that increased insulin signaling can increase levels of IDE [44] which can be abolished by pharmacological inhibition of PI3K. Aβ can decrease PI3K activity, [342] and thus is able to prevent its own degradation. In cases of hyperinsulinemia, excess insulin blocks IDE binding sites which further diminishes Aβ degradation [115].

In summary, Aβ contributes to insulin resistance [297, 332] by occupying binding sites on insulin receptors [297] and is associated with decreased insulin receptor numbers in neurons [332]. Decreases in insulin signaling result in increased Aβ processing as well as activation of GSK-3β which promotes Aβ processing [160, 338]. Insulin signaling impairment also leads to decreased IDE, which is needed to degrade Aβ [339-341, 343]. IDE deficiencies are exacerbated in hyperinsulinemic conditions as IDE binding sites are overloaded with excess insulin and made unavailable for Aβ [115]. Lack of insulin signaling and IDE availability allows for continued accumulation of Aβ, further depression of insulin signaling systems, increased neuronal vulnerability and further neurodegeneration.

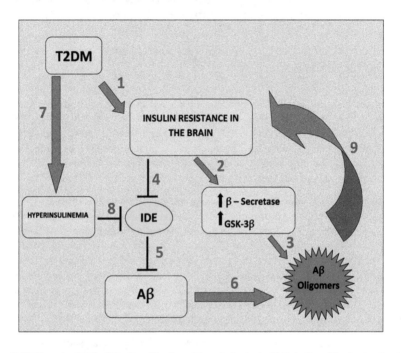

Figure 3. T2DM can lead to the induction of insulin resistance in the brain. (2) Reduction of insulin signaling in the brain increases the activities of GSK-3β and β secretases which (3) increase levels of toxic Aβ oligomers. Furthermore, (4) insulin resistance lowers the expression of Aβ-degrading IDE. (5) Reduced IDE then leads to increased Aβ and (6) accumulation of Aβ oligomers. T2DM also causes (7) hyperinsulinemia which exacerbates IDE deficiencies because (8) excess insulin occupies IDE binding sites rendering them unavailable for Aβ. The increased amyloidogenic processing that occurs in insulin resistance combined with decreased Aβ clearance by IDE results in a deleterious positive-feed-back cycle as (9) Aβ oligomers contribute to insulin resistance in the brain. As Aβ levels continue to rise, insulin resistance worsens leading to further production of the toxic peptide.

6. Conclusion

By 2050 it's estimated that over 100 million people worldwide will have AD [344] causing a substantial financial burden for health care systems. In that same time span, the annual cost of treating AD is predicated to exceed $1 trillion in the United States alone [345]. These crippling social and economical effects place increased priority for advancement of AD research.

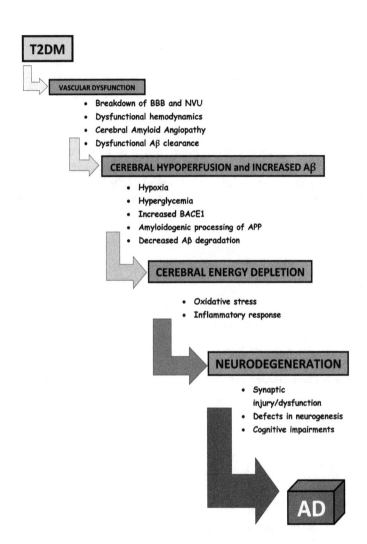

Figure 4. Vascular hypothesis of AD. The vascular complications have been casually linked to the progression of AD. Vascular dysfunction resulting from type 2 diabetes results in a state of cerebral hypoperfusion, leading to significant energy depletion in the brain. Neurodegeneration results in cognitive impairments and ultimately AD.

While AD remains a disease of more questions than answers, a wide array of evidence suggests a close relationship between AD and T2DM. T2DM has been characterized as having both macrovascular and microvascular complications that result in CVD. It is the vasculature that provides the tangible pathological link between T2DM and AD. Significant data has been collected in favor of the vascular hypothesis of AD, which is founded on the idea that pre-existing CVD sets into motion pathological cascades that ultimately result in AD.

AD and T2DM also share commonality in the form of insulin resistance. Lack of insulin neurotrophic support in the brain leaves neurons defenseless against oxidative stress, Aβ toxicity and apoptosis. Aβ is especially dangerous to neurons because it further depresses insulin signaling and can alter levels of protective enzymes involved in its degradation such as IDE. AD is a disease that not only causes death in weakened cells but also further depresses protective mechanisms making recovery unattainable.

Because AD affects multiple structures and pathways, it is likely that successful treatment will involve a comprehensive battery of therapeutics rather than a single therapy. T2DM plays a major role in vascular abnormalities and insulin resistance which parallel AD pathologies. As a result, further exploration of the relationship between T2DM and AD may be a promising direction of future research. Moreover, preventative measures against T2DM such as proper diet and dedication to an active lifestyle may take center stage as a means of curbing the AD epidemic.

Author details

Brent D. Aulston[1,2], Gary L. Odero[1], Zaid Aboud[1,2] and Gordon W. Glazner[1,2]

1 St. Boniface Hospital Research Centre, Winnipeg, MB, Canada

2 Department of Pharmacology and Therapeutics, University of Manitoba, Winnipeg, MB, Canada

References

[1] Ott, A, et al. Diabetes mellitus and the risk of dementia: The Rotterdam Study. Neurology, (1999). , 1937-1942.

[2] Ritchie, K, & Lovestone, S. The dementias. Lancet, (2002). , 1759-1766.

[3] Frolich, L, et al. A disturbance in the neuronal insulin receptor signal transduction in sporadic Alzheimer's disease. Ann N Y Acad Sci, (1999). , 290-293.

[4] Rivera, E. J, et al. Insulin and insulin-like growth factor expression and function deteriorate with progression of Alzheimer's disease: link to brain reductions in acetylcholine. J Alzheimers Dis, (2005). , 247-268.

[5] Steen, E, et al. Impaired insulin and insulin-like growth factor expression and signaling mechanisms in Alzheimer's disease--is this type 3 diabetes? J Alzheimers Dis, (2005). , 63-80.

[6] Sinclair, A. J, Girling, A. J, & Bayer, A. J. Cognitive dysfunction in older subjects with diabetes mellitus: impact on diabetes self-management and use of care services. All Wales Research into Elderly (AWARE) Study. Diabetes Res Clin Pract, (2000)., 203-212.

[7] Peila, R, Rodriguez, B. L, & Launer, L. J. Type 2 diabetes, APOE gene, and the risk for dementia and related pathologies: The Honolulu-Asia Aging Study. Diabetes, (2002)., 1256-1262.

[8] Kannel, W. B, & Mcgee, D. L. Diabetes and cardiovascular disease. The Framingham study. JAMA, (1979)., 2035-2038.

[9] Stratton, I. M, et al. Association of glycaemia with macrovascular and microvascular complications of type 2 diabetes (UKPDS 35): prospective observational study. BMJ, (2000)., 405-412.

[10] Defronzo, R. A. Pharmacologic therapy for type 2 diabetes mellitus. Ann Intern Med, (2000)., 73-74.

[11] Buse, J. B, et al. Primary prevention of cardiovascular diseases in people with diabetes mellitus: a scientific statement from the American Heart Association and the American Diabetes Association. Diabetes Care, (2007)., 162-172.

[12] Bell, R. D, et al. SRF and myocardin regulate LRP-mediated amyloid-beta clearance in brain vascular cells. Nat Cell Biol, (2009)., 143-153.

[13] De La Torre, J. C. Is Alzheimer's disease a neurodegenerative or a vascular disorder? Data, dogma, and dialectics. Lancet Neurol, (2004)., 184-190.

[14] Formichi, P, et al. CSF Biomarkers Profile in CADASIL-A Model of Pure Vascular Dementia: Usefulness in Differential Diagnosis in the Dementia Disorder. Int J Alzheimers Dis, 2010. (2010).

[15] Jagust, W. J, et al. The Alzheimer's Disease Neuroimaging Initiative positron emission tomography core. Alzheimers Dement, (2010)., 221-229.

[16] Pakrasi, S, & Brien, J. T. O. Emission tomography in dementia. Nucl Med Commun, (2005)., 189-196.

[17] Kahn, A. M, et al. Insulin acutely inhibits cultured vascular smooth muscle cell contraction by a nitric oxide synthase-dependent pathway. Hypertension, (1997)., 928-933.

[18] Bolotina, V. M, et al. Nitric oxide directly activates calcium-dependent potassium channels in vascular smooth muscle. Nature, (1994)., 850-853.

[19] Potenza, M. A, et al. Insulin resistance in spontaneously hypertensive rats is associated with endothelial dysfunction characterized by imbalance between NO and ET-1 production. Am J Physiol Heart Circ Physiol, (2005)., H813-H822.

[20] Potenza, M. A, et al. Treatment of spontaneously hypertensive rats with rosiglitazone and/or enalapril restores balance between vasodilator and vasoconstrictor actions of

insulin with simultaneous improvement in hypertension and insulin resistance. Diabetes, (2006). , 3594-3603.

[21] Formoso, G, et al. Dehydroepiandrosterone mimics acute actions of insulin to stimulate production of both nitric oxide and endothelin 1 via distinct phosphatidylinositol 3-kinase- and mitogen-activated protein kinase-dependent pathways in vascular endothelium. Mol Endocrinol, (2006). , 1153-1163.

[22] Wild, S, et al. Global prevalence of diabetes: estimates for the year 2000 and projections for 2030. Diabetes Care, (2004). , 1047-1053.

[23] Biessels, G. J, et al. Risk of dementia in diabetes mellitus: a systematic review. Lancet Neurol, (2006). , 64-74.

[24] Lu, F. P, Lin, K. P, & Kuo, H. K. Diabetes and the risk of multi-system aging phenotypes: a systematic review and meta-analysis. PLoS One, (2009). , e4144.

[25] Profenno, L. A, Porsteinsson, A. P, & Faraone, S. V. Meta-analysis of Alzheimer's disease risk with obesity, diabetes, and related disorders. Biol Psychiatry, (2012). , 505-512.

[26] Ahtiluoto, S, et al. Diabetes, Alzheimer disease, and vascular dementia: a population-based neuropathologic study. Neurology, (2010). , 1195-1202.

[27] Kalaria, R. N. Neurodegenerative disease: Diabetes, microvascular pathology and Alzheimer disease. Nat Rev Neurol, (2009). , 305-306.

[28] Zlokovic, B. V. The blood-brain barrier in health and chronic neurodegenerative disorders. Neuron, (2008). , 178-201.

[29] Zlokovic, B. V. Neurovascular pathways to neurodegeneration in Alzheimer's disease and other disorders. Nat Rev Neurosci, (2011). , 723-738.

[30] Moskowitz, M. A, Lo, E. H, & Iadecola, C. The science of stroke: mechanisms in search of treatments. Neuron, (2010). , 181-198.

[31] Beckman, J. A, Creager, M. A, & Libby, P. Diabetes and atherosclerosis: epidemiology, pathophysiology, and management. JAMA, (2002). , 2570-2581.

[32] Masters, S. L, Latz, E, & Neill, L. A. O. The inflammasome in atherosclerosis and type 2 diabetes. Sci Transl Med, (2011). , 81ps17.

[33] Klein, R. Hyperglycemia and microvascular and macrovascular disease in diabetes. Diabetes Care, (1995). , 258-268.

[34] Turner, R. C, et al. Risk factors for coronary artery disease in non-insulin dependent diabetes mellitus: United Kingdom Prospective Diabetes Study (UKPDS: 23). BMJ, (1998). , 823-828.

[35] Kuusisto, J, et al. NIDDM and its metabolic control predict coronary heart disease in elderly subjects. Diabetes, (1994). , 960-967.

[36] Lehto, S, et al. Predictors of stroke in middle-aged patients with non-insulin-dependent diabetes. Stroke, (1996). , 63-68.

[37] Cheng, G, et al. Diabetes as a risk factor for dementia and mild cognitive impairment: a meta-analysis of longitudinal studies. Intern Med J, (2012). , 484-491.

[38] Janson, J, et al. Increased risk of type 2 diabetes in Alzheimer disease. Diabetes, (2004). , 474-481.

[39] Leibson, C. L, et al. Risk of dementia among persons with diabetes mellitus: a population-based cohort study. Am J Epidemiol, (1997). , 301-308.

[40] Pansari, K, Gupta, A, & Thomas, P. Alzheimer's disease and vascular factors: facts and theories. Int J Clin Pract, (2002). , 197-203.

[41] De La Monte, S. M. Insulin resistance and Alzheimer's disease. BMB Rep, (2009). , 475-481.

[42] Kim, B, & Feldman, E. L. Insulin resistance in the nervous system. Trends Endocrinol Metab, (2012). , 133-141.

[43] Kim, B, et al. Cortical neurons develop insulin resistance and blunted Akt signaling: a potential mechanism contributing to enhanced ischemic injury in diabetes. Antioxid Redox Signal, (2011). , 1829-1839.

[44] Zhao, Z, et al. Insulin degrading enzyme activity selectively decreases in the hippocampal formation of cases at high risk to develop Alzheimer's disease. Neurobiol Aging, (2007). , 824-830.

[45] Stocker, R, & Keaney, J. F. Jr., Role of oxidative modifications in atherosclerosis. Physiol Rev, (2004). , 1381-1478.

[46] Jiang, Z. Y, et al. Characterization of selective resistance to insulin signaling in the vasculature of obese Zucker (fa/fa) rats. J Clin Invest, (1999). , 447-457.

[47] Cusi, K, et al. Insulin resistance differentially affects the PI 3-kinase- and MAP kinase-mediated signaling in human muscle. J Clin Invest, (2000). , 311-320.

[48] Piatti, P. M, et al. Hypertriglyceridemia and hyperinsulinemia are potent inducers of endothelin-1 release in humans. Diabetes, (1996). , 316-321.

[49] Sarkar, R, et al. Nitric oxide reversibly inhibits the migration of cultured vascular smooth muscle cells. Circ Res, (1996). , 225-230.

[50] Kubes, P, Suzuki, M, & Granger, D. N. Nitric oxide: an endogenous modulator of leukocyte adhesion. Proc Natl Acad Sci U S A, (1991). , 4651-4655.

[51] Zeiher, A. M, et al. Nitric oxide modulates the expression of monocyte chemoattractant protein 1 in cultured human endothelial cells. Circ Res, (1995). , 980-986.

[52] Nomura, S, et al. Significance of chemokines and activated platelets in patients with diabetes. Clin Exp Immunol, (2000). , 437-443.

[53] Collins, T, & Cybulsky, M. I. NF-kappaB: pivotal mediator or innocent bystander in atherogenesis? J Clin Invest, (2001). , 255-264.

[54] Petersen, K. F, & Shulman, G. I. Etiology of insulin resistance. Am J Med, (2006). Suppl 1): , S10-S16.

[55] Roden, M, et al. Mechanism of free fatty acid-induced insulin resistance in humans. J Clin Invest, (1996). , 2859-2865.

[56] Steinberg, H. O, & Baron, A. D. Vascular function, insulin resistance and fatty acids. Diabetologia, (2002). , 623-634.

[57] Wang, X. L, et al. Free fatty acids inhibit insulin signaling-stimulated endothelial nitric oxide synthase activation through upregulating PTEN or inhibiting Akt kinase. Diabetes, (2006). , 2301-2310.

[58] Naruse, K, et al. Activation of vascular protein kinase C-beta inhibits Akt-dependent endothelial nitric oxide synthase function in obesity-associated insulin resistance. Diabetes, (2006). , 691-698.

[59] Kim, F, et al. Free fatty acid impairment of nitric oxide production in endothelial cells is mediated by IKKbeta. Arterioscler Thromb Vasc Biol, (2005). , 989-994.

[60] Muniyappa, R, et al. Cardiovascular actions of insulin. Endocr Rev, (2007). , 463-491.

[61] Du, X. L, et al. Hyperglycemia inhibits endothelial nitric oxide synthase activity by posttranslational modification at the Akt site. J Clin Invest, (2001). , 1341-1348.

[62] Schnyder, B, et al. Rapid effects of glucose on the insulin signaling of endothelial NO generation and epithelial Na transport. Am J Physiol Endocrinol Metab, (2002). , E87-E94.

[63] Barba, R, et al. Poststroke dementia : clinical features and risk factors. Stroke, (2000). , 1494-1501.

[64] Breteler, M. M. Vascular risk factors for Alzheimer's disease: an epidemiologic perspective. Neurobiol Aging, (2000). , 153-160.

[65] Hofman, A, et al. Atherosclerosis, apolipoprotein E, and prevalence of dementia and Alzheimer's disease in the Rotterdam Study. Lancet, (1997). , 151-154.

[66] Barnes, D. E, & Yaffe, K. The projected effect of risk factor reduction on Alzheimer's disease prevalence. Lancet Neurol, (2011). , 819-828.

[67] Arenillas, J. F, et al. Metabolic syndrome and resistance to IV thrombolysis in middle cerebral artery ischemic stroke. Neurology, (2008). , 190-195.

[68] De Angelis, M, et al. Prevalence of carotid stenosis in type 2 diabetic patients asymptomatic for cerebrovascular disease. Diabetes Nutr Metab, (2003). , 48-55.

[69] Letonja, M. S, et al. Association of the C242T polymorphism in the NADPH oxidase phox gene with carotid atherosclerosis in Slovenian patients with type 2 diabetes. Mol Biol Rep, (2012). , 22.

[70] Palomo, I, et al. Hemostasis alterations in metabolic syndrome (review). Int J Mol Med, (2006). , 969-974.

[71] Alessi, M. C, & Juhan-vague, I. Metabolic syndrome, haemostasis and thrombosis. Thromb Haemost, (2008). , 995-1000.

[72] Kalaria, R. N, & Ballard, C. Overlap between pathology of Alzheimer disease and vascular dementia. Alzheimer Dis Assoc Disord, (1999). Suppl 3: , S115-S123.

[73] Henon, H, et al. Preexisting dementia in stroke patients. Baseline frequency, associated factors, and outcome. Stroke, (1997). , 2429-2436.

[74] Kokmen, E, et al. Dementia after ischemic stroke: a population-based study in Rochester, Minnesota (1960-1984). Neurology, (1996). , 154-159.

[75] Pasquier, F, Leys, D, & Scheltens, P. The influence of coincidental vascular pathology on symptomatology and course of Alzheimer's disease. J Neural Transm Suppl, (1998). , 117-127.

[76] Ferrucci, L, et al. Cognitive impairment and risk of stroke in the older population. J Am Geriatr Soc, (1996). , 237-241.

[77] Gale, C. R, Martyn, C. N, & Cooper, C. Cognitive impairment and mortality in a cohort of elderly people. BMJ, (1996). , 608-611.

[78] Cai, Y, et al. beta-Secretase-1 elevation in aged monkey and Alzheimer's disease human cerebral cortex occurs around the vasculature in partnership with multisystem axon terminal pathogenesis and beta-amyloid accumulation. Eur J Neurosci, (2010). , 1223-1238.

[79] Beach, T. G, et al. Circle of Willis atherosclerosis: association with Alzheimer's disease, neuritic plaques and neurofibrillary tangles. Acta Neuropathol, (2007). , 13-21.

[80] Roher, A. E, et al. Circle of willis atherosclerosis is a risk factor for sporadic Alzheimer's disease. Arterioscler Thromb Vasc Biol, (2003). , 2055-2062.

[81] Honig, L. S, Kukull, W, & Mayeux, R. Atherosclerosis and AD: analysis of data from the US National Alzheimer's Coordinating Center. Neurology, (2005). , 494-500.

[82] Grammas, P. Neurovascular dysfunction, inflammation and endothelial activation: implications for the pathogenesis of Alzheimer's disease. J Neuroinflammation, (2011). , 26.

[83] Kawai, M, et al. The relationship of amyloid plaques to cerebral capillaries in Alzheimer's disease. Am J Pathol, (1990). , 1435-1446.

[84] Kalaria, R. N. The role of cerebral ischemia in Alzheimer's disease. Neurobiol Aging, (2000). , 321-330.

[85] Kalaria, R. N, & Hedera, P. Differential degeneration of the cerebral microvasculature in Alzheimer's disease. Neuroreport, (1995). , 477-480.

[86] De La Torre, J. C. Cerebromicrovascular pathology in Alzheimer's disease compared to normal aging. Gerontology, (1997). , 26-43.

[87] Buee, L, et al. Pathological alterations of the cerebral microvasculature in Alzheimer's disease and related dementing disorders. Acta Neuropathol, (1994). , 469-480.

[88] Christov, A, et al. Structural changes in Alzheimer's disease brain microvessels. Curr Alzheimer Res, (2008). , 392-395.

[89] Davies, D. C, & Hardy, J. A. Blood brain barrier in ageing and Alzheimer's disease. Neurobiol Aging, (1988). , 46-48.

[90] Kalaria, R. N, & Pax, A. B. Increased collagen content of cerebral microvessels in Alzheimer's disease. Brain Res, (1995). , 349-352.

[91] Masters, C. L, & Beyreuther, K. The blood-brain barrier in Alzheimer's disease and normal aging. Neurobiol Aging, (1988). , 43-44.

[92] Claudio, L. Ultrastructural features of the blood-brain barrier in biopsy tissue from Alzheimer's disease patients. Acta Neuropathol, (1996). , 6-14.

[93] Yan, S. D, et al. RAGE and amyloid-beta peptide neurotoxicity in Alzheimer's disease. Nature, (1996). , 685-691.

[94] Van Beek, A. H, et al. Cerebral autoregulation: an overview of current concepts and methodology with special focus on the elderly. J Cereb Blood Flow Metab, (2008). , 1071-1085.

[95] Rancillac, A, Geoffroy, H, & Rossier, J. Impaired neurovascular coupling in the APPxPS1 mouse model of Alzheimer's disease. Curr Alzheimer Res, (2012).

[96] Claassen, J. A, et al. Transcranial Doppler estimation of cerebral blood flow and cerebrovascular conductance during modified rebreathing. J Appl Physiol, (2007). , 870-877.

[97] Lee, S. T, Jung, K. H, & Lee, Y. S. Decreased vasomotor reactivity in Alzheimer's disease. J Clin Neurol, (2007). , 18-23.

[98] Menendez-gonzalez, M, et al. Vasomotor reactivity is similarly impaired in patients with Alzheimer's disease and patients with amyloid hemorrhage. J Neuroimaging, (2011). , e83-e85.

[99] Barone, F. C, et al. Vascular cognitive impairment: dementia biology and translational animal models. Curr Opin Investig Drugs, (2009). , 624-637.

[100] Farkas, E, Luiten, P. G, & Bari, F. Permanent, bilateral common carotid artery occlusion in the rat: a model for chronic cerebral hypoperfusion-related neurodegenerative diseases. Brain Res Rev, (2007). , 162-180.

[101] Vicente, E, et al. Astroglial and cognitive effects of chronic cerebral hypoperfusion in the rat. Brain Res, (2009). , 204-212.

[102] Liu, H, et al. Regulation of beta-amyloid level in the brain of rats with cerebrovascular hypoperfusion. Neurobiol Aging, (2011). e31-42., 826.

[103] Zhiyou, C, et al. Upregulation of BACE1 and beta-amyloid protein mediated by chronic cerebral hypoperfusion contributes to cognitive impairment and pathogenesis of Alzheimer's disease. Neurochem Res, (2009). , 1226-1235.

[104] Kalaria, R. N, et al. The amyloid precursor protein in ischemic brain injury and chronic hypoperfusion. Ann N Y Acad Sci, (1993). , 190-193.

[105] Stephenson, D. T, Rash, K, & Clemens, J. A. Amyloid precursor protein accumulates in regions of neurodegeneration following focal cerebral ischemia in the rat. Brain Res, (1992). , 128-135.

[106] Wen, Y, et al. Increased beta-secretase activity and expression in rats following transient cerebral ischemia. Brain Res, (2004). , 1-8.

[107] Zhang, X, et al. Hypoxia-inducible factor 1alpha (HIF-1alpha)-mediated hypoxia increases BACE1 expression and beta-amyloid generation. J Biol Chem, (2007). , 10873-10880.

[108] Tesco, G, et al. Depletion of GGA3 stabilizes BACE and enhances beta-secretase activity. Neuron, (2007). , 721-737.

[109] Zhang, Y, et al. Mutant ubiquitin-mediated beta-secretase stability via activation of caspase-3 is related to beta-amyloid accumulation in ischemic striatum in rats. J Cereb Blood Flow Metab, (2010). , 566-575.

[110] Li, L, et al. Hypoxia increases Abeta generation by altering beta- and gamma-cleavage of APP. Neurobiol Aging, (2009). , 1091-1098.

[111] Okamoto, Y, et al. Cerebral hypoperfusion accelerates cerebral amyloid angiopathy and promotes cortical microinfarcts. Acta Neuropathol, (2012). , 381-394.

[112] Deane, R, et al. RAGE mediates amyloid-beta peptide transport across the blood-brain barrier and accumulation in brain. Nat Med, (2003). , 907-913.

[113] Miners, J. S, et al. Decreased expression and activity of neprilysin in Alzheimer disease are associated with cerebral amyloid angiopathy. J Neuropathol Exp Neurol, (2006). , 1012-1021.

[114] Weeraratna, A. T, et al. Alterations in immunological and neurological gene expression patterns in Alzheimer's disease tissues. Exp Cell Res, (2007). , 450-461.

[115] Qiu, W. Q, & Folstein, M. F. Insulin, insulin-degrading enzyme and amyloid-beta peptide in Alzheimer's disease: review and hypothesis. Neurobiol Aging, (2006). , 190-198.

[116] Hayashi, S, et al. Alzheimer disease-associated peptide, amyloid beta40, inhibits vascular regeneration with induction of endothelial autophagy. Arterioscler Thromb Vasc Biol, (2009). , 1909-1915.

[117] Donnini, S, et al. Abeta peptides accelerate the senescence of endothelial cells in vitro and in vivo, impairing angiogenesis. FASEB J, (2010). , 2385-2395.

[118] Gentile, M. T, et al. Mechanisms of soluble beta-amyloid impairment of endothelial function. J Biol Chem, (2004). , 48135-48142.

[119] Huang, Z, et al. Enlarged infarcts in endothelial nitric oxide synthase knockout mice are attenuated by nitro-L-arginine. J Cereb Blood Flow Metab, (1996). , 981-987.

[120] Christie, R, et al. Structural and functional disruption of vascular smooth muscle cells in a transgenic mouse model of amyloid angiopathy. Am J Pathol, (2001). , 1065-1071.

[121] Merlini, M, et al. Vascular beta-amyloid and early astrocyte alterations impair cerebrovascular function and cerebral metabolism in transgenic arcAbeta mice. Acta Neuropathol, (2008). , 293-311.

[122] Tong, P, et al. Insulin-induced cortical actin remodeling promotes GLUT4 insertion at muscle cell membrane ruffles. J Clin Invest, (2001). , 371-381.

[123] Arvanitakis, Z, et al. Diabetes is related to cerebral infarction but not to AD pathology in older persons. Neurology, (2006). , 1960-1965.

[124] Luchsinger, J. A. Type 2 diabetes, related conditions, in relation and dementia: an opportunity for prevention? J Alzheimers Dis, (2010). , 723-736.

[125] Curb, J. D, et al. Longitudinal association of vascular and Alzheimer's dementias, diabetes, and glucose tolerance. Neurology, (1999). , 971-975.

[126] Xu, W. L, et al. Diabetes mellitus and risk of dementia in the Kungsholmen project: a 6-year follow-up study. Neurology, (2004). , 1181-1186.

[127] Brookmeyer, R, Gray, S, & Kawas, C. Projections of Alzheimer's disease in the United States and the public health impact of delaying disease onset. Am J Public Health, (1998). , 1337-1342.

[128] Clark, C. M, et al. Earlier onset of Alzheimer disease symptoms in latino individuals compared with anglo individuals. Arch Neurol, (2005). , 774-778.

[129] Korczyn, A. D. Mixed dementia--the most common cause of dementia. Ann N Y Acad Sci, (2002). , 129-134.

[130] Goldberg, I, et al. Microembolism, silent brain infarcts and dementia. J Neurol Sci, (2012).

[131] Erkinjuntti, T. Clinical deficits of Alzheimer's disease with cerebrovascular disease and probable VaD. Int J Clin Pract Suppl, (2001). , 14-23.

[132] Roman, G. C, & Royall, D. R. Executive control function: a rational basis for the diagnosis of vascular dementia. Alzheimer Dis Assoc Disord, (1999). Suppl 3: , S69-S80.

[133] Barber, R, et al. White matter lesions on magnetic resonance imaging in dementia with Lewy bodies, Alzheimer's disease, vascular dementia, and normal aging. J Neurol Neurosurg Psychiatry, (1999). , 66-72.

[134] Cordonnier, C, et al. Prevalence and severity of microbleeds in a memory clinic setting. Neurology, (2006). , 1356-1360.

[135] Zarei, M, et al. Regional white matter integrity differentiates between vascular dementia and Alzheimer disease. Stroke, (2009). , 773-779.

[136] Cacabelos, R, et al. Cerebrovascular risk factors in Alzheimer's disease: brain hemodynamics and pharmacogenomic implications. Neurol Res, (2003). , 567-580.

[137] Gorelick, P. B. Risk factors for vascular dementia and Alzheimer disease. Stroke, (2004). Suppl 1): , 2620-2622.

[138] Sabayan, B, et al. Cerebrovascular hemodynamics in Alzheimer's disease and vascular dementia: a meta-analysis of transcranial Doppler studies. Ageing Res Rev, (2012). , 271-277.

[139] Altman, R, & Rutledge, J. C. The vascular contribution to Alzheimer's disease. Clin Sci (Lond), (2010). , 407-421.

[140] Vinters, H. V. Cerebral amyloid angiopathy. A critical review. Stroke, (1987). , 311-324.

[141] Kalaria, R. N, et al. Production and increased detection of amyloid beta protein and amyloidogenic fragments in brain microvessels, meningeal vessels and choroid plexus in Alzheimer's disease. Brain Res Mol Brain Res, (1996). , 58-68.

[142] Kosunen, O, et al. Diagnostic accuracy of Alzheimer's disease: a neuropathological study. Acta Neuropathol, (1996). , 185-193.

[143] Olichney, J. M, et al. Cerebral infarction in Alzheimer's disease is associated with severe amyloid angiopathy and hypertension. Arch Neurol, (1995). , 702-708.

[144] Premkumar, D. R, et al. Apolipoprotein E-epsilon4 alleles in cerebral amyloid angiopathy and cerebrovascular pathology associated with Alzheimer's disease. Am J Pathol, (1996). , 2083-2095.

[145] Kalaria, R. Similarities between Alzheimer's disease and vascular dementia. J Neurol Sci, (2002). , 29-34.

[146] Frisoni, G. B, et al. Apolipoprotein E epsilon 4 allele in Alzheimer's disease and vascular dementia. Dementia, (1994). , 240-242.

[147] Snowdon, D. A, et al. Brain infarction and the clinical expression of Alzheimer disease. The Nun Study. JAMA, (1997). , 813-817.

[148] Bondy, C. A, & Cheng, C. M. Signaling by insulin-like growth factor 1 in brain. Eur J Pharmacol, (2004). , 25-31.

[149] Yamaguchi, Y, et al. Ligand-binding properties of the two isoforms of the human insulin receptor. Endocrinology, (1993). , 1132-1138.

[150] Kasuga, M, Karlsson, F. A, & Kahn, C. R. Insulin stimulates the phosphorylation of the 95,000-dalton subunit of its own receptor. Science, (1982). , 185-187.

[151] Jacobs, S, et al. Somatomedin-C stimulates the phosphorylation of the beta-subunit of its own receptor. J Biol Chem, (1983). , 9581-9584.

[152] Rubin, J. B, Shia, M. A, & Pilch, P. F. Stimulation of tyrosine-specific phosphorylation in vitro by insulin-like growth factor I. Nature, (1983). , 438-440.

[153] Schechter, R, et al. Developmental regulation of insulin in the mammalian central nervous system. Brain Res, (1992). , 27-37.

[154] Schechter, R, et al. Preproinsulin I and II mRNAs and insulin electron microscopic immunoreaction are present within the rat fetal nervous system. Brain Res, (1996). , 16-27.

[155] Schechter, R, & Abboud, M. Neuronal synthesized insulin roles on neural differentiation within fetal rat neuron cell cultures. Brain Res Dev Brain Res, (2001). , 41-49.

[156] Coker, G. T, et al. Analysis of tyrosine hydroxylase and insulin transcripts in human neuroendocrine tissues. Brain Res Mol Brain Res, (1990). , 93-98.

[157] Devaskar, S. U, et al. Insulin gene expression and insulin synthesis in mammalian neuronal cells. J Biol Chem, (1994). , 8445-8454.

[158] Banks, W. A. The source of cerebral insulin. Eur J Pharmacol, (2004). , 5-12.

[159] Burns, J. M, et al. Peripheral insulin and brain structure in early Alzheimer disease. Neurology, (2007). , 1094-1104.

[160] Salkovic-petrisic, M, & Hoyer, S. Central insulin resistance as a trigger for sporadic Alzheimer-like pathology: an experimental approach. J Neural Transm Suppl, (2007). , 217-233.

[161] Erol, A. An integrated and unifying hypothesis for the metabolic basis of sporadic Alzheimer's disease. J Alzheimers Dis, (2008). , 241-253.

[162] Park, C. R. Cognitive effects of insulin in the central nervous system. Neurosci Biobehav Rev, (2001). , 311-323.

[163] Ebina, Y, et al. The human insulin receptor cDNA: the structural basis for hormone-activated transmembrane signalling. Cell, (1985). , 747-758.

[164] Ullrich, A, et al. Human insulin receptor and its relationship to the tyrosine kinase family of oncogenes. Nature, (1985). , 756-761.

[165] Frasca, F, et al. Insulin receptor isoform A, a newly recognized, high-affinity insulin-like growth factor II receptor in fetal and cancer cells. Mol Cell Biol, (1999). , 3278-3288.

[166] Mosthaf, L, et al. Functionally distinct insulin receptors generated by tissue-specific alternative splicing. Embo J, (1990). , 2409-2413.

[167] Hedo, J. A, et al. Direct demonstration of glycosylation of insulin receptor subunits by biosynthetic and external labeling: evidence for heterogeneity. Proc Natl Acad Sci U S A, (1981). , 4791-4795.

[168] Massague, J, Pilch, P. F, & Czech, M. P. A unique proteolytic cleavage site on the beta subunit of the insulin receptor. J Biol Chem, (1981). , 3182-3190.

[169] Siegel, T. W, et al. Purification and properties of the human placental insulin receptor. J Biol Chem, (1981). , 9266-9273.

[170] Kanzaki, M. Insulin receptor signals regulating GLUT4 translocation and actin dynamics. Endocr J, (2006). , 267-293.

[171] Frattali, A. L, & Pessin, J. E. Relationship between alpha subunit ligand occupancy and beta subunit autophosphorylation in insulin/insulin-like growth factor-1 hybrid receptors. J Biol Chem, (1993). , 7393-7400.

[172] Lee, J, et al. Insulin receptor autophosphorylation occurs asymmetrically. J Biol Chem, (1993). , 4092-4098.

[173] Lee, J, & Pilch, P. F. The insulin receptor: structure, function, and signaling. Am J Physiol, (1994). Pt 1): , C319-C334.

[174] White, M. F, et al. Mutation of the insulin receptor at tyrosine 960 inhibits signal transmission but does not affect its tyrosine kinase activity. Cell, (1988). , 641-649.

[175] White, M. F. The IRS-signalling system: a network of docking proteins that mediate insulin action. Mol Cell Biochem, (1998). , 3-11.

[176] Myers, M. G, et al. IRS-1 activates phosphatidylinositol 3'-kinase by associating with src homology 2 domains of Proc Natl Acad Sci U S A, (1992). p. 10350-4., 85.

[177] Virkamaki, A, Ueki, K, & Kahn, C. R. Protein-protein interaction in insulin signaling and the molecular mechanisms of insulin resistance. J Clin Invest, (1999). , 931-943.

[178] Mayer, B. J, et al. A putative modular domain present in diverse signaling proteins. Cell, (1993). , 629-630.

[179] Yenush, L, et al. The pleckstrin homology domain is the principal link between the insulin receptor and IRS-1. J Biol Chem, (1996). , 24300-24306.

[180] Coffer, P. J, & Woodgett, J. R. Molecular cloning and characterisation of a novel putative protein-serine kinase related to the cAMP-dependent and protein kinase C families. Eur J Biochem, (1991). , 475-481.

[181] Burgering, B. M, & Coffer, P. J. Protein kinase B (c-Akt) in phosphatidylinositol-3-OH kinase signal transduction. Nature, (1995). , 599-602.

[182] Andjelkovic, M, et al. Activation and phosphorylation of a pleckstrin homology domain containing protein kinase (RAC-PK/PKB) promoted by serum and protein phosphatase inhibitors. Proc Natl Acad Sci U S A, (1996). , 5699-5704.

[183] Kohn, A. D, Takeuchi, F, & Roth, R. A. Akt, a pleckstrin homology domain containing kinase, is activated primarily by phosphorylation. J Biol Chem, (1996). , 21920-21926.

[184] Bellacosa, A, et al. Akt activation by growth factors is a multiple-step process: the role of the PH domain. Oncogene, (1998). , 313-325.

[185] Soskic, V, et al. Functional proteomics analysis of signal transduction pathways of the platelet-derived growth factor beta receptor. Biochemistry, (1999). , 1757-1764.

[186] Alessi, D. R, et al. Phosphoinositide-dependent protein kinase-1 (PDK1): structural and functional homology with the Drosophila DSTPK61 kinase. Curr Biol, (1997). , 776-789.

[187] Stokoe, D, et al. Dual role of phosphatidylinositol-3,4,5-trisphosphate in the activation of protein kinase B. Science, (1997). , 567-570.

[188] Currie, R. A, et al. Role of phosphatidylinositol 3,4,5-trisphosphate in regulating the activity and localization of 3-phosphoinositide-dependent protein kinase-1. Biochem J, (1999). Pt 3): , 575-583.

[189] Alessi, D. R, et al. Mechanism of activation of protein kinase B by insulin and IGF-1. EMBO J, (1996). , 6541-6551.

[190] Alessi, D. R, et al. Characterization of a 3-phosphoinositide-dependent protein kinase which phosphorylates and activates protein kinase Balpha. Curr Biol, (1997). , 261-269.

[191] Sarbassov, D. D, et al. Phosphorylation and regulation of Akt/PKB by the rictor-mTOR complex. Science, (2005). , 1098-1101.

[192] Yang, J, et al. Crystal structure of an activated Akt/protein kinase B ternary complex with GSK3-peptide and AMP-PNP. Nat Struct Biol, (2002). , 940-944.

[193] Cardone, M. H, et al. Regulation of cell death protease caspase-9 by phosphorylation. Science, (1998). , 1318-1321.

[194] Datta, S. R, et al. Akt phosphorylation of BAD couples survival signals to the cell-intrinsic death machinery. Cell, (1997). , 231-241.

[195] del PesoL., et al., Interleukin-3-induced phosphorylation of BAD through the protein kinase Akt. Science, (1997). , 687-689.

[196] Blume-jensen, P, Janknecht, R, & Hunter, T. The kit receptor promotes cell survival via activation of PI 3-kinase and subsequent Akt-mediated phosphorylation of Bad on Ser136. Curr Biol, (1998). , 779-782.

[197] Wang, H. G, et al. Ca2+-induced apoptosis through calcineurin dephosphorylation of BAD. Science, (1999). , 339-343.

[198] Du, K, & Montminy, M. CREB is a regulatory target for the protein kinase Akt/PKB. J Biol Chem, (1998). , 32377-32379.

[199] Kane, L. P, et al. Induction of NF-kappaB by the Akt/PKB kinase. Curr Biol, (1999). , 601-604.

[200] Biggs, W. H, et al. Protein kinase B/Akt-mediated phosphorylation promotes nuclear exclusion of the winged helix transcription factor FKHR1. Proc Natl Acad Sci U S A, (1999). , 7421-7426.

[201] Brunet, A, et al. Akt promotes cell survival by phosphorylating and inhibiting a Forkhead transcription factor. Cell, (1999). , 857-868.

[202] Kops, G. J, et al. Direct control of the Forkhead transcription factor AFX by protein kinase B. Nature, (1999). , 630-634.

[203] Read, D. E, & Gorman, A. M. Involvement of Akt in neurite outgrowth. Cell Mol Life Sci, (2009). , 2975-2984.

[204] Bhat, R. V, et al. Regulation and localization of tyrosine216 phosphorylation of glycogen synthase kinase-3beta in cellular and animal models of neuronal degeneration. Proc Natl Acad Sci U S A, (2000). , 11074-11079.

[205] Llambi, F, et al. A unified model of mammalian BCL-2 protein family interactions at the mitochondria. Mol Cell, (2011). , 517-531.

[206] Green, D. R, & Reed, J. C. Mitochondria and apoptosis. Science, (1998). , 1309-1312.

[207] Reed, J. C. Bcl-2 family proteins. Oncogene, (1998). , 3225-3236.

[208] Pastorino, J. G, et al. Functional consequences of the sustained or transient activation by Bax of the mitochondrial permeability transition pore. J Biol Chem, (1999). , 31734-31739.

[209] Antonsson, B, et al. Bax oligomerization is required for channel-forming activity in liposomes and to trigger cytochrome c release from mitochondria. Biochem J, (2000). Pt 2: , 271-278.

[210] Rong, Y, & Distelhorst, C. W. Bcl-2 protein family members: versatile regulators of calcium signaling in cell survival and apoptosis. Annu Rev Physiol, (2008). , 73-91.

[211] Lemasters, J. J, et al. Mitochondrial calcium and the permeability transition in cell death. Biochim Biophys Acta, (2009). , 1395-1401.

[212] Paradies, G, et al. Role of cardiolipin peroxidation and Ca2+ in mitochondrial dysfunction and disease. Cell Calcium, (2009). , 643-650.

[213] Bossy-wetzel, E, & Green, D. R. Apoptosis: checkpoint at the mitochondrial frontier. Mutat Res, (1999). , 243-251.

[214] Tornero, D, Posadas, I, & Cena, V. Bcl-x(L) blocks a mitochondrial inner membrane channel and prevents Ca2+ overload-mediated cell death. PLoS One, (2011). , e20423.

[215] Yang, E, et al. Bad, a heterodimeric partner for Bcl-XL and Bcl-2, displaces Bax and promotes cell death. Cell, (1995). , 285-291.

[216] Ottilie, S, et al. Dimerization properties of human BAD. Identification of a BH-3 domain and analysis of its binding to mutant BCL-2 and BCL-XL proteins. J Biol Chem, (1997). , 30866-30872.

[217] Zha, J, et al. BH3 domain of BAD is required for heterodimerization with BCL-XL and pro-apoptotic activity. J Biol Chem, (1997). , 24101-24104.

[218] Datta, S. R, Brunet, A, & Greenberg, M. E. Cellular survival: a play in three Akts. Genes Dev, (1999). , 2905-2927.

[219] Tsujimoto, Y. Role of Bcl-2 family proteins in apoptosis: apoptosomes or mitochondria? Genes Cells, (1998). , 697-707.

[220] Cryns, V, & Yuan, J. Proteases to die for. Genes Dev, (1998). , 1551-1570.

[221] Pettmann, B, & Henderson, C. E. Neuronal cell death. Neuron, (1998). , 633-647.

[222] Merry, D. E, & Korsmeyer, S. J. Bcl-2 gene family in the nervous system. Annu Rev Neurosci, (1997). , 245-267.

[223] Murphy, A. N, et al. Bcl-2 potentiates the maximal calcium uptake capacity of neural cell mitochondria. Proc Natl Acad Sci U S A, (1996). , 9893-9898.

[224] Vercesi, A. E, et al. The role of reactive oxygen species in mitochondrial permeability transition. Biosci Rep, (1997). , 43-52.

[225] Ellerby, L. M, et al. Shift of the cellular oxidation-reduction potential in neural cells expressing Bcl-2. J Neurochem, (1996). , 1259-1267.

[226] Esposti, M. D, et al. Bcl-2 and mitochondrial oxygen radicals. New approaches with reactive oxygen species-sensitive probes. J Biol Chem, (1999). , 29831-29837.

[227] Singleton, J. R, Dixit, V. M, & Feldman, E. L. Type I insulin-like growth factor receptor activation regulates apoptotic proteins. J Biol Chem, (1996). , 31791-31794.

[228] Minshall, C, et al. IL-4 and insulin-like growth factor-I inhibit the decline in Bcl-2 and promote the survival of IL-3-deprived myeloid progenitors. J Immunol, (1997). , 1225-1232.

[229] Tamatani, M, Ogawa, S, & Tohyama, M. Roles of Bcl-2 and caspases in hypoxia-induced neuronal cell death: a possible neuroprotective mechanism of peptide growth factors. Brain Res Mol Brain Res, (1998). , 27-39.

[230] Pugazhenthi, S, et al. Insulin-like growth factor-I induces bcl-2 promoter through the transcription factor cAMP-response element-binding protein. J Biol Chem, (1999). , 27529-27535.

[231] Shieh, P. B, et al. Identification of a signaling pathway involved in calcium regulation of BDNF expression. Neuron, (1998). , 727-740.

[232] Tao, X, et al. Ca2+ influx regulates BDNF transcription by a CREB family transcription factor-dependent mechanism. Neuron, (1998). , 709-726.

[233] Hu, Y, & Russek, S. J. BDNF and the diseased nervous system: a delicate balance between adaptive and pathological processes of gene regulation. J Neurochem, (2008)., 1-17.

[234] Fu, W, Lu, C, & Mattson, M. P. Telomerase mediates the cell survival-promoting actions of brain-derived neurotrophic factor and secreted amyloid precursor protein in developing hippocampal neurons. J Neurosci, (2002). , 10710-10719.

[235] Rohe, M, et al. Brain-derived neurotrophic factor reduces amyloidogenic processing through control of SORLA gene expression. J Neurosci, (2009). , 15472-15478.

[236] Arancibia, S, et al. Protective effect of BDNF against beta-amyloid induced neurotoxicity in vitro and in vivo in rats. Neurobiol Dis, (2008). , 316-326.

[237] Laske, C, et al. BDNF serum and CSF concentrations in Alzheimer's disease, normal pressure hydrocephalus and healthy controls. J Psychiatr Res, (2007). , 387-394.

[238] Lee, J. G, et al. Decreased serum brain-derived neurotrophic factor levels in elderly korean with dementia. Psychiatry Investig, (2009). , 299-305.

[239] Forlenza, O. V, Diniz, B. S, & Gattaz, W. F. Diagnosis and biomarkers of predementia in Alzheimer's disease. BMC Med, 20108: , 89.

[240] Forlenza, O. V, et al. Clinical and biological predictors of Alzheimer's disease in patients with amnestic mild cognitive impairment. Rev Bras Psiquiatr, (2010). , 216-222.

[241] Forlenza, O. V, et al. Effect of brain-derived neurotrophic factor Val66Met polymorphism and serum levels on the progression of mild cognitive impairment. World J Biol Psychiatry, (2010). , 774-780.

[242] Gunstad, J, et al. Serum brain-derived neurotrophic factor is associated with cognitive function in healthy older adults. J Geriatr Psychiatry Neurol, (2008). , 166-170.

[243] Maggirwar, S. B, et al. Nerve growth factor-dependent activation of NF-kappaB contributes to survival of sympathetic neurons. J Neurosci, (1998). , 10356-10365.

[244] Riccio, A, et al. Mediation by a CREB family transcription factor of NGF-dependent survival of sympathetic neurons. Science, (1999). , 2358-2361.

[245] Mincheva, S, et al. The canonical nuclear factor-kappaB pathway regulates cell survival in a developmental model of spinal cord motoneurons. J Neurosci, (2011). , 6493-6503.

[246] Maehara, K, Hasegawa, T, & Isobe, K. I. A NF-kappaB subunit is indispensable for activating manganese superoxide: dismutase gene transcription mediated by tumor necrosis factor-alpha. J Cell Biochem, (2000). p. 474-86., 65.

[247] Rojo, A. I, et al. Regulation of Cu/Zn-superoxide dismutase expression via the phosphatidylinositol 3 kinase/Akt pathway and nuclear factor-kappaB. J Neurosci, (2004). , 7324-7334.

[248] Tamatani, M, et al. Tumor necrosis factor induces Bcl-2 and Bcl-x expression through NFkappaB activation in primary hippocampal neurons. J Biol Chem, (1999). , 8531-8538.

[249] May, M. J, Ghosh, S, Rel, N. F-k. a. p. p. a B, Kappa, I, & Proteins, B. an overview. Semin Cancer Biol, (1997). , 63-73.

[250] Mercurio, F, & Manning, A. M. Multiple signals converging on NF-kappaB. Curr Opin Cell Biol, (1999). , 226-232.

[251] Perkins, N. D. Integrating cell-signalling pathways with NF-kappaB and IKK function. Nat Rev Mol Cell Biol, (2007). , 49-62.

[252] Ozes, O. N, et al. NF-kappaB activation by tumour necrosis factor requires the Akt serine-threonine kinase. Nature, (1999). , 82-85.

[253] Van Der Heide, L. P, Hoekman, M. F, & Smidt, M. P. The ins and outs of FoxO shuttling: mechanisms of FoxO translocation and transcriptional regulation. Biochem J, (2004). Pt 2): , 297-309.

[254] Miyashita, T, & Reed, J. C. Tumor suppressor is a direct transcriptional activator of the human bax gene. Cell, (1995). p. 293-9., 53.

[255] Reif, K, Burgering, B. M, & Cantrell, D. A. Phosphatidylinositol 3-kinase links the interleukin-2 receptor to protein kinase B and S6 kinase. J Biol Chem, (1997). p. 14426-33., 70.

[256] Stahl, M, et al. The forkhead transcription factor FoxO regulates transcription of and Bim in response to IL-2. J Immunol, (2002). p. 5024-31., 27Kip1.

[257] Dijkers, P. F, et al. Expression of the pro-apoptotic Bcl-2 family member Bim is regulated by the forkhead transcription factor FKHR-L1. Curr Biol, (2000). , 1201-1204.

[258] Graham, S. H, & Chen, J. Programmed cell death in cerebral ischemia. J Cereb Blood Flow Metab, (2001). , 99-109.

[259] Yamaguchi, H, & Wang, H. G. Bcl-XL protects BimEL-induced Bax conformational change and cytochrome C release independent of interacting with Bax or BimEL. J Biol Chem, (2002). , 41604-41612.

[260] Yamaguchi, A, et al. Akt activation protects hippocampal neurons from apoptosis by inhibiting transcriptional activity of J Biol Chem, (2001). p. 5256-64., 53.

[261] Kowaltowski, A. J, Vercesi, A. E, & Fiskum, G. Bcl-2 prevents mitochondrial permeability transition and cytochrome c release via maintenance of reduced pyridine nucleotides. Cell Death Differ, (2000). , 903-910.

[262] Aloyz, R. S, et al. is essential for developmental neuron death as regulated by the TrkA and p75 neurotrophin receptors. J Cell Biol, (1998). p. 1691-703., 53.

[263] Jaworski, J, et al. Control of dendritic arborization by the phosphoinositide-3'-kinase-Akt-mammalian target of rapamycin pathway. J Neurosci, (2005). , 11300-11312.

[264] Kumar, V, et al. Regulation of dendritic morphogenesis by Ras-PI3K-Akt-mTOR and Ras-MAPK signaling pathways. J Neurosci, (2005). , 11288-11299.

[265] Yoshimura, T, et al. Ras regulates neuronal polarity via the PI3-kinase/Akt/GSK-3beta/CRMP-2 pathway. Biochem Biophys Res Commun, (2006). , 62-68.

[266] Lim, C. S, & Walikonis, R. S. Hepatocyte growth factor and c-Met promote dendritic maturation during hippocampal neuron differentiation via the Akt pathway. Cell Signal, (2008). , 825-835.

[267] Zheng, J, et al. Clathrin-dependent endocytosis is required for TrkB-dependent Akt-mediated neuronal protection and dendritic growth. J Biol Chem, (2008). , 13280-13288.

[268] Markus, A, Zhong, J, & Snider, W. D. Raf and akt mediate distinct aspects of sensory axon growth. Neuron, (2002). , 65-76.

[269] Mills, J, et al. Role of integrin-linked kinase in nerve growth factor-stimulated neurite outgrowth. J Neurosci, (2003). , 1638-1648.

[270] Tucker, B. A, Rahimtula, M, & Mearow, K. M. Laminin and growth factor receptor activation stimulates differential growth responses in subpopulations of adult DRG neurons. Eur J Neurosci, (2006). , 676-690.

[271] Tucker, B. A, Rahimtula, M, & Mearow, K. M. Src and FAK are key early signalling intermediates required for neurite growth in NGF-responsive adult DRG neurons. Cell Signal, (2008). , 241-257.

[272] Cross, D. A, et al. Inhibition of glycogen synthase kinase-3 by insulin mediated by protein kinase B. Nature, (1995). , 785-789.

[273] Salas, T. R, et al. Alleviating the suppression of glycogen synthase kinase-3beta by Akt leads to the phosphorylation of cAMP-response element-binding protein and its transactivation in intact cell nuclei. J Biol Chem, (2003). , 41338-41346.

[274] Asnaghi, L, et al. Bcl-2 phosphorylation and apoptosis activated by damaged micro-tubules require mTOR and are regulated by Akt. Oncogene, (2004). , 5781-5791.

[275] Konishi, H, et al. Identification of peripherin as a Akt substrate in neurons. J Biol Chem, (2007). , 23491-23499.

[276] Kim, H, et al. Delta-catenin-induced dendritic morphogenesis. An essential role of interaction through Akt1-mediated phosphorylation. J Biol Chem, (2008). p. 977-87., 190RhoGEF.

[277] Konishi, H, et al. Activation of protein kinase B (Akt/RAC-protein kinase) by cellular stress and its association with heat shock protein Hsp27. FEBS Lett, (1997). , 493-498.

[278] Murashov, A. K, et al. Crosstalk between Hsp25 and Akt in spinal motor neurons after sciatic nerve injury. Brain Res Mol Brain Res, (2001). p. 199-208., 38.

[279] Frame, S, & Cohen, P. GSK3 takes centre stage more than 20 years after its discovery. Biochem J, (2001). Pt 1): , 1-16.

[280] Grimes, C. A, & Jope, R. S. The multifaceted roles of glycogen synthase kinase 3beta in cellular signaling. Prog Neurobiol, (2001). , 391-426.

[281] Doble, B. W, & Woodgett, J. R. GSK-3: tricks of the trade for a multi-tasking kinase. J Cell Sci, (2003). Pt 7): , 1175-1186.

[282] Hooper, C, Killick, R, & Lovestone, S. The GSK3 hypothesis of Alzheimer's disease. J Neurochem, (2008). , 1433-1439.

[283] Iqbal, K, et al. Mechanisms of tau-induced neurodegeneration. Acta Neuropathol, (2009). , 53-69.

[284] Mandelkow, E. M, et al. Clogging of axons by tau, inhibition of axonal traffic and starvation of synapses. Neurobiol Aging, (2003). , 1079-1085.

[285] Brewster, J. L, et al. Endoplasmic reticulum stress and trophic factor withdrawal activate distinct signaling cascades that induce glycogen synthase kinase-3 beta and a caspase-9-dependent apoptosis in cerebellar granule neurons. Mol Cell Neurosci, (2006). , 242-253.

[286] Duyckaerts, C, Delatour, B, & Potier, M. C. Classification and basic pathology of Alzheimer disease. Acta Neuropathol, (2009). , 5-36.

[287] Takashima, A. Amyloid-beta, tau, and dementia. J Alzheimers Dis, (2009). , 729-736.

[288] Wang, J. M, et al. Reduction of ischemic brain injury by topical application of insulin-like growth factor-I after transient middle cerebral artery occlusion in rats. Brain Res, (2000). , 381-385.

[289] St-pierre, J, et al. Topology of superoxide production from different sites in the mitochondrial electron transport chain. J Biol Chem, (2002). , 44784-44790.

[290] Barthel, A, Schmoll, D, & Unterman, T. G. FoxO proteins in insulin action and metabolism. Trends Endocrinol Metab, (2005). , 183-189.

[291] Zetterberg, H, Wahlund, L. O, & Blennow, K. Cerebrospinal fluid markers for prediction of Alzheimer's disease. Neurosci Lett, (2003). , 67-69.

[292] Lacor, P. N, et al. Synaptic targeting by Alzheimer's-related amyloid beta oligomers. J Neurosci, (2004). , 10191-10200.

[293] Walsh, D. M, et al. Naturally secreted oligomers of amyloid beta protein potently inhibit hippocampal long-term potentiation in vivo. Nature, (2002). , 535-539.

[294] Tillement, L, Lecanu, L, & Papadopoulos, V. Alzheimer's disease: effects of beta-amyloid on mitochondria. Mitochondrion. 11(1): , 13-21.

[295] Abramov, A. Y, Canevari, L, & Duchen, M. R. Calcium signals induced by amyloid beta peptide and their consequences in neurons and astrocytes in culture. Biochim Biophys Acta, (2004). , 81-87.

[296] Mattson, M. P, et al. beta-Amyloid peptides destabilize calcium homeostasis and render human cortical neurons vulnerable to excitotoxicity. J Neurosci, (1992). , 376-389.

[297] Xie, L, et al. Alzheimer's beta-amyloid peptides compete for insulin binding to the insulin receptor. J Neurosci, (2002). , RC221.

[298] Messier, C, & Teutenberg, K. The role of insulin, insulin growth factor, and insulin-degrading enzyme in brain aging and Alzheimer's disease. Neural Plast, (2005). , 311-328.

[299] Thinakaran, G, & Koo, E. H. Amyloid precursor protein trafficking, processing, and function. J Biol Chem, (2008). , 29615-29619.

[300] Rocchi, A, et al. Causative and susceptibility genes for Alzheimer's disease: a review. Brain Res Bull, (2003). , 1-24.

[301] Zhang, Y. W, et al. APP processing in Alzheimer's disease. Mol Brain. 4: , 3.

[302] De Strooper, B, & Annaert, W. Proteolytic processing and cell biological functions of the amyloid precursor protein. J Cell Sci, (2000). Pt 11): , 1857-1870.

[303] Zheng, H, & Koo, E. H. The amyloid precursor protein: beyond amyloid. Mol Neurodegener, (2006). , 5.

[304] Loffler, J, & Huber, G. Beta-amyloid precursor protein isoforms in various rat brain regions and during brain development. J Neurochem, (1992). , 1316-1324.

[305] Tominaga-yoshino, K, et al. Neurotoxic and neuroprotective effects of glutamate are enhanced by introduction of amyloid precursor protein cDNA. Brain Res, (2001). , 121-130.

[306] Wasco, W, et al. Isolation and characterization of APLP2 encoding a homologue of the Alzheimer's associated amyloid beta protein precursor. Nat Genet, (1993). , 95-100.

[307] Wasco, W, et al. Identification of a mouse brain cDNA that encodes a protein related to the Alzheimer disease-associated amyloid beta protein precursor. Proc Natl Acad Sci U S A, (1992). , 10758-10762.

[308] Coulson, E. J, et al. What the evolution of the amyloid protein precursor supergene family tells us about its function. Neurochem Int, (2000). , 175-184.

[309] Goate, A, et al. Segregation of a missense mutation in the amyloid precursor protein gene with familial Alzheimer's disease. Nature, (1991). , 704-706.

[310] Rohan de SilvaH.A., et al., Cell-specific expression of beta-amyloid precursor protein isoform mRNAs and proteins in neurons and astrocytes. Brain Res Mol Brain Res, (1997). , 147-156.

[311] Kang, J, & Muller-hill, B. Differential splicing of Alzheimer's disease amyloid A4 precursor RNA in rat tissues: PreA4(695) mRNA is predominantly produced in rat and human brain. Biochem Biophys Res Commun, (1990). , 1192-1200.

[312] Menendez-gonzalez, M, et al. APP processing and the APP-KPI domain involvement in the amyloid cascade. Neurodegener Dis, (2005). , 277-283.

[313] Xu, H, et al. Generation of Alzheimer beta-amyloid protein in the trans-Golgi network in the apparent absence of vesicle formation. Proc Natl Acad Sci U S A, (1997). , 3748-3752.

[314] Hartmann, T, et al. Distinct sites of intracellular production for Alzheimer's disease A beta40/42 amyloid peptides. Nat Med, (1997). , 1016-1020.

[315] Greenfield, J. P, et al. Endoplasmic reticulum and trans-Golgi network generate distinct populations of Alzheimer beta-amyloid peptides. Proc Natl Acad Sci U S A, (1999). , 742-747.

[316] Cupers, P, et al. The discrepancy between presenilin subcellular localization and gamma-secretase processing of amyloid precursor protein. J Cell Biol, (2001). , 731-740.

[317] Kovacs, D. M, et al. Alzheimer-associated presenilins 1 and 2: neuronal expression in brain and localization to intracellular membranes in mammalian cells. Nat Med, (1996). , 224-229.

[318] Perez, A, et al. Degradation of soluble amyloid beta-peptides 1-40, 1-42, and the Dutch variant 1-40Q by insulin degrading enzyme from Alzheimer disease and control brains. Neurochem Res, (2000). , 247-255.

[319] Sinha, S, et al. Purification and cloning of amyloid precursor protein beta-secretase from human brain. Nature, (1999). , 537-540.

[320] Vassar, R, et al. Beta-secretase cleavage of Alzheimer's amyloid precursor protein by the transmembrane aspartic protease BACE. Science, (1999). , 735-741.

[321] Yan, R, et al. Membrane-anchored aspartyl protease with Alzheimer's disease beta-secretase activity. Nature, (1999). , 533-537.

[322] Lau, K. F, et al. X11 alpha and x11 beta interact with presenilin-1 via their PDZ domains. Mol Cell Neurosci, (2000). , 557-565.

[323] Dominguez, D, et al. Phenotypic and biochemical analyses of BACE1- and BACE2-deficient mice. J Biol Chem, (2005). , 30797-30806.

[324] Hu, X, et al. Bace1 modulates myelination in the central and peripheral nervous system. Nat Neurosci, (2006). , 1520-1525.

[325] Chow, V. W, et al. An overview of APP processing enzymes and products. Neuromolecular Med. 12(1): , 1-12.

[326] Nikolaev, A, et al. APP binds DR6 to trigger axon pruning and neuron death via distinct caspases. Nature, (2009). , 981-989.

[327] Kimberly, W. T, et al. Gamma-secretase is a membrane protein complex comprised of presenilin, nicastrin, Aph-1, and Pen-2. Proc Natl Acad Sci U S A, (2003). , 6382-6387.

[328] Takasugi, N, et al. The role of presenilin cofactors in the gamma-secretase complex. Nature, (2003). , 438-441.

[329] Burdick, D, et al. Assembly and aggregation properties of synthetic Alzheimer's A4/beta amyloid peptide analogs. J Biol Chem, (1992). , 546-554.

[330] Scheuner, D, et al. Secreted amyloid beta-protein similar to that in the senile plaques of Alzheimer's disease is increased in vivo by the presenilin 1 and 2 and APP mutations linked to familial Alzheimer's disease. Nat Med, (1996). , 864-870.

[331] Borchelt, D. R, et al. Familial Alzheimer's disease-linked presenilin 1 variants elevate Abeta1-42/1-40 ratio in vitro and in vivo. Neuron, (1996). , 1005-1013.

[332] Zhao, W. Q, et al. Amyloid beta oligomers induce impairment of neuronal insulin receptors. FASEB J, (2008). , 246-260.

[333] Gasparini, L, et al. Stimulation of beta-amyloid precursor protein trafficking by insulin reduces intraneuronal beta-amyloid and requires mitogen-activated protein kinase signaling. J Neurosci, (2001). , 2561-2570.

[334] Gouras, G. K, et al. Intraneuronal Abeta42 accumulation in human brain. Am J Pathol, (2000). , 15-20.

[335] Oddo, S, et al. Triple-transgenic model of Alzheimer's disease with plaques and tangles: intracellular Abeta and synaptic dysfunction. Neuron, (2003). , 409-421.

[336] Oddo, S, et al. A dynamic relationship between intracellular and extracellular pools of Abeta. Am J Pathol, (2006). , 184-194.

[337] Oakley, H, et al. Intraneuronal beta-amyloid aggregates, neurodegeneration, and neuron loss in transgenic mice with five familial Alzheimer's disease mutations: potential factors in amyloid plaque formation. J Neurosci, (2006). , 10129-10140.

[338] Phiel, C. J, et al. GSK-3alpha regulates production of Alzheimer's disease amyloid-beta peptides. Nature, (2003). , 435-439.

[339] Farris, W, et al. Partial loss-of-function mutations in insulin-degrading enzyme that induce diabetes also impair degradation of amyloid beta-protein. Am J Pathol, (2004). , 1425-1434.

[340] Vekrellis, K, et al. Neurons regulate extracellular levels of amyloid beta-protein via proteolysis by insulin-degrading enzyme. J Neurosci, (2000). , 1657-1665.

[341] Farris, W, et al. Insulin-degrading enzyme regulates the levels of insulin, amyloid beta-protein, and the beta-amyloid precursor protein intracellular domain in vivo. Proc Natl Acad Sci U S A, (2003). , 4162-4167.

[342] Takashima, A, et al. Exposure of rat hippocampal neurons to amyloid beta peptide (25-35) induces the inactivation of phosphatidyl inositol-3 kinase and the activation of tau protein kinase I/glycogen synthase kinase-3 beta. Neurosci Lett, (1996). , 33-36.

[343] Zhao, L, et al. Insulin-degrading enzyme as a downstream target of insulin receptor signaling cascade: implications for Alzheimer's disease intervention. J Neurosci, (2004). , 11120-11126.

[344] Brookmeyer, R, et al. Forecasting the global burden of Alzheimer's disease. Alzheimers Dement, (2007). , 186-191.

[345] Vellas, B, et al. Disease-modifying trials in Alzheimer's disease: a European task force consensus. Lancet Neurol, (2007). , 56-62.

Chapter 5

Apathy as a Key Symptom in Behavior Disorders: Difference Between Alzheimer's Disease and Subcortical Vascular Dementia

Rita Moretti, Paola Torre, Francesca Esposito,
Enrica Barro, Paola Tomietto and
Rodolfo M. Antonello

Additional information is available at the end of the chapter

1. Introduction

There is currently no consensus on the nosological position of apathy in clinical practice. The clinical significance of negative symptoms such as apathy is increasingly recognized in neurological and psychiatric disorders, particularly those associated with frontal-subcortical dysfunction (Starkstein et al., 2008; Moretti et al., 2012). Apathy is defined as lack of motivation as manifested by diminished goal-directed behavior, reduced goal-directed cognition, and decreased emotional engagement, a reduced interest and participation in normal purposeful behavior, problems in initiation or sustaining an activity, lack of concern or indifference, and a flattening of affect. The prevalence of apathy in neurodegenerative disorders, such as Parkinson's disease vary between 16.5% and 51%, depending upon the instrument for assessment and on the samples examined. Apathy is quite common also in sVAD; different studies try to define its role in AD, but, even the most recent and well-conducted did not distinguish between early and advanced stages of AD, or even between AD and AD with parkinsonism (Starkstein et al., 2008; Stuss et al., 2000; Dujardin et al., 2009). It has been hypothesized that dysfunction of the nigro-striatal pathway may play an important role in the pathophysiology of apathy in neuro-degenerative disorders. In fact, apathy seems to be independent of disease duration, disability and severity of parkinsonism, and levodopa dose in PD, indicating that the brain changes underlying apathy differ from those associated with motor symptoms. Much more interesting is that not all the PD patients become apathetic, indicating that apathy should not entirely be considered a dopamine-dependent syndrome in PD, and is in fact present even in not-purely dopaminergic alterations, such as AD or sVAD (Moretti et al., 2012; Levy et al., 1998; Brown and Pluck, 2000). Existing evidence suggests that apathy can be related to depression, as a key symptom of major depression or side-effect of antidepressant or antipsychotic drugs (Chase et al., 2011). Though, apathy and depression clearly dissociate in specific motor disorders, such as progressive supranuclear palsy, in which there is a high incidence of apathy but a low incidence of depression (Aarsland et al., 2001). Other Authors suggested that apathy might be a consequence of chronic disabling disease and its impact on mobility and opportunity for participation in normal activities. Thus, many Authors used the term "premature social aging" to describe the findings that patients with apathy have little in the way of interests or social activities, spending more time in solitary activities such as watching television or just sitting doing nothing (Starkstein et al., 1992). If apathy is a primary consequence of physical disability or impairment in daily living, then similar changes might be predicted for patients with articular/orthopedic impairment. Surprisingly, the osteoarthritis sample population, despite the motor disability, showed no evidence of apathy. It is thus likely that the physiopathology of apathy is a multifaceted entity. The aim of this preliminary was to assess the behavior spectrum of Alzheimer's Disease (AD) and that of subcortical Vascular Dementia (sVAD), with a particular concern for apathy, and to assess its possible role in the differential clinical diagnosis, as compared to other behavioral changes and different neuropsychological patterns.

We decided to conduct a prospective cohort study, designed to investigate behavioural alterations, and in particular apathy of an AD and of a sVAD population. Therefore, our group recruited 75 men and women aged 65–94 years, entering in Cognitive Disorder Unit Evaluation of the University of Trieste, with Mini-Mental State Examination (MMSE) scores of at least 14 and satisfying DSM-IV for dementia, and suffering from Alzheimer's Disease, according to NINDCS-ADRDA criteria (McKAhn et al., 1984) and 317 patients suffered from from subcortical vascular dementia, in accordance with the NINDS-AIREN criteria (Román et al., 1993); the patients have been selected from June 1st 2008 to June 1st 2011. In order to be enrolled into the study subjects had to show on brain MRI the classical pattern of atrophy of AD (hippocampal atrophy) and display hypoperfusion in temporoparietal and precuneus regions (AD) on HMPAO-SPECT. A patient was diagnosed as having subcortical VaD (sVaD) when the CT/MRI scan showed moderate to severe ischaemic white matter changes (Erkinjuntti et al., 1997) and at least one lacunar infarct. Brain CT-scans or MRI images were randomized and assessed independently, after the radiologist's opinion, by neurologists (RM, PT, RMA). The diagnosis was confirmed after 6 and 12 months of clinical follow-up.

Patients were not included in the study if they showed signs of normal pressure hydrocephalus, previous brain tumours, previous diagnosis of major stroke or brain haemorrhage. We did not include patients with white matter lesions, caused by specific aetiologies, such as multiple sclerosis, brain irradiation, collagen vascular disease, and genetic forms of vascular dementia (such as CADASIL or CARASIL). Patients with previous major psychiatric illness (i.e. schizophrenia, bipolar disorders, psychosis, compulsive-obsessive disorders, etc) or central nervous system disorders and alcoholism were excluded too. Exclusion criteria were, in addition to those provided by the corresponding diagnostic criteria, the absence of an informed caregiver, unavailability of neuroradiological examination, and/or the assumption of psychotropic drugs within two months prior to the clinical assessment. Therefore, five patients were excluded in consequence of lack of a sufficiently informed caregiver and twelve subjects were excluded because they assumed psychotropic drugs during the two months prior to our assessment.

Study subjects underwent a standardized baseline assessment that included a detailed history, a physical examination, laboratory tests and psychiatric evaluations. The physical examination included evaluations of pulse rate and rhythm, blood pressure, heart size and sounds, peripheral pulses, retinal vessel and carotid artery evaluation, electrocardiographic evaluation, and chest X-ray. All patients were followed with periodical neurological and neuropsychological examinations. A complete neuropsychological examination was conducted at baseline, and at 12 months' results were compared.

Main outcomes of the study were: Global performance, which was assessed using the Mini Mental State Examination (Folstein et al., 1975), Frontal Assessment Battery (FAB) (Dubois et al., 2000); Semantic and Phonological Fluency, Digit span subtest (digit span forward and backward) and arithmetic subtest (from Wechsler Adult Intelligent Scale-WAIS; Wechsler, 1981); global behavioral symptoms, assessed by the NeuroPsychiatric Inventory, NPI (Cummings et al., 1994); the caregiver stress, assessed by the Relative Stress Scale, RSS (Green et al., 1992). In addition to these main outcome measures, three further scales were used. The Cornell Scale for Depression in Dementia (Alexopoulos et al., 1988); the Behavioral Pathology in Alzheimer's Disease Rating Scale (BEHAVE-AD) (Greene et al., 1982), and the Clinical Insight Rating Scale (CIR) (Ott et al., 1986) (which provides a measure of its four comprising items – awareness, cognitive deficit, disease progression and functional deficit) were performed. In order to evaluate the apathy, as an independent scale (it is tested as specific item in NPI, and in BEHAVE-AD), we employed the Clinician/Researcher Rated Version of the Apathy Evaluation Scale (AES-C) (Marin et al., 1991). Statistical analyses were performed using the Statistical Package for the Social Sciences (SPSS, version 16.0). Within Groups comparisons were performed by Wilcoxon Signed Rank tests. Between-group comparisons of changes were tested using the marginal homogeneity test, employing the Stewart Maxwell test. This was done for the overall scores for each efficacy variable. In addition, sub-analyses of Spearmann's rho correlation, 2-tailed analyses were performed between behavioral data obtained using the Apathy scores (AES-C), the FAB scores, Cornell's Depression Scores, RSS, CIR, and NPI scores. Results are presented as mean changes from baseline with standard deviations, and P-values are presented where appropriate.

The study subjects were 61 AD patients and 310 sVAD patients. All the patients could be fully studied (mean age 71.1 ± 7.3 years, range= 65-94 years). A synopsis of the cognitive performances obtained by the two groups has been reported in Table 1-2; a synoptic summary of the behavior scores has been reported in Table 3-4; the differential reappraisal of Apathy-scores (AES-C) has been reported in table 5-6. In summary, it can be stated that there are some important cognitive differences in the two groups: AD patients did worse in MMSE; they produced lower in phonological and semantic tasks, in arithmetic calculation and in digit tasks of WAIS; sVAD patients did generally worse in FAB tests. From the behavioral perspective, the following aspects merged from the study: at baseline, the AD group had a worse score of NPI and BEHAVE-AD, and their caregivers did have a heavier stress, as stated by RSS. On the contrary, sVAD patients, at baseline did feel much more depressed (as stated by Cornell'Scale) and did have a better insight in their situation. After 12 months, AD patients showed higher NPI and Behave scores; sVAD patients did show more insight and remained more depressed. Surprisingly, the stress of the caregivers was not significantly different in the two groups. Very interestingly, sVAD patients did manifest more overt apathy, which merged from the AES-C scores, which increase during follow-up and remained a major key point in behavior disturbances of these patients. Spearman's rank correlation analyses indicated that there was a significant correlation between AES-C scores and RSS in sVAD (r=0.88, p<0.01); a negative correlation with FAB scores (r=-0.81, p<0.01); analyzing the sub-items, it can be stated a negative relationship between AES-S and C scores and the go/no-go strategies (r=-0.71, p<0.05); there was no relationship between apathy and depression and insight ratio.

baseline	sVAD	AD	P value (between group)
MMSE	25.8 (2.4)	22.1 (1.9)	<0.05
Word phonological fluency (WAIS)**	34.5 (7.9)	31.2 (3.6)	ns
Semantic category (WAIS)***	37.7 (5.6)	24.5 (3.2)	<0.01
Arithmetic calculations (WAIS) §	6.3 (1.6)	8.6 (1.2)	<0.05
Digit span forward (WAIS)	5.8 (1.5)	5.1 (0.6)	<0.05
Digit span backward (WAIS)	4.4 (2.5)	2.6 (0.8)	<0.05
FAB total score	11.2 (2.1)	10.8 (1.2)	ns
Analogies	2 (0.9)	1.6 (0.2)	ns
Phonemic fluency	1.6 (0.2)	1.8 (0.2)	ns
Motor series	2.2 (0.1)	2.7 (0.4)	ns
Contrast Instructions	2.3 (0.3)	2.2 (0.2)	ns
Go/no-go	0.8 (0.5)	0.9 (0.3)	ns
Comprehension	1.9 (0.1)	0.9 (0.2)	<0.05

Values are mean (SD). NS = not significant.. *Number of items in 45 seconds.; ** Total number of words produced, beginning with T, P, C;

*** Total number of words produced, comprised in the following categories: animal, fruits, professions ; § Number of mistakes

Table 1. Cognitive synoptical results obtained by the two groups studied

12 months follow-up	sVAD within group (12 months vs baseline)	AD within group (12 months vs baseline)	P value (between group)
MMSE	23.8 (2.1) (-2 (.0.3); p<0.05)	17.1 (1.7) (-5 (0.2); p<0.01)	<0.01
Word phonological fluency (WAIS)**	29.5 (2.3) (-5 (5.6); p<0.01)	16.2 (3.1) (-15 (0.5); p<0.01)	<0.01
Semantic category (WAIS)***	27.1 (2.1) (-10.6 (3.5); p<0.01)	12.6 (1.3) (-9.9 (1.9); p<0.01)	<0.01
Arithmetic calculations (WAIS) §	5.4 (1.1) (-0.9 (0.5); ns)	3.4 (1.7) (-5.2 (0.5); p<0.01)	<0.05
Digit span forward (WAIS)	4.1 (1.4) (-1.7 (0.1); p<0.05)	3.2 (0.2) (-1.9 (0.4); p<0.05)	<0.05
Digit span backward (WAIS)	3.6 (0.3) (-0.8 (2.2); ns)	1.9 (0.1) (-0.5 (0.7); p<0.05)	<0.01
FAB total score	5.7 (1.5) (-5.5 (0.6); p<0.01)	7.5 (0.2) (-3.3 (1.0); p<0.05)	<0.01
Analogies	1.2 (0.1) (-0.8 (0.8); p<0.05)	1.4 (0.1) (-0.2 (0.2); ns)	ns
Phonemic fluency	(0.1) (-0.5 (0.1); p<0.05)	1.4 (0.1) (-0.4 (0.1); p<0.05)	ns
Motor series	1.1 (0.3) (-1.1 (0.5); p<0.01)	1.6 (0.2) (-0.9 (0.2); p<0.05)	ns
Contrast Instructions	1.2 (0.5) (-1.1 (0.3); p<0.01)	2.0 (0.1) (-0.2 (0.1); ns)	ns
Go/no-go	0.1 (0.3) (-0.7 (0.2); p<0.05)	0.8 (0.1) (-0.1 (0.2); ns)	ns
Comprehension	1.0 (0.9) (-0.9 (0.8); p<0.05)	0.3 (0.1) (-0.6 (0.1); p<0.05)	<0.05

Values are mean (SD). NS = not significant.. *Number of items in 45 seconds.; ** Total number of words produced, beginning with T, P, C;

*** Total number of words produced, comprised in the following categories: animal, fruits, professions ; § Number of mistakes

In brackets, in each column, comparison within group, 12 months vs baseline, reported as mean, SD, and p

Table 2. Cognitive synoptical results obtained by the two groups studied, at 12 months

baseline	sVAD	AD	P value
RSS	24.7 (8.7)	36.1 (8.5)	(p<0.01)
NPI	14.9 (0.3)	24.4 (5.2)	(p<0.01)
CIR	3 (0.2)	2 (0.5)	(p<0.05)
Cornell	18.5 (3.5)	13.5 (4)	(p<0.05)
BEHAVE	9.5 (2.1)	12.6 (4.1)	(p<0.05)

Values are mean (SD). NS = not significant..

Table 3. Behavioral synoptical results

	sVAD	AD	P value
RSS	44.5 (1.6)	43.9 (2.1)	ns
	(+20.2 (5.9), <0.01)	(+7.8 (6.8), <0.05)	
NPI	24.1 (0.8)	56.3 (4.5)	(p<0.01)
	(+10.8 (0.5), <0.01)	(+31.9 (1.1), <0.01)	
CIR	2.7 (0.3)	(0.3)	(p<0.01)
	(+0.3 (0.1), ns)	(+1.0 (0.3), <0.05)	
Cornell	22.1 (1.2)	12.3 (1.1)	(p<0.01)
	(+4.4 (2.3), <0.05)	(-0.8 (3.1), ns)	
BEHAVE	22.7 (1.3)	43.1 (2.3)	(p<0.01)
	(+13.2 (0.8), <0.01)	(+30.5 (0.8), <0.01)	

Values are mean (SD). NS = not significant.; In brackets, in each column, comparison within group, 12 months vs baseline, reported as mean, SD, and p

Table 4. Behavioral synoptical results

baseline	sVAD	AD	P value
AES-C	48.5 (7.2)	28.0 (4.9)	<0.01

Values are mean (SD). NS = not significant.

Table 5. Apathy scores, by the researcher evaluation (AES-C)

	sVAD	AD	P value
AES-C	67.2 (3.5)	33.4 (6.1)	<0.01
	(+18.7 (3.7); p<0.01)	(5.4 (1.2); ns)	

Apathy scores, by the researcher evaluation (AES-C)

Table 6. Values are mean (SD). NS = not significant.. In brackets, in each column, comparison within group, 12 months vs baseline, reported as mean, SD, and p

What merged from this study is a confirmation of the wide known rule, that behavioral disorders are the most problematic in the follow-up of dementia. Among them, apathy is one of the most concerning. Frequency and severity of apathy vary across different dementia subtypes; it is the most common behavioral symptom of behavioral variant of frontotemporal dementia (bvFTD), with reported prevalence ranging from 62 to 89% of patients (Mendez et al., 2008); the prevalence of apathy in AD ranges from 25 to 88% with a trend to increase with disease severity (Starkestein et al., 2006). The prevalence of apathy in other neuro-degenerative disorders, such as Parkinson's disease vary between 16.5% and 51%, depending upon the instrument for assessment and on the samples examined (Moretti et al., 2012). Apathy may be associated with an increased risk of cognitive decline. Symptoms of apathy, but not symptoms of depressive affect, increase the risk of progression from MCI to AD (Richard et al., 2012). Conversely, patients with or without apathy had an increase of similar magnitude in anosognosia scores. In conclusion, anosognosia is a significant predictor of apathy in Alzheimer's disease (Starkstein et al., 2010).

The aim of our study was to assess the behavior spectrum of Alzheimer's Disease (AD) and that of subcortical Vascular Dementia (sVAD), with a particular concern for apathy, and to assess the possible role of apathy in the differential clinical diagnosis, as compared to other behavioral changes and different neuropsychological patterns. Our results showed that there are some important cognitive differences in the two groups. Obviously, the AD patients did worse in MMSE; they produced lower in phonological and semantic tasks, they did many mistakes in arithmetic calculation and their digit span were lower; sVAD patients did generally worse in FAB tests, as a sensitive measure of executive dysfunction. And their behavior problems were different. At baseline, the AD group had a worse score of NPI and BEHAVE-AD, and their caregivers did have a heavier stress, as stated by RSS. On the contrary, sVAD patients, at baseline did feel much more depressed (as stated by Cornell'Scale) and did have a better insight in their situation. After 12 months, AD patients showed higher NPI and Behave scores; sVAD patients did show more insight and remained more depressed. Surprisingly, the stress of the caregivers was not significantly different in the two groups. Very interestingly, sVAD patients did manifest more overt apathy, which merged from the AES-C scores, which increased during follow-up.

So far, it can be argued that sVAD patients have higher insight, more depression and more apathy than AD, and the two last aspects are the major causative factors for an increase of caregiver stress in the one-year follow-up. At that time, the significant difference which was noted at the beginning of the study for the RSS of AD patients, is practically cancelled out, and there is no difference between RSS in AD and sVAD patients. The main reason for what observed is that apathy increases, and caregivers do not know how to manage it. Apathy is one of the greatest stressors for caregivers, and the second most common is disinhibition (Massimo et al., 2009).

As a general observation (Quaranta et al., 2012), the occurrence of apathy is connected to damage of prefrontal cortex (PFC) and basal ganglia (Chase, 2011); "emotional affective" apathy may be related to the orbitomedial PFC and ventral striatum; "cognitive apathy" may be associated with dysfunction of lateral PFC and dorsal caudate nuclei; deficit of "autoactivation" may be due to bilateral lesions of the internal portion of globus pallidus, bilateral paramedian thalamic lesions, or the dorsomedial portion of PFC (Chow et al. 2009). Trying to compare apathy in AD and in the behavior form of Frontal dementia (bvFTD), Quaranta et al (2012) lead to an observation of a different distribution of apathetic symptoms; they stated that subjects affected by bvFTD displayed higher frequency of "affective" symptoms, and a reduction of "auto-activation" (Levy and Dubois, 2006) (or "behavioral apathy," (Marin, 1991)) in comparison with AD sample. The different clinical expression of apathy, among the two groups of patients probably reflects the involvement of different anatomic substrates. Previous studies have reported that in bvFTD apathy is associated with changes in orbitofrontal cortex (Zamboni et al., 2008; Peters et al., 2006), which, in turn, has been postulated to be the anatomical correlate of "affective" apathy (Levy and Dubois, 2006), and with volume loss in the dorsal anterior cingulate and dorsolateral prefrontal cortex (Massimo et al., 2009). Thus, it is possible that the observation by Quaranta et al (2012) may reflect an alteration of orbitofrontal cortex and its connections with subcortical nuclei (ventral striatum), that could be specific of bvFTD. "Affective apathy" may be also regarded as the clinical expression of personality changes in bvFTD; for example, Sollberger et al. (2009) reported that subjects with FTD and semantic dementia displayed a reduction in affiliative behavior (lack of warmth) and showed, in a large sample of subjects aff ected by different neurodegenerative diseases, an association between "warmth" and several cortical and subcortical right hemisphere structures (viz. orbitofrontal cortex, insular cortex, amygdala, and hippocampal and parahippocampal regions). This finding is of particular interest, since the authors reported an association between lack of warmth and cerebral structures related to reward mechanisms, and "affective apathy" has been regarded as consequence of the inability to associate emotions to behaviors (Marin, 1991; 1996). Analogously, affective apathy may be related to an impairment of the so-called prosocial sentiments (such as guilt, pity, and embarrassment), connected to lack of empathy; Moll et al. (2011) reported reduced social sentiments in bvFTD subjects; this deficit was related to hypometabolism in medial frontal polar cortex and septal area.

On the other hand, in AD, apathy severity has been connected to neurofibrillary tangles density in the anterior cingulate gyrus (Marshall et al., 2006) and to grey matter atrophy in the anterior cingulate and in the left medial frontal cortex (Apostolova et al, 2007; Tekin et al., 2001; Marshall et al., 2006). These findings were confirmed by a PET study showing the association of apathy with hypometabolism in the bilateral anterior cingulate gyrus and medial orbitofrontal cortex (Marshall et al., 2007). Many studies tried to identify the neuroanatomical correlates of apathy in AD (Tunnard et al., 2011). Functional imaging studies have tended to find impaired functioning measured by either reduced blood flow or reduced metabolism in the anterior cingulate cortex (ACC) and medial frontal or orbitofrontal cortical (OFC) brain regions (Robert et al., 2006; Lanctot et al., 2007; Marshall et al., 2007). However, it is uncertain whether these regions are unilaterally or bilaterally affected. Others have found reduced function limited to the OFC alone (Holthoff et al., 2005) or the ACC alone (Migneco et al., 2001), suggesting that impaired functioning of both regions is not necessary for apathy to result. MRI studies investigating the structural correlates of apathy in AD patients have, for the most part, replicated findings from functional studies implicating the ACC and OFC most consistently (Apostolova et al., 2007;Laveretsky et al., 2007; Bruen et al., 2008). Additional regions of atrophy in the superior frontal gyrus, specifically BA 9, are also reported (Apostolova et al., 2007; Bruen et al., 2008) as is atrophy of frontopolar (BA 10) and ventrolateral prefrontal regions, including BA 45 (pars triangularis; Bruen et al., 2008).

Also of note, is some evidence that subcortical nuclei which project to prefrontal regions, including the caudate and putamen have shown greater atrophy in apathy in AD (Bruen et al., 2008). Overall then, functional, structural and pathological studies point towards a specific involvement of the ACC and OFC in mediating symptoms of apathy, with a suggestion of wider involvement of frontocortical networks.

One pathophysiological model for apathy in Alzheimer's disease which addresses both structural and biochemical disruption is that of Guimaraes et al. (2008). Their model proposes that the ACC and OFC are part of a broader fronto striatal circuit, which is involved in decision-making. Specifically, these regions are involved in evaluating action and outcomes and, via the basolateral amygdala and nucleus accumbens, feed into an ascending frontostriatal pathway to the dorsolateral prefrontal cortex, which is ultimately responsible for selecting and executing behavioural responses. Damage to the ACC and OFC leads to a disruption of this circuit resulting in impaired decision-making and impaired response initiation, which presents as apathy.

This model resembles quite well our idea of apathy in sVAD. There is good evidence of high levels of apathy subcortical disease, such as Parkinson's Disease, resulting from dysfunction at the striatal level (Pluck and Brown, 2002), and our data suggest than in AD the locus of dysfunction is at the cortical level, namely the ACC and the OFC.

In sVAD, apathy might be the result of a wider prefrontal disease process, or may suggest a putative role for these regions in mediating apathy, namely due to an involvement of the pars triangularis, of the superior frontal gyrus and of the orbital operculum may suggest that degeneration of the OFC is part of. Ventrolateral and superior frontal regions are also involved in the selection and execution of willed action, and so may contribute to the diminished behavioural responses to everyday challenges displayed by apathetic patients. Recently, increased incidence of white matter hyperintensities in the frontal lobe has been associated with apathy (Starkstein et al., 2009); however, some studies have found no evidence of frontal involvement in apathy (Rosen et al., 2005). A recent and well conducted study examined the relationship between behavior alterations and subcortical lesions (white-matter lesions and lacunes) in AD (Palmqvist et al., 2011). Lacunes in the basal ganglia resulted in a 2- to 3-fold increased risk of delusions, hallucinations and depression, when adjusting for cognition and atrophy. This suggests that basal ganglia lesions can contribute to BPSD in patients with AD, independently of the AD process (Palmqvist et al., 2011).

Being that we have chosen sVAD and AD patients, we have tried to avoid the spurious cases of AD/sVAD coexistence. What we have found is a major involvement of subcortical frontal circuits in sVAD, than in AD, and deriving from that, major evidence of apathy in sVAD, than in AD. In normal conditions, one may propose that the prefrontal cortex internalizes the information from the external and internal environments needed to make a decision about possible actions to be elaborated and performed. Neural signals corresponding to the thoughts or actions are then processed by the basal ganglia in order to validate the most relevant signal. Validation processing may be translated into the extraction of the relevant signal from noise to be readdressed to the output target, namely the prefrontal cortex (Levy and Dubois, 2006), where a clear-cut signal can be detected and contributes to disambiguating decision-making and maintaining or modifying the ongoing behaviour. In pathological situations, if there is a focal destruction within the basal ganglia sub-regions, the signal emerging from the basal ganglia is diminished, the ongoing behaviour is not validated (i.e. not amplified) at the level of the cortex and could be difficult to maintain, and the forthcoming one (if it is not reflexive) is not activated (Levy and Dubois, 2006). In sum, an 'auto-activation' deficit results from the inability of voluntary thoughts or actions to reach the activation threshold due to a decreased signal-to-noise ratio at the level of the prefrontal cortex (Levy and Dubois, 2006).

Thus, in that way, we can justify apathy in sVAD due to the major involvement of cortical-subcortical neural pathways. Many studies should be done to differentiate the anatomical, biological, and physiological eventual different substrate in the subcortical vascular forms, and in degenerative disorders, in order to better differentiate them, if necessary, and eventually to treat them.

Acknowledgements

The Authors wish to thank Andrew Wright Smithson, PhD for the careful reading and corrections of the manuscript.

Author details

Rita Moretti[1], Paola Torre[1], Francesca Esposito[1], Enrica Barro[1], Paola Tomietto[2] and Rodolfo M. Antonello[1]

*Address all correspondence to: moretti@univ.trieste.it

1 Medicina Clinica, Ambulatorio Complicanze Internistiche Cerebrali, Dipartimento Universitario Clinico di Scienze Mediche Tecnologiche e Traslazionali, Università degli Studi di Trieste, Italy

2 Reumatologia-Clinica Medica, AOUTS, Ospedale di Cattinara, Italy

References

[1] Aarsland D, Litvan I, Larsen JP. Neuropsychiatric symptoms of patients with progressive supranuclear palsy and Parkinson's disease. J Neuropsychiatry Clin Neurosci 2001;13:42–9.

[2] Alexopoulos GS, Abrams RC, Young RC, Shamoian CA. Cornell Scale for Depression in Dementia. Biol Psychiatry 1988; 23: 271–84.

[3] American Psychiatric Association. DSM-IV (4th ed.) 1994; Washington, DC: American Psychiatric Association.

[4] Brown RG, Pluck G. Negative symptoms: the "pathology" of motivation and goal-directed behaviour. Trends Neurosci 2000;23:412–17.

[5] Cummings JL, Mega M, Gray K, et al. The Neuropsychiatric Inventory: comprehensive assessment of psychopathology in dementia. Neurology 1994; 44: 2308–14.

[6] Dubois B, Slachevsky A, Litvan I, Pillon B. The FAB: a Frontal Assessment Battery at bedside. Neurology. 2000 Dec 12;55(11):1621-6.

[7] Dujardin K, Sockeel P, elliaux M, DESTEE A, Defebvre L. Apathy may herald cognitive decline and dementia in Parkinsons's Disease. Movement Disorders, 2009 (24); 16: 2391-2397.

[8] Erkinjuntti T. Vascular dementia: challenge of clinical diagnosis. Int Psychogeriatr 1997;9: 77–83.

[9] Folstein M, Folstein S, McHugh P. Mini-Mental state. A practical method for grading the cognitive state of patients for the clinician. J Psychiatr Res 1975;12:189–98.

[10] G. McKhann, D. Drachman, M. Folstein, R. Katzman, D. Price, and E. M. Stadlan, "Clinical diagnosis of Alzheimer's disease: Report of the NINCDS-ADRDA Work Group under the auspices of Department of Health and Human Services Task Force on Alzheimer's Disease," Neurology, 1984; 34, 7. 939–944.

[11] Greene JG, Smith R, Gardiner M, Timburg GC. Measuring behavioural disturbance of elderly demented in patients in the community and its effects on relatives: a factor analytic study. Age Ageing 1982; 11: 121–6.

[12] Levy ML, Cummings JL, Fairbanks LA, et al. Apathy is not depression. J Neuropsychiatry Clin Neurosci 1998;10: 314–19.

[13] Marin RS, Biedrzycki RC, Firinciogullari S. Reliability and validity of the apathy evaluation scale. Psychiatr Res 1991; 38:143–62.

[14] Moretti R, Torre P., Antonello RM, Vidus rosin M, Esposito F, Rubelli Furman M, Bellini G. Apathy: a complex symptom, specific to the clinical pattern pf presentation of Parkinson's Disease. Am. J .Alzheimer's Disease and other Dementias, 2012; Volume 27 (3) 2012 pp. 196 - 201.

[15] Ott BR, Lafleche G, Whelihan WM, et al. Impaired awareness of deficits in Alzheimer's Disease. Alzheimer Dis Assoc Disord 1996; 10: 68–76.

[16] Reisberg B, Borenstein J, Salob SP, et al. Behavioral symptoms in Alzheimer's disease: phenomenology and treatment. J Clin Psychiatr 1987; 48(S1): 9–15.

[17] Roman GC, et al. Vascular dementia: Diagnostic criteria for research studies. (Report of the NINDS-AIREN International Workshop) Neurology,1993; 43, 250-260.

[18] Starkstein SE, Leentjens AF. The nosological position of apathy in clinical practice. J Neurol Neurosurg Psychiatr 2008; 10; 202-209.

[19] Starkstein SE, Mayberg SE, Preziosi TJ, et al. Reliability, validity and clinical correlates of apathy in Parkinson's disease. J Neuropsychiatry 1992;4:134–9.

[20] Stuss DT, Van Reekum R, Murphy KJ. Differentiation of states and causes of apathy. In: Borod JC(ed.): The Neuropsychology of emotion. Oxford: Oxford University Press. 2000. Pp. 340--363.

[21] Chase T. N. "Apathy in neuropsychiatric disease: diagnosis, pathophysiology, and treatment," Neurotoxicity Research, 2011; vol. 19, no. 2: pp. 266–278.

[22] Wechsler D. Wechsler adult intelligence scale manual-R. New York: Grune & Stratton. 1981.

[23] Mendez M. F., Lauterbach E. C., Sampson S. M. An evidence-based review of the psychopathology of frontotemporal dementia: a report of the ANPA Committee on Research Journal of Neuropsychiatry and Clinical Neurosciences, 2008; vol. 20, no. 2: 130–149

[24] Starkstein S. E., Jorge R., Mizrahi R., Robinson R. G. A prospective longitudinal study of apathy in Alzheimer's Disease Journal of Neurology, Neurosurgery & Psychiatry, 2006; vol. 77, no. 1: 8–11.

[25] Chow T. W., Binns M. A., Cummings J. L. et al. Apathy symptom profile and behavioral associations in frontotemporal dementia vs dementia of Alzheimer type," Archives of Neurology, 2009; vol. 66, no. 7: 888–893.

[26] Zamboni G., Huey E.D., Krueger F., Nichelli P. F., Grafman J. Apathy and disinhibition in frontotemporal dementia: insights into their neural correlates, Neurology, 2008; vol. 71, no. 10: 736–742.

[27] Peters F., Perani D., Herholz K. et al. Orbitofrontal dysfunction related to both apathy and disinhibition in frontotemporal Dementia. Dementia and Geriatric Cognitive Disorders, 2006; vol. 21, no. 5-6: 373–379.

[28] Massimo L., Powers C., Moore P. et al. Neuroanatomy of apathy and disinhibition in frontotemporal lobar degeneration. Dementia and Geriatric Cognitive Disorders, 2009; vol. 27, no. 1: 96–104.

[29] Marshall G. A., Fairbanks L. A., Tekin S., Vinters H. V., Cummings J. L. Neuropathologic correlates of apathy in Alzheimer's disease. Dementia and Geriatric Cognitive Disorders, 2006; vol. 21, no. 3: 144–147.

[30] Apostolova L.G., Akopyan G. G., Partiali N. et al. Structural correlates of apathy in Alzheimer's disease. Dementia and Geriatric Cognitive Disorders, 2007; vol. 24, no. 2: 91–97.

[31] Marshall G. A., Monserratt L., Harwood D., Mandelkern M., Cummings J. L., Sultzer
      D. L. Positron emission tomography metabolic correlates of apathy in Alzheimer dis-
      ease. Archives of Neurology, 2007; vol. 64, no. 7: 1015–1020.

[32] Marin R. S. Apathy: a neuropsychiatric syndrome. Journal of Neuropsychiatry and
      Clinical Neurosciences, 1991; vol. 3, no. 3: pp. 243–254.

[33] Marin R. S. Apathy: Concept, Syndrome, Neural Mechanisms, and Treatment," Semi-
      nars in Clinical Neuropsychiatry, 1996; vol. 1, no. 4: 304–314.

[34] Moll J., Zahn R., de Oliveira-Souza R. et al. Impairment of prosocial sentiments is as-
      sociated with frontopolar and septal damage in frontotemporal dementia," Neuro-
      Image, 2011; vol. 54, no. 2: 1735–1742.

[35] Quaranta D, Marra C, Rossi C, Gainotti G, Masullo C. Different Apathy Profile in Be-
      havioral Variant of Frontotemporal Dementia and Alzheimer's Disease: A Prelimina-
      ry Investigation. Current Gerontology and Geriatrics Research, 2012; Article ID
      719250, 8 pages; doi:10.1155/2012/719250

[36] Tunnard C., Whitehead D., Hurt C., Wahlund L.O., Mecocci P., Tsolaki M., Vellas B.,
      Spenger C., Kłoszewska I., Soininen H., Lovestone S., Simmons A., on behalf of the
      AddNeuroMed Consortium. Apathy and cortical atrophy in Alzheimer's disease. Int
      J Geriatr Psychiatry 2011; 26: 741–748.

[37] Apostolova LG, Akopyan GG, Partiali N, et al. Structural correlates of apathy in Alz-
      heimer's disease. Dement Geriartr Cogn Disord. 2007; 24: 91–97.

[38] Bruen PD, McGeown WJ, Shanks MF, Vennner A. Neuroanatomical correlates of
      neuropsychiatric sypmptoms in Alzheimer's disease. Brain 2008; 131: 2455–2463.

[39] Guimara͂es HC, Levy R, Teixeira AL, Beato RG, Caramelli P. Neurobiology of apa-
      thy in Alzheimer's disease. Arq Neuro-Psiquiatr. 2008; 66: 436–443.

[40] Holthoff VA, Beuthien-Bauman B, Kalbe E, et al. Regional cerebral metabolism in
      early Alzheimer's disease with clinically significant apathy or depression. Biol. Psy-
      chiatry 2005; 57: 412–421.

[41] Lanctot KL, Moosa S, Herrmann N, et al. A SPECT study of apathy in Alzheimer's
      disease. Dement Geriartr Cogn Disord. 2007; 24: 65–72.

[42] Laveretsky H, Ballmaier M, Pham D, Toga A, Kumar A. Neuroanatomical character-
      istics of geriatric apathy and depression: a magnetic resonance imaging study. Am J
      Geriatr Psychiatry 2007; 15: 386–394.

[43] Marshall GA, Fairbanks LA, Tekin S, Vinters HV, Cummings JL. Neuropathologic
      correlates of apathy in Alzheimer's disease. Dement Geriatr Cogn Disord. 2006; 21:
      144–147.

[44] Marshall GA, Monserratt L, Harwood D, et al. Positron emission tomography meta-
      bolic correlates of apathy in Alzheimer's disease. Arch Neurol. 2007; 64: 1015–1020.

[45] Migneco O, BenoitM, Koulibaly PM, et al. Perfusion brain SPECT and statistical para-
      metric mapping analysis indicate that apathy is a cingulate syndrome: a study in
      Alzheimer's disease and nondemented patients. Neuroimage 2001; 13: 896–902.

[46] Pluck GC, Brown RG. Apathy in Parkinson's disease. J Neurol Neurosurg Psychiatr
      2002; 73: 636–642.

[47] Robert PH, Darcourt G, Koulibaly MP, et al. Lack of initiative and interest in Alz-
      heimer's disease: a single photon emission computed tomography study. Eur J Neu-
      rol 2006; 13: 729–735.

[48] Rosen HJ, Allison SC, Schaeur GF, et al. Neuroanatomical correlates of behavioral
      disorders in dementia. Brain 2005; 128: 2612–2625.

[49] Starkstein SE, Mizrahi R, Capizzano AA, et al. Neuroimaging correlates of apathy
      and depression in Alzheimer's Disease. J Neuropsychiatry Clin Neurosci. 2009; 21:
      259–265.

[50] Tekin S, Mega MS, Masterman DM, et al. Orbitofrontal and anterior cingulate cortex
      neurofibrillary tangle burden is associated with agitation in Alzheimer's disease.
      Ann Neurol 2001; 49: 355–361.

[51] Starkstein SE, Petracca G, Chemerinski E, Kremer J. Syndrome validity of apathy in
      Alzheimer's disease. Am. J. Psychiatry 2001; 158: 872–577.

[52] Marin RS, Firinciogullari S, Biedrzycki RC. The sources of convergence between
      measures of apathy and depression. J. Affect. Disord. 1993; 28: 7–14.

[53] Clarke DE, Van Reekum R, Patel J, Simard M, Gomez E, Streiner DL. An appraisal of
      the psychometric properties of the clinician version of the Apathy Evaluation Scale
      (AESC)- Int. J. Methods Psychiatr. Res. 2007; 16: 97–110.Resnick B, Zimmerman SI,
      Magaziner J et al. Use of the Apathy Evaluation Scale as a measure of motivation in
      elderly people. Rehabil. Nurs. 1998; 23: 141–147.

[54] Tatsch M, Bottino CM, Azevedo D et al. Neuropsychiatric symptoms in Alzheimer
      disease and cognitively impaired, non-demented elderly from a community-based
      sample in Brazil: Prevalence and relationship with dementia severity. Am. J. Geriatr.
      Psychiatry 2006; 14: 438–445.

[55] Jung Hsieh C, Chu H, Jror-Serk Cheng J, Shen WW, Lin CC. Validation of apathy
      evaluation scale and assessment of severity of apathy in Alzheimer's dis-
      ease.pcn_Psychiatry and Clinical Neurosciences 2012; 66: 227–234

[56] Starkstein SE, Brockman S, Bruce D, Petracca G. Anosognosia Is a Significant Predic-
      tor ofApathy in Alzheimer's Disease. The Journal of Neuropsychiatry and Clinical
      Neurosciences 2010; 22:378 –383

[57] Richard E, Schmand B, Eikelenboom P, Yang SC, Ligthart SA, Moll van Charante EP,
      van Gool WA. Symptoms of apathy are associated with progression from mild cogni-

tive impairment to Alzheimer's disease in non-depressed subjects. Dement Geriatr Cogn Disord. 2012;33(2-3):204-9.

[58] Palmqvist S, Sarwari A, Wattmo C, Bronge L, Zhang Y, Wahlund LO, Nägga K. Association between subcortical lesions and behavioral and psychological symptoms in patients with Alzheimer's disease. Dement Geriatr Cogn Disord. 2011;32(6):417-23.

[59] Massimo L, Powers C, Moore P, Vesely L, Avants B, Gee J, Libon DJ, Grossman M. Neuroanatomy of apathy and disinhibition in frontotemporal lobar degeneration. Dement Geriatr Cogn Disord. 2009;27(1):96-104.

[60] Levy R., Dubois B. Apathy and the functional anatomy of the prefrontal cortex-basal ganglia circuits. Cerebral Cortex, 2006; 16, 7: 916–928.

[61] Moretti R, Torre P, Antonello RM (Eds). Basal Ganglia and Thalamus: their role in cognition and behavior. Novascience Editor, NewYork. 2009.

Chapter 6

Predicting Cognitive Decline in Alzheimer's Disease (AD): The Role of Clinical, Cognitive Characteristics and Biomarkers

Mei Sian Chong and Tih-Shih Lee

Additional information is available at the end of the chapter

1. Introduction

Given the rapid ageing of the population worldwide, global estimates of AD - generally considered to be the commonest subtype of dementia - are expected to increase from the current estimated 25 million to 63 million in 2030, and by 2050, a staggering 114 million [1]. Over the last two decades in particular, significant but modest breakthroughs in pharmacological treatment of this devastating condition have occurred. Presently, there is increasing conviction that intervention (especially disease-modifying therapy) will have to be instituted at the earliest possible stage of the illness to confer the greatest benefit.

Prevailing clinical criteria for Mild Cognitive Impairment (MCI) have low to moderate diagnostic accuracy in identifying and predicting progression to dementia. MCI is an unstable clinical construct where some patients convert (MCI-converters) while others remain relatively stable (MCI non-converters). As observed from neuropathological and recent biomarker studies, the accumulation of AD pathology (β-amyloid plaques and neurofibrillary tangles) may precede the onset of clinical disease by as long as 20-30 years [2,3]. This suggests that functional and structural brain changes may occur prior to apparent clinical manifestations of cognitive impairment (Figure 1). However, the current definition of MCI is based primarily on clinical and neuropsychological criteria, and this may have contributed to limited demonstration of efficacy in therapeutic and disease-modifying trials thus far. Supplementing existing criteria with information about biomarkers may enrich the definition of MCI This provided the impetus for the development of reliable biomarkers such as cerebrospinal fluid (CSF), neuroimaging and blood biomarkers to complement clinical approaches in early diagnosis and predicting progression. In support of this, the recent proposed criteria for symptomatic pre-dementia phase of AD (MCI), preclinical AD and presymptomatic AD have included biomarkers reflecting molecular pathology, downstream measures of structural and functional/metabolic changes, and associated biochemical changes in their research diagnostic armamentarium [4].

Longitudinal studies in AD subjects have also noted variability in disease progression. In one study, 11.9% of subjects exhibit rapid cognitive decline while some remained relatively stable [5]. Other studies that utilized parameters such as the decline in Mini Mental State Examination (MMSE) scores [6, 7] (≥3 point decline) also reported a distinctive difference in the clinical course between the fast-progressors and slow-progressors.

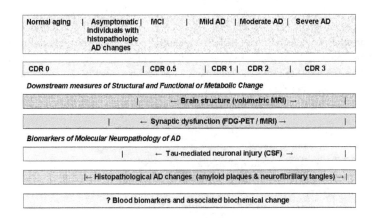

Figure 1. Clinical Continuum of Alzheimer's disease and hypothetical biomarker model

In this chapter, we will review the body of evidence on the use of various clinical and co-morbid factors, alone and/or in combination with biomarkers, on predicting rapid cognitive decline across the spectrum of cognitive impairment – defined in terms of AD progression in MCI subjects and rapid cognitive decline in AD subjects. We will also look at longitudinal biomarker measurements as well as their role (alone and/ in combination with clinical and comorbid factors) in predicting cognitive decline and disease trajectories. We will discuss the implications of current research findings to their application in clinical and therapeutic trials. The chapter is not intended to be an exhaustive review of this burgeoning literature, but instead to highlight integrative and potentially novel lines of inquiry.

2. Clinical and cognitive/ behavioural characteristics (table 1)

A number of socio-demographic factors and vascular risk factors have been found to increase risk of development of AD.

Increased risk of cognitive decline in diabetes may reflect a dual pathologic process involving both cerebrovascular damage and neurodegenerative changes. Several possible pathophysiological mechanisms may include hyperglycemia, insulin resistance [8], oxidative stress, advanced glycation end products, and inflammatory cytokines. A shared clinicopathologic study alluded to the potential shared predisposition for developing amyloid in both the pancreas and brain [9]. This is supported by a study of intranasal insulin preventing cognitive decline, cerebral atrophy and white matter changes in mouse models [10]. Diabetes and pre-diabetes have been found to be associated with AD progression in MCI subjects, with pro-gression from MCI to dementia accelerated by 3.18 years[11]. The stronger effect of pre-diabetes on MCI conversion may be caused by high glycemic level in pre-diabetes and increased insulin resistance [12]. Although antihypertensive therapy has been shown to be associated with reduced rate of conversion to AD in midregional proatrial natriuretic peptide-stratified subjects with MCI [13], there has been a paucity of data with regard to the individual effect of hypertension on MCI-converters[14]. A non-significant trend was found for cerebro-vascular disease as a risk factor for MCI-converters[15]. Diabetes, hypertension and cerebro-vascular disease have been found to be associated with faster progression rate in dementia [16-19]. Although mid-life hypercholesterolemia has been repeatedly shown to increase risk of late-life dementia, there is relatively little evidence of its influence on MCI-converters and the rate of AD decline [20].

Study variable	Population	Results	Key findings
Predicting AD conversion in MCI subjects			
Diabetes and pre-diabetes [11]	302 aMCI and 182 CIND subjects aged ≥ 75 years over 9 years	155 subjects had AD progression	HR 2.87 diabetes (95%CI 1.3-6.34) HR 4.96 pre-diabetes (95% CI 2.27 -10.84) Accelerated progression by 3.18 years
Vascular risk factors [21]	837 MCI subjects followed annually over 5 years	298 converters 352 stable	HR 2.04 (95% CI 1.33-3.11) Hypertension HR 1.84 (95% CI 1.19-2.84) Diabetes HR 1.62 (95% CI 1.00 – 2.62) Hypercholesterolemia HR 1.11 (95% CI 1.04-1.18) Cerebrovascular disease HR 1.60 (95% CI 1.03 – 2.49)
Diabetes, baseline white matter severity, baseline moderate-to-severe carotid stenosis and carotid stenosis change [22]	257 MCI subjects over 3 years	MCI conversion to AD 7.05%/year	Diabetes HR 2.92 (95% CI 1.12-7.6) Baseline WMC severity (mild vs severe) HR 0.04 (95% CI 0.006-0.242) Baseline carotid stenosis (moderate vs mild) HR 8.46 (95% CI 2.1-34.14) Carotid stenosis change HR 124.1 (95% CI 0.95- 16,209.68)
Stroke [15]	121 MCI subjects over 3 years	MCI conversion to AD based on age strata rate (per 100 person-years) Total 2.3 65-69y 0 70-74y 0 75-79 3.1 80-84y 2.0	Stroke RR 4.0 (95% CI 0.92-13.87)
Metabolic syndrome [8]	49 MCI subjects with metabolic syndrome and 72 without metabolic syndrome	Progression to dementia	67.6 (95% CI 35.17 – 129.93) Rate 1000 per person-years
Age [23]	97 amnestic MCI 88 cognitively-unimpaired controls followed up mean 38.8 mths	Annual rate of progression to AD	Odds ratio = 4.5 of AD progression Older age [exp(β)=1.11, SE(β)=0.7, WALD=4.2, p=0.040] predictors of AD conversion
Empirically weighted and Combined neuropsycho-gical battery [42]	43 MCI subjects	14 subsequently converted to AD	Multivariate combinations achieved 84% accuracy, 86% Sn, 83%Sp in predicting AD progression (using episodic memory, speeded executive function, recognition memory (false positives). recognition memory (true positives), speed in visuospatial memory, visuospatial episodic memory
Learning measure and retention measure [43]	607 MCI and HC patients in ADNI cohort divided into 4 groups: (based on learning and retention)	Conversion to AD at 2 years	Low-learning, Low retention OR17.84, 95%CI 7.37-43.10, p<0.001; Low-learning, High reten-tion OR 9.01, 95%CI2.98-27.21,p<0.001; High learning, low retention OR8.48, 95%CI 3.45-20.86, p<0.001 (high learning, high retention as reference group)
MISplus [44]	40MCI subjects	Conversion to to AD at 18 months (n=7)	OR 0.28, 95%CI 0.099-0.79) At cut-off of 2, PPV 71.5%, NPV 91.5%, Accuracy 87%

Hypertension [16]	135 incident AD Patients in Cache Country Dementia Progression Study	Rapid decline on CDR-sum of boxes and MMSE using linear mixed models	Systolic BP ≥160 versus <160mmHg (controlling for other vascular variables) for CDR-SB coeff X time 1.78 (95% CI 1.20-2.36) for MMSE coeff X time -2.38 (-3.23,-1.53)
Hypertension [17]	719 AD patients In multi-center Trial	ADAS-cog increase by ≥1 standard deviation of baseline ADAS-cog score of	OR 6.9 (95% CI 1.5-31.1, p=0.005)
Diabetes [18]	154 AD patients attending Dementia center	Disease progression of decrease of 5 pts or more on MMSE	Crude OR 0.38 (95% CI 0.2-0.9) Multivariate OR 0.36 (95% CI 0.1-0.9)
Cerebrovascular disease[19]	224 AD patients	Decline in MMSE, ADAS-cog and SIB difference	No difference in vascular risk factors except cerebrovascular disease (mean difference in MMSE 13.6 (-14.3—7.6); ADAS-cog 27 (-30.1- -13.7); SIB 54.4 (-62.3—29.9)
Vascular risk factors including heart disease, stroke, diabetes, hypertension), smoking, pre-diagnosis blood lipid and LDL-C [20]	156 AD patients living in community mean age 83 y	AD decline using generalized estimating equation models	Only higher LDL-cholesterol was independently associated with faster cognitive decline. Stratified according to APOEe4 showed higher total cholesterol, higher LDL, stroke and heart disease associated with faster decline.
Age [24]	201 Caucasian Probable/Possible AD subjects at ADRC, Pittsburgh	Latent class mixture models of quadratic trajectories including random intercept and concomitant variables (MMSE)	Best latent trajectory model: Initial MMSE and age. Parameter estimate 0.85, p<.001 for MMSE, Parameter estimate 0.04,p =0.04 for age.
Education [27]	127 persons in Bronx Aging study developed dementia (out of 488 community dwelling subjects)	Change point models to test predictions of cognitive reserve hypothesis using Buschke Selective Reminding Test (SRT)	Prior to diagnosis, lower levels of formal education associated with poorer performance on memory and verbal fluency. Accelerated decline in SRT shown by estimated annual rates of decline for 16 years, 9.5 years and 4 years of formal education was 3.22, 2.57 and 2.03 points/year respectively.
Neuropsychiatric symptoms [30]	177 memory-clinic AD outpatients	Rapid disease progression defined as loss of ≥1 ability in ADL or drop of ≥ 5 points on MMSE	Affective syndrome increased risk of functional decline (HR2.0, 95%CI 1.1-3.6) AND Manic syndrome (HR 3.2, 95% CI 1.3-7.5)
Pre-progression rate- Clinician estimate of of duration and baseline MMSE [28]	798 probable AD subjects from Alzheimer's Disease and Memory Disorders Centre	Random effects linear regression to calculate pre-progression categories and of change in ADAS-cog, VSAT Time, VSAT Errors, CDR Sum of boxes, PSMS and IADL scores	Slopes of ADAScog and PSMS change for slow pre-progression smaller than fast pre-progression. Rates of change on ADAScog slower for Intermediate pre-progression group. Slow progressors survived longer.
Memory and executive Functioning [45]	154 newly diagnosed AD Patients	Rapid progression of ≥ 5MMSE decrease over 2yrs	Memory moderate deficits: HR 1.3 (95%CI: 0.4-4.5); severe deficits: HR 2.3 (95%CI: 0.6-9.0). Executive functions moderate deficits: HR 3.5 (95%CI 0.9-13.7); severe deficits: HR 5.7 (95%CI 1.4-23.2)

HR = Hazards ratio; PPV = Positive predictive value

95% CI= 95% confidence interval; NPV= Negative predictive value

WMC= White matter severity; MMSE =Mini Mental State Examination

RR= Relative risk; SIB = Severe Impairment Battery

OR= Odds ratio

Table 1. Clinical and cognitive/ behavioural characteristics in predicting AD conversion in MCI patients and rapid AD progression/ decline

Vascular risk factors, as a composite entity, have been shown to be associated with MCI conversion [21]. The individual risk factors of hypertension, diabetes, cerebrovascular disease and hypercholesterolemia in the study were associated with high risk of MCI conversion. Treatment of hypertension, diabetes and hypercholesterolemia showed reduced risk of MCI conversion. In the same Chongqing study, the authors showed separately the association of diabetes, baseline white matter changes (WMC), baseline moderate-to-severe carotid stenosis and carotid stenosis change during follow-up to be predictors of MCI conversion [22]. A separate longitudinal community study (ILSA- Italian Longitudinal Study on Aging) showed MCI progression to AD of 2.3 per 100 person-years with stroke as the only vascular risk factor associated with progression [15].

The heterogeneity of AD syndrome is likely related to, other than amyloid and tau pathology, a number of other factors, such as impaired energy metabolism, oxidative stress, neuro-inflammation, insulin and insulin growth factor (IGF) resistance, and insulin/ IGF-deficiency. These factors are often included as variables of interest in studies attempting to develop diagnostic and therapeutic targets for this disease. Brain insulin resistance promotes oxidative stress, reactive oxygen species (ROS) generation, DA damage and mitochondrial dysfunction, all of which drive pro-apoptosis, pro-inflammatory and pro-AβPP-Aβ cascades. Also, hyperinsulinaemia increases AβPP-Aβ and inflammatory indices in the brain, also promoting formation of advanced glycation end-products which lead to increased generation of ROS. Tau gene expression and phosphorylation are also regulated by insulin and IGF stimulation, where brain insulin and IGF resistance may result in decreased signaling through phosphoinositol-3-kinase (PI3K), Akt and Wnt/β-catenin and increased activation of GSK-3β – which is partly responsible for tau hyperphosphorylation. Hence, the focus on vascular factors in AD is justified based on chronic hyperglycemia, hyperinsulinemia, oxidative stress, advanced glycation end-products and inflammation promoting vascular disease [8].

The metabolic syndrome defined by the Third Adults Treatment Panel of the National Cholesterol Education Program as a combination of three or more of the following components: abdominal obesity (waist circumference >102cm for men and >88 cm for women; elevated plasma triglycerides ($\geq$150mg/dl); low HDL cholesterol (<40mg/dl for men and <50mg/dl for women); high blood pressure ($\geq$130/ $\geq$85mmHg) or being in hypertensive treatment; and high fasting plasma glucose ($\geq$110mg/dl). This represents a clustering of vascular risk factors for morbidity and mortality. In addition, these factors may interact synergistically to influence cognition in a negative manner. Among MCI patients the presence of metabolic syndrome independently predicted an increased risk of progression to dementia over 3.5 years of follow-up. [23]

Older age has been shown to predict MCI-converters [24]. Latent class modeling methods and disease system analysis approach to characterize trajectories of cognitive decline in AD cohorts have also shown initial MMSE and age to best predict decline [25,26]. However, separate studies using AD clinical trial data with subjects on Donepezil have shown younger age to predict faster decline in placebo-treated patients [27]. Low education is a risk factor for AD. The cognitive reserve hypothesis predicts that persons with higher education delay the onset of accelerated cognitive decline; however, once AD disease process begins, it takes a more rapid course due to increased disease burden [28]. Pre-progression rate (calculated using clinician's standardized assessment of symptom duration in years and baseline MMSE) has also been shown to predict cognitive decline trajectory [29]. Neuropsychiatric symptoms have also been shown to predict faster cognitive and functional decline [25,30,31].

Prospective studies of amnestic MCI (a-MCI) subjects have shown that episodic memory (such as delayed recall of word lists [32-34], spatial short term memory and visual recognition memory [35], and paired-associates learning [36,37]), semantic memory [37,38], attentional processing [39] and mental speed consistently predicted MCI converters. Within a very mild cognitive impairment group, higher CDR-sum of boxes and lower executive function predicted AD conversion [40]. Similarly, in a retrospective study of MCI-converters, verbal and visual memory, associative learning, vocabulary, executive functioning and other verbal tests of general intelligence were impaired at baseline [41]. An empirically weighted and combined set of neuropsychological tests involving domains of episodic memory, speeded executive functioning, recognition memory (false and true positives), visuospatial memory processing speed, and visual episodic memory together were strong predictors of MCI conversion to AD [42]. A recent study demonstrated that MCI individuals with learning deficits on the Rey Auditory Verbal Learning test showed widespread pattern of gray matter loss at baseline, as compared to retention deficits which was associated with more focal gray matter loss. However, impaired learning had modestly better predictive power than impaired retention, highlighting the importance of including learning measures in addition to retention measures when predicting outcomes in MCI subjects [43]. Verbal cued recall measured using the Memory Impairment Screen plus (MISplus) has also been shown to predict MCI conversion [44].

In subjects with AD, rapid disease progression was noted more frequently in subjects with higher education and those with moderate severity of global impairment. More severe memory impairment and executive dysfunctioning were associated with higher probabilities of progression at 2 years [45].

Longitudinally, follow-up of those who developed AD versus those who were non-demented prior to AD diagnosis, showed no evidence for accelerated decline of episodic memory from 6 to 3 years prior to incident dementia diagnosis [46]. Working memory (using digit span backward and forward as well as digit ordering) also did not show temporal change as a potentially useful marker of progression [47].

2.1. Summary

Age, vascular risk factors and metabolic syndrome affect AD conversion in MCI subjects. However, there is currently a lack of data on the effect of intensive vascular risk factor treatment in delaying/halting the rate of progression in MCI subjects. Educational attainment plays an interesting role in AD. In support of the cognitive reserve hypothesis, higher educational attainment predicts delay of the onset of accelerated cognitive decline; however, once AD disease process begins, it takes a more rapid course due to increased disease burden.

Neuropsychological tests, especially episodic memory and executive functioning tests, seem to predict MCI-converters. When assessing MCI subjects, the inclusion of impaired learning in addition to retention measures may improve predictive power of AD progression from MCI. More severe cognitive impairment is associated with rapid AD progression.

3. Cerebrospinal fluid biomarkers (tables 2)

The most widely studied candidate CSF biomarkers include CSF total tau (t-tau), 42 amino acid form of Aβ (Aβ$_{1-42}$) and phosphorylated tau protein (p-tau) [48]. They reflect respectively the corresponding central pathogenetic process of neuronal degeneration, amyloid-β peptide deposition in plaques, and hyperphosphorylation of tau with subsequent tangle formation. Fagan et al has also recently demonstrated that CSF Aβ and tau protein measurements, performed using INNOTEST enzyme-linked immunosorbent assay (ELISA) and INNO-BIA AlzBio3, were highly correlated with brain amyloid load, as assessed by PET and Pittsburgh compound B amyloid-imaging (r value from 0.77 to 0.94)[49]. This was further suggested, by a study of antemortem CSF concentrations of Aβ$_{1-42}$ and t-tau/ Aβ$_{1-42}$ ratio in an autopsy-confirmed AD cohort, that the standardization of biomarker techniques could potentially replace autopsy-confirmed AD for future diagnosis of definite AD [50].

3.1. Established CSF biomarkers

CSF biomarkers of elevated t-tau [51-56], high p-tau [52,53,57,58], low Aβ$_{1-42}$ [52,53], and combinations of high t-tau/ p-tau and low Aβ$_{1-42}$ concentrations [59-64], have been shown to be predictive of MCI-conversion to AD. The consistent feature in all of these studies is that increased CSF t-tau and p-tau concentrations are highly sensitive while low Aβ$_{1-42}$ concentration is more specific. A recent longitudinal study showed that subjects with the lowest baseline Aβ42, highest tau and and p-tau concentration exhibited the most rapid MMSE decline. In addition, while there was little difference in the levels of these CSF biomarkers between stable MCI and cognitively healthy subjects, MCI-AD converters had the highest total tau concentrations [65].

High CSF t-tau and p-tau concentration (but not Aβ42) was associated with more rapid MMSE decline in a 3-year prospective longitudinal study. This suggests that increased t-tau levels reflect intensity of disease and hence rapidity of AD progression, while Aβ42 is more a diagnostic state marker, not associated with rate or stage of AD [65,66]. Another study showed p-tau to poorly differentiate between AD and vascular dementia, but to correlate with MMSE progression [67]. In contrast, another recent report showed lower Aβ42 levels to be associated with rapid-progressors compared with slow-progressors [68]. Wallin et al showed that AD subjects with a combination of low Aβ42 and very high CSF t-tau and p-tau levels performed worse on baseline cognitive tests, with faster deterioration, poorer outcome to cholinesterase inhibitor treatment and increased mortality [69].

With respect to serial biomarker measurements with disease progression, we found studies showing increasing p-tau 231 levels with disease progression in MCI subjects [70, 71] compared to controls over a period of 12-24 months. No definite trends were observed with Aβ40 and Aβ42 in the same studies [70,71]. A recent longitudinal study showed that nonspecific CSF biomarkers, in particular isoprostane, demonstrated an increase over time, which was correlated with AD conversion in MCI subjects and cognitive decline (as assessed by MMSE) [72].

Study variable	Population	Results	Key findings
Predicting AD conversion in MCI subjects			
Combination CSF biomarkers [64]	137 MCI subjects compared to 39 healthy controls	42% converted to AD	- t-tau >350ng/L & Aβ42 <530 ng/L: Sn: 95%, Sp 83% of AD conversion HR 30, 95% CI 9.32-96.8, p<0.001 - p-tau >60ng/L & Aβ42 <530 ng/L: Sn 95%, Sp 81% of AD conversion HR 26.3, 95% CI 8.16-83.4, p<0.001 - t-tau/ Aβ42 ratio < 6.5 (t-tau>350ng/L) Sn 95%, Sp 87% of AD conversion HR 32.8 (10.2-105.6,p<0.001)
Predicting rapid AD progression/ decline			
CSF biomarker concentration [66]	142 AD subjects followed-up over 5 years	35 subjects had t-tau>800ng/L	- High levels of t-tau correlated with lower baseline MMSE scores. More rapid decline in MMSE score correlated with higher baseline t-tau (r_s=-0.23,p=008). - p-tau>110ng/L showed lower baseline MMSE scores but no difference in progression. - Aβ42 showed no difference in baseline scores or progression.
CSF p-tau concentration [67]	70 AD and VD subjects with 36 age-matched healthy controls	Cognitive decline assessed 12 mth (MMSE ≥ 5 point decline after 1yr)	58% of probable AD patients showed p-tau concentration higher than 36.08ng/L. Cognitive decline correlated with p-tau concentration (x^2 =12.442, p=0.001).
CSF Aβ42 concentration [68]	74 AD subjects	Rapid progressors defined at MMSE decline >4/years	Lower Aβ42 CSF concentration (mean 292 pg/ ml) in fast-progressors compared to slow-progressors (mean 453 pg/ml) (p=0.042)
Low CSF Aβ42 and high CSF t-tau and p-tau levels [69]	151 AD subjects	k-means cluster analysis done. Cluster 1 low Aβ42 and low t-tau, p-tau Cluster 2 low Aβ42 and intermediate t-tau, p-tau Cluster 3 low Aβ42 and high t-tau, p-tau	Cluster 3 performed poorer on baseline cognitive tests. They exhibited poorer outcome of cholinesterase inhibitor treatment. Cognition deterioriated faster over time with substantially increased mortality rate.

HR = Hazards ratio

CRP = C-reactive protein

MMSE =Mini Mental State Examination

OR = Odds ratio

Sn = Sensitivity

Sp= Specific

LR+ = positive Likelihood ratio

LR - = negative Likelihood ratio

HR = Hazards ratio

95% CI= 95% confidence interval

Table 2. Cerebrospinal fluid biomarkers in predicting AD conversion in MCI patients and rapid AD progression/ decline

Faster progression of brain atrophy (in terms of regional cortical thinning) has been found in the presence of lower Aβ1-42 levels and higher p-tau in Alzheimer's Disease Neuroimaging Initiative (ADNI) data [73].

3.2. Novel CSF approaches

In a study in which novel CSF biomarkers were identified through mass spectrometry and re-evaluated by ELISA, it was found that NrCAM, YKL-40, chromogranin A and Carnosinase I were potentially able to improve the diagnostic accuracy of existing Aβ42 and tau CSF biomarkers. This could potentially improve characterization of clinic-pathological stages of the cognitive continuum from cognitive normalcy to mild dementia, with the promise of potential utility in clinical trials and monitoring disease progression [74]. Other potential CSF biomarkers include nanoparticle-based amyloid-β-derived diffusible ligands (ADDLs)[75], as well as a multiplexed immunoassay panel of a combination of a subset of markers, in particular, calbindin, which showed significant prognostic potential [76]. Preliminary data have also shown that soluble Aβ oligomers might inhibit long-term potentiation and hence, play an important role in AD pathogenesis. The increasing appreciation of Aβ oligomers (as compared to its native forms) in the pathogenesis of AD may suggest novel pathways to biomarkers, such as anti-oligomer antibodies that are specific for the soluble oligomeric state (as opposed to the fibrillar states). By quantifying Aβ oligomer formation, anti-oligomer antibodies may provide a promising strategy for monitoring disease progression [77,78].

Concerns with CSF biomarkers include measurement variability occurring through lack of standardization of CSF assays [79], high inter-laboratory and between-assay variance, sampling-handling factors, post lumbar-puncture headache, and poor acceptability to patients, especially if repeated measurements are involved. In an attempt to overcome these, the Alzheimer's Association has launched a global quality-control program for AD CSF biomarkers, which will be administered from the Clinical Neurochemistry Laboratory in Molndal, Sweden. This includes reference samples for use in studies, allowing normalization of biomarker levels and meta-analyses of published papers [80].

3.3. Summary

Elevated CSF total tau, p-tau, low Aβ and high tau: Aβ concentrations have been consistently shown to highly predict MCI-converters and AD progression. CSF Aβ and tau may reach a plateau at a relatively early stage of disease and remain fairly constant thereafter, limiting its utility for longitudinal measurement and in monitoring therapeutic response at the more advanced/ established stage of AD. However, it remains an important biomarker during the preclinical and prodromal stages of AD, reflecting the central pathogenic neurodegenerative process. Novel CSF biomarkers hold promise of circumventing this current limitation, especially Aβ oligomers and their potential use in documenting disease progression as well as being a potential therapeutic target. The invasive nature of lumbar puncture and standard-ization issues preclude its current routine clinical use.

4. Blood markers (table 3)

Peripheral blood is one of the most convenient sources of biomarkers. While the quest for a marker with high sensitivity and specificity has been ongoing for decades, no single blood-derived biomarker has been particularly outstanding in the diagnosis of AD, in predicting conversion from MCI to AD and in predicting slow and fast progression. The following are some of the most studied biomarkers. One should note that negative studies are usually not published and hence publication bias is possible.

Study variable	Population	Results	Key findings
Predicting AD conversion in MCI subjects			
Abeta Hansson [82]	Cohort 1: 117 MCI subjects followed up for 4 -7 years; Cohort 2: 110 followed up for 2 – 4 years	48 (41%) subjects of cohort 1 developed AD; 15 (14%) subjects of cohort 2 developed AD	No difference in plasma Abeta levels between MCI subjects that subsequently developed AD and HC or stable MCI subjects. HR (per SD decrease adjusted for age, sex): Aβ40 1.08 (0.78-1.51), Aβ42 0.95 (0.71-1.27), Aβ42/42 ratio 0.83 (0.64-1.08)
Koyama [84]	Meta-analysis with 10,303 subjects	Summary risk ratio of 1.60 and 1.67 for AD and dementia respectively	Association of low plasma Abeta42/Abeta40 ratio with AD and dementia.
C Reactive Protein [86]	168 MCI subjects followed up over 2 years	58 subjects developed dementia	Association of high plasma CRP level with accelerated cognitive deterioration and increased risk of AD. MMSE score was significantly lower for patients with high CRP levels than those with low CRP levels (-4.9 ± 5.4 vs -3.2 ±4.2, $p < 0.05$)
APOE [90]	35 prospective cohort studies of MCI subjects, including 6095 subjects over 2.9 years of follow-up	1236 developed AD.	APOE-ε4 allele is associated with a moderately increased risk for progression from MCI to AD-type dementia. OR for MCI subjects with APOE ε4 progression to AD 2.29 (95% CI 1.88 to 2.80).Sn 0.53 (95% CI 0.4 to 0.61), Sp 0.67 (95% CI 0.62 to 0.71), PPV 0.57 (95% CI 0.48 to 0.66), NPV 0.75 (95% CI 0.70 to 0.80). LR+ 1.60 (95% CI 1.48 to 1.72), and LR- 0.75 (95% CI 0.67 t o0.82). Meta-regression showed that Sn,Sp and NPV were dependent on age, APOE-ε4 allele background prevalence or follow-up length
Predicting rapid AD progression/ decline			
APP isoforms in platelets [85]	48 AD subjects followed up over 1 year	Progression of AD	Association of low APPr at baseline in predicting cognitive decline in AD. APPr <0.40, ΔMMSE = -2.8 ± 3.0, $p < 0.05$ APPr ≥0.40, ΔMMSE = -0.9 ±2.3, $p < 0.05$

Combination of Aβ and CRP [87]	122 AD subjects	Followed up 4.2 years	Low plasma levels of Abeta40, Abeta42, and high-sensitivity CRP were associated with a significantly more rapid cognitive decline. Plasma biomarkers contributed to 5-12% variance on Blessed Dementia Scale and Activities of Daily Living.
Ceramides [89]	120 probable AD subjects	Follow-up 2.3y	Highest tertiles of DHSM/DHCer and SM/ceramide ratios declined1.35 points (p=0.001) and 1.19 (p=0.004) less per year on the MMSE and increased 3.18 points (p=0.001) and 2.42 (p=0.016) less per year on ADAS-Cog.
APOEε4 Martins [91]	218 AD subjects	In the non-linear model, possession of an APOEε4 allele was related to earlier and faster cognitive decline. APOEε2 allele related to slower decline.	APOE genotype strongly predicts the rate of cognitive decline in AD. APOEε4 homozygotes showed faster cognitive decline than heterozygotes.
Cosentino [92]	199 population-based incident AD subjects, 215 population-based prevalent AD subjects, 156 clinic-based AD subjects followed up for an average of 4 years	Presence of at least one ε4 allele associated with faster cognitive decline in the population-based incident AD group ($p = 0.01$). However, this association is absent in prevalent AD subjects in population or clinic based group.	APOEε4 influences cognitive decline most significantly in the earliest stages of AD.

HC = Healthy controls

SD = Standard deviation

OR = Odds ratio

95% CI= 95% confidence interval

Sn = Sensitivity

Sp= Specificity

OR = Odds ratio

PPV = Positive predictive value

NPV= Negative predictive value

LR+ = positive Likelihood Ratio

LR- = negative Likelihood Ratio

Table 3. Blood biomarkers in predicting AD conversion in MCI patients and rapid AD progression/ decline

4.1. Plasma proteins/ peptides

Teleologically the most logical candidate is plasma Amyloid-beta (Aβ) and its derivatives, Aβ40 and Aβ42. They are the most studied of blood markers.

As Aβ accumulation is an early step in AD pathogenesis, such a biomarker would be potentially suitable for identifying patients in the earliest stage of disease process when intervention might be more effective.

Circulating Aβ is composed of Aβ produced by brain and peripheral tissue, and can be transported across the blood-brain barrier. They are derived from the amyloid precursor protein (APP). APP is catabolized via 2 pathways, one of which is amyloidogenic, and involves 3 enzyme systems, alpha, beta and gamma secretases. In the amyloidogenic pathway, APP is first cleaved by beta secretase to generate a secreted form of APP (sAPPbeta) and a C99 fragment. The C99 is then cleaved by gamma secretase to yield Aβ. Different cleavage sites on the C99 fragment produces two forms of Aβ – Aβ40 and Aβ42. While Aβ40 is the more common product, Aβ42 aggregates into amyloid fibrils more rapidly and is contained in both early diffuse plaques and fully formed neuritic plaques. In the non-amyloidogenic pathway, alpha secretase is involved and does not lead to Aβ formation [81].

Since elevation appears to be before or just at the onset of the clinically diagnosed disease, it has been hypothesized that high plasma Aβ42 is an antecedent risk indicator for AD, and its plasma levels declines with onset and progression. There have been many studies involving Aβ40 and Aβ42, though results have been inconclusive and at times contradictory refer to Table 1 [82, 83]. These inconsistent results may reflect variability due to technical reasons, such as timing of sample collection with reference to AD onset, the assay methods, and differential affinities of the antibodies used for different Aβ species. Koyama [84], in a large systematic review, concluded that plasma levels of Aβ40 and Aβ42 individually were not associated with development of AD and dementia. However the *ratio of Aβ42:Aβ40* could predict development of AD and dementia, although the evidence is limited in MCI conversion and AD progression.

APP isoforms in platelets have been suggested to predict cognitive decline. APP metabolism has been found to be altered in the platelets of AD patients, specifically a reduced ratio of the upper (130kDa) to the lower (110-106 kDa) immunoreactivity band (APPr) [85].

The level of plasma C-reactive protein (CRP) rises in response to inflammation. Its role is primarily to activate the complement system. CRP by itself has been reported to be associated with accelerated cognitive deterioration and increased risk of conversion in MCI patients [86]. A combination of raised CRP with low Aβ has been associated with a significantly more rapid cognitive decline [87].

Homocysteine has been reported to be associated with human disease states, notably cardiovascular disease. Deficiencies of the B vitamins – B6(pyridoxine), B9(folic acid) and B12(cobalamin) are associated with high homocysteine levels. However, there is no data on homocysteine with MCI conversion and AD progression.

Clusterin, also called apolipoprotein J and coded by gene CLU, has been reported in genome-wide association studies (GWAS) to be associated with AD [83]. Clusterin is functionally associated with apoptosis and the clearance of cellular debris, including amyloid. Thambiesetty [88] found that higher clusterin levels were associated with slower brain atrophy in normal subjects who developed MCI during a 6-year follow-up. However, there is no current data with MCI conversion and AD progression.

Ceramides are a family of lipid molecules that are made up of sphingosine and a fatty acid. They are also constituent of sphinomyelin (SM). In addition to their structural function, they play a role as signaling molecules in regulating cell differentiation, proliferation, and programmed cell death. Mielke [89] found that high plasma levels of dihydroceramides (DHCer) and ceramide were associated with AD progression, though results did not reach significance. Nevertheless, higher plasma levels of SM, dihydrosphingomyelin (DHSM), SM/ceramide, and DHSM/DHCer ratios were associated with less progression on the MMSE and ADAS-Cog with the ratios being the strongest predictors of clinical progression. There is no current data on MCI progression.

4.2. Genetic and transcriptomic markers

APOEε4 is the best-established genetic risk factor for AD. APOE genotyping is not recommended for the routine diagnosis of AD. However many studies have investigated whether APOEε4 has a predictive value for progression from MCI to AD.

In a large meta-analysis, Elias-Sonnenschein [90] and co-workers found that APOEε4 is associated with a moderately increased risk of progression from MCI to AD.

Martins [91] found that the APOEε4 genotype predicts the age of onset of AD and neuropathic progression in a non-linear fashion. In their non-linear model, possession of an APOEε4 allele was related to earlier and faster cognitive decline, while possession of an APOEε4 was associated with slower decline. Homozygous APOEε4 showed faster cognitive decline than APOEε4 heterozygotes. The linear model was less sensitive and did not detect differences between APOEε4 homo- and heterozygotes.

Cosentino [92] also showed that the presence of at least one allele of APOEε4 was associated with faster decline in the incident population-based AD group. However the findings could not be extrapolated to prevalent AD in population or clinic-based samples. Hence APOEε4 influence may be more stage-dependent, with its effect on cognitive decline most evident in the earliest stages of disease and less so in moderate to severe stages.

Other genetic markers that have been identified in genome-wide association studies (GWAS) have not yet been shown to aid in diagnosis of AD or predict progression of disease in MCI or AD.

Unlike the static genome, the transcriptome comprises the dynamic expression of the genome over the course of the disease. Transcriptomic, or genome-wide gene expression studies, have been used to distinguish AD from healthy controls. One of the genes identified from transcriptomic studies is TOMM40, which has also been identified in GWAS studies [93]. We found that TOMM40 remained significantly downregulated over three time points in a longitudinal study (manuscript submitted for review). Transcriptomic products would ideally be used to track the progression of disease, identify markers that predict conversion of MCI to AD, and distinguish between fast and slow progressors. Hence this is a potential area of biomarker development in predicting MCI conversion and rapid AD progression.

4.3. Multiple marker arrays

Given the disappointing results achieved by single markers despite tremendous efforts, the field has now moved towards multiple markers that are obtained through high throughput technologies, sophisticated statistical analysis and bioinformatics. Ray [94] published a blood plasma-based proteomic screening tool to identify patients with AD and also to identify those likely to progress from MCI to AD. Biological analysis of the 18 proteins points to systemic dysregulation of hematopoiesis, immune responses, apoptosis and neuronal support. However efforts at independent validation of Ray's findings have been discouraging [95].

Based on current literature, no single marker has been found to be significant in all the multiple marker arrays. Moreover one can expect that utilizing high throughput array technology, more multiple marker arrays will appear and dominate the blood biomarker landscape. To sound a note of caution, however, some panels may be derived from 'over-fitting' the dataset and may not survive generalization and independent validation. To date, multiple marker arrays have not been employed to study the conversion of MCI to AD and to differentiate between fast and slow progressors. This would be a logical next step for investigation.

4.4. Summary

Plasma Aβ is an appealing biomarker since many AD interventions under investigation are directed against Aβ. Thus an Aβ-based biomarker is attractive for those who will benefit from such treatments. However, many studies involving various blood biomarkers have conflicting and/or inconclusive results.

APOEε4 influence may be more stage-dependent, with its effect on disease trajectory most evident in the earliest stages of disease and less so in moderate to severe stages. Hence it should be included as a covariate in various clinical progression and therapeutic trials. A major challenge is that the literature thus far has focused on the use of blood biomarkers for diagnosis (requiring the identification of dichotomous - disease versus normal- states), which may not be applicable to the use of such biomarkers for tracking disease progression (for which an effective biomarker must show continuous change rather than merely being present or absent). Nevertheless blood biomarkers should be employed in combination with clinical assessment and neuroimaging to improve diagnostic and prognostic accuracy, especially given the peripheral nature and ease of blood sampling.

5. Neuroimaging (Table 4)

5.1. Structural imaging

Neuroimaging is now one of the most common tools used to aid the diagnosis of AD. It is a huge and burgeoning field and only select modalities and important studies on longitudinal imaging are discussed here.

Study variable	Population	Results	Key findings
Predicting AD conversion in MCI subjects			
Structural Imaging			
Jack et al. [96]	55 NC, 41 MCI, 64 AD subjects; 1-5 years follow-up	Atrophy rates of four structures (hippocampus, entorhinal cortex, whole brain, and ventricle)	Rates of change from serial MRI studies together with standard clinical/psychometric measures can be used as surrogate markers of disease progression in AD. Atrophy rates greater among MCI converters. Atrophy rates greater among AD fast progressors
Jack et al. [97]	133 MCI subjects	52 subjects developed AD (45 were APOEε4 carriers). Mean time to conversion 556 day in APOE carriers.	MRI brain atrophy rate measures can be used as indicators of disease progression in a multi-site therapeutic MCI setting. APC was greater in converters than non-converters. APCs greater in APOE ε4 non-carriers. APCs and changes in cognitive test performance uniformly correlated in expected direction (p<0.000)
Jack et al. [98]	72 aMCI subjects, 91 HC; 1-2 years follow-up.	13 HC developed MCI or AD; 39 MCI subjects developed AD	Larger ventricular APC (HR for a 1-SD increase 1.4, p=0.007) increased risk of AD conversion. Both ventricular APC (HR for a 1-SD increase 1.59, p=0.001) and whole brain APC (HR for 1-SD increase 1.32, p=0.009) provided additional predictive information to covariate-adjusted sectional HC volume at baseline about risk of AD conversion. However, overlap present among those converters and non-converters indicate that these measures are unlikely to provide absolute prognosis for MCI-converters.
Apostolova et al. [99]	20 MCI subjects followed up over 3 years	6 subjects developed AD (MCI-c), 7 remained stable (MCI-nc), and 7 improved (MCI- i).	Smaller hippocampi and specifically CA1 and subicular subfields are associated with increased risk for conversion from MCI to AD. Larger hippocampal volumes and relative preservation of both the subiculum and CA1 are associated with cognitive stability or improvement.
Risascher et al. [101]	339 MCI (277 MCI-stable, 62 MCI-converters) subjects, 206 HC, 148 AD subjects	62 MCI developed AD	Degree of neurodegeneration of MTL structures is the best antecedent MRI marker of imminent conversion, with decreased hippocampal volume (left > right) being the most robust structural MRI feature. Effect sizes of hippocampus (0.6) and MTL structures (0.53) comparing MCI-stable and converters.
Querbes et al. [103]	122 aMCI (50 stable MCI, 72 progressive MCI), 130 HC, 130 AD followed up over 24 months.	72 aMCI developed AD.	Normalised cortical thickness can predict AD conversion with 76% cross-validated accuracy.
Molecular Imaging			
Lo et al. [105]	229 normal ,397 MCI and 193 AD subjects followed up 3 years	Rates of change in CSF Aβ42 , glucose metabolism and hippocampal volume	Amyloid deposition is an early event before hypometabolism or hippocampal atrophy, suggesting that biomarker prediction for cognitive change is stage dependent. Positive APOE4 status accelerated hippocampal atrophy changes in MCI and AD.
Okello et al. [106]	31 aMCI subjects, 26 HC followed up over 3 years	17 out of 31 MCI (55%) had increased [11C]PIB retention at baseline (PIB-positive). 14 of these 17 PIB-positive MCI (82%) developed AD. Half (47%) converted to AD within 1 year.	PIB-positive MCI subjects are more likely to develop AD than PIB-negative subjects. Fast converters have higher PIB retention levels at baseline than slower converters in anterior cingulate, (p=0.027) and frontal cortex (p=0.031). Only 1 out of 14 PIB-negative subjects develop AD. 7 of 17 PIB-positive MCI, APOEε4 carriers associated with faster conversion rates (p=0.035)
Koivunen et al. [107]	29 MCI, 13 HC followed up over 2 years	17 MCI developed AD	Hippocampal atrophy increases and amyloid deposition changes modestly during conversion to AD, suggesting dissociation between the two during evolution of MCI. AD converters had greater [11C]PIB retention at baseline in posterior cingulate (p=0.022), putamen (p=0.041), caudate nucleus (p=0.025). Greater hippocampal atrophy in MCI converters at baseline.

Small et al. [108]	22 HC and 21 MCI followed up over 2 years	Increases in frontal, posterior cingulate, and global binding at follow-up correlated with progression of memory decline (r = -0.32 to -0.37, P = 0.03 to 0.01).	[18F]FDDNP PET scanning may be useful in identifying people at risk for future cognitive decline. Higher [18F]FDDNP binding at baseline is associated with future decline in most cognitive domains (r = -0.31 to -0.56, P = 0.05 to 0.002). Frontal and parietal [18F]FDDNP binding yielded highest diagnostic accuracy. ROC 0.88 (95% CI 0.72-1.00) compared with 0.68 (95% CI 0.45-0.91) for medial temporal binding.
Doraiswamy et al. [109]	51 MCI, 69 HC, and 31 AD followed up over 18 months.	MCI Aβ+ and HC Aβ+ associated with greater clinical worsening on ADAS-Cog and CDR-SB. MCI Aβ+ associated With greater decline in memory, DSS and MMSE (p < 0.05).	Florbetapir PET, which detects Aβ pathology, may be helpful in identifying individuals at increased risk for progression to AD. Higher SUVr in MCI associated with greater decline on ADAS-Cog, CDR-SB, memory measure (DSS) and MMSE (all p<0.05). MCI Aβ+ had higher risk of developing AD.
Ossenkoppele et al. [110]	11 HC, 12 MCI, and 8 AD followed up over 2.5 years.	Global cortical [11C]PIB BPND is significantly increased in MCI subjects, but no changes was observed in AD subjects or HC. Increase most prominent in lateral temporal lobe (p < 0.05). No changes in global [18F] FDDNP.	[11C]PIB and [18F] FDG track molecular changes in different stages of AD. MCI subjects were found to have an increased amyloid load while AD subjects had increased progressive metabolic impairment. [18F]FDDNP is less useful for examining disease progression. Reduction in [18F]FDG uptake at follow-up observed in AD subjects only (esp frontal, parietal, temporal lobes (all p<0.01). Changes in global [11C]PIB binding (p=-0.42, p<0.05) and cingulate [18F]FDG uptake (p=0.43, p<0.01) correlated with changes in MMSE score over time across groups but not for [18F] FDDNP binding (p=-0.18, p=0.35).
Zhang et al. [111]	Meta-analysis of 13 research studies (7 FDG-PET)	FDG-PET pooled estimates: 78.7% Sn (95% CI 68.7-86.6%) 74% Sp (95%CI 67.0-80.3%) PIB-PET pooled estimates: 93.5% Sn (95% CI 71.3-99.9%) 56.2% Sp (95% CI 47.2-64.8%)	Both FDG-PET and PIB-PET are valuable techniques for prediction of AD progression in MCI subjects.

Predicting rapid AD progression/ decline

Thompson et al. [100]	12 AD subjects, 14 HC	Followed up 3 years	Cortical atrophy occurred in a well defined sequence (temporal- frontal- sensorimotor) as the disease progressed. Mirroring the sequence of neurofibrillary tangle accumulation observed in cross sections at autopsy. Left hemisphere degenerates faster (5.3 ± 2.3% per year in AD v.s. 0.9 ± 0.9% per year in controls; p<0.029) than the right
Kinkingnéhun et al.[103]	23 mild AD subjects and 18 HC followed up	Followed up 3 years	Fast decliners had a more extensive cortical atrophy than slow decliners, especially in the medial occipitoparietal areas (specifically precuneus, Lingual gyrus and cuneus which was not yet detected by clinical and neuropsychological assessment.

Functional Imaging

Silverman et al. [107]	284 patients presenting symptoms of dementia	Progressive dementia in 59%	In patients presenting symptoms of dementia, regional brain metabolism was a sensitive indicator of AD. A negative PET scan indicated that pathologic progression of cognitive impairment during the mean 3-year follow-up was unlikely to occur. Sn 93%, Sp 76%. –LR 0.1 (95% CI 0.06-0.16) experiencing progressive course after a single negative PET scan.

NC = Normal Controls

MRI = Magnetic Resonance Imaging

APC = Annual percent change

HC = Healthy Controls

SD = Standard deviation

MTL = Medial Temporal Lobe

aMCI = amnestic MCI

PIB = Pittsburgh Compound B

FDDNP = Fluoroethyl)methylamino]-2-napthyl}ethylidene) malononitrile

PET = Positron Emission Tomography

MMSE =Mini Mental State Examination

Sn = Sensitivity

Sp= Specific

-LR = negative Likelihood ratio

Table 4. Neuroimaging methods in predicting AD conversion in MCI patients and rapid AD progression/ decline

With technological advances over the past three decades, MRI is now readily available and relatively economical. Currently it is widely used as a diagnostic tool, to complement clinical assessment and neuropsychological testing. Moreover, MRI has also been considered for longitudinal tracking of the disease progression and to predict whether a MCI patient may go on to develop AD, or whether an AD patient will have an indolent or rapid course. Advances in technology have led to automated data-driven methods, such as automated measurement of whole brain volume over time, voxel-based morphometry (VBM), deformation-based morphometry (DBM) and analysis of cortical thickness. These technologies ameliorate the previous problems associated with manual measurement, inter-rater reliability and difficulties in cross-study comparisons.

In a seminal paper, Jack [96] studied annualized changes in volume of four structures in serial MRI studies: hippocampus, entorhinal cortex, whole brain and ventricles of normal, MCI and AD subjects. All four atrophy rates were greater among MCI-converters compared to non-converters and fast-progressors versus slow progressors. Although the differences in atrophy rates have been replicated consistently in several follow-up studies [97,98], given the overlap among those who did and did not convert, the authors cautioned that these measures were unlikely to provide absolute prognostic information for individual patients.

Using hippocampal volumetry, a prospective longitudinal cohort study found that greater atrophy in the CA1 hippocampal and subicular subfields predicted MCI conversion, whereas larger hippocampal volumes predicted cognitive stability and/or improvement [99].

Employing a 3-dimensional cortical mapping approach, Thompson [100], demonstrated a temporal-frontal-sensorimotor sequence of cortical atrophy with AD progression in a longitudinal series of 12 AD subjects, where left brain was found to degenerate faster than right.

Employing VBM technique, Risacher [101] found that AD and MCI converters demonstrated high atrophy across regions as compared to HC in global and hippocampal grey matter (GM)

density, hippocampal and amygdalar volumes, and cortical thickness values from entorhinal cortex and other temporal and parietal lobe regions. MCI-stable showed intermediate atrophy. Degree of atrophy of medial temporal structures, especially the hippocampi, was found to be the best antecedent MRI marker of imminent conversion.

A separate study also showed that occipitoparietal (specifically precuneus, lingual gyrus and cuneus) atrophy at baseline better anticipated the rate of progression (fast decliners from slow decliners) over 3 years compared to clinical and neuropsychological assessment [102].

Cortical thickness is another measure of interest in structural neuroimaging where a normalized thickness index was computed using a subset of these regions, namely the right medial temporal, left lateral temporal and right posterior cingulate. Normalized thickness index at baseline differed significantly among all the four diagnosis groups (HC, stable MCI, progressive MCI and AD). Furthermore, normalized thickness index also correctly predicted evolution to AD for 76% of aMCI subjects after cross-validation [103].

5.2. Functional and molecular imaging

There are many functional imaging studies for AD though only a few specifically investigate longitudinal progression of MCI and AD using Fluorodeoxyglucose (18F) (FDG)-Positron Emission Tomography (PET) [104].

Lo [105] found that the rate of change of glucose metabolism and hippocampal volume accelerated as cognitive function deteriorated. Moreover, glucose metabolic decline and hippocampal atrophy were significantly slower in subjects with normal cognition compared to those with MCI or AD. Positive APOE4 status was also associated with accelerated hippocampal atrophy.

Molecular imaging utilizes small molecule ligands that bind with nanomolar affinity to amyloid and enters the brain for imaging with PET. It is a measure to detect and quantify cerebral beta-amyloidosis. It should be noted that besides AD, there are other disease conditions that may have cerebral Aβ. The most commonly used ligand is the carbon-11(11C)-based Pittsburgh compound B (PIB), which binds specifically to fibrillar Aβ but exhibits no demonstrable binding to neurofibrillary tangles. However, fluorine-18 (18F)-based tracers, e.g. 2-(1-{6-[(2-fluorine 18-labeled fluoroethyl)methylamino]-2-napthyl}ethylidene) malononitrile ([(18)F]FDDNP) have a considerably longer half-life compared to [11(C)]PIB and some types have been shown to also bind to neurofibrillary tangles.

Okello [106] showed that PIB-positive subjects with MCI are significantly more likely to convert to AD than PIB-negative ones. A separate longitudinal study showed that hippocampal atrophy and amyloid deposition (in posterior cingulate, lateral frontal cortex, temporal cortex, putamen and caudate nucleus) seem to dissociate during the evolution of MCI, the atrophy increasing clearly and [(11)C] PIB retention changing modestly when conversion to AD occurs [107]. Using [(18)F]FDDNP PET, higher baseline binding was associated with future decline in most cognitive domains. Specifically, frontal and parietal [(18)F]FDDNP binding yielded the greatest diagnostic accuracy in identifying MCI-converters versus non-converters [108]. With 18F florbetapir (18F-AV-45) tracer, baseline Aβ + scans were associated with greater clinical worsening on the AD Assessment Scale-Cognitive subscale (ADAS-Cog) and Clinical Dementia Rating-sum of boxes (CDR-SB). In MCI, $A\beta$ + scans were also associated with greater decline in memory, Digit Symbol Substitution (DSS) and MMSE. $A\beta$ + MCI subjects again tended to convert to AD at a higher rate than $A\beta$- subjects [109].

In a seminal comparison study of three modalities [110], using [(11)C]PIB, [(18)F]FDDNP and [18F]FDG, there was a significant increase in global cortical [(11)C]PIB binding (most prominent in the lateral temporal lobe) in MCI patients, but no changes in AD patients or controls. Interestingly, [(18)F]FDDNP did not show any changes in global binding potential. Moreover, changes in global [(11)C]PIB binding and posterior cingulate [(18)F]FDG uptake were correlated with changes in MMSE score over time across groups, but not with [(18)F]FDDNP binding. Hence it was postulated that [(11)C]PIB and [(18)F]FDDNP track molecular changes in different stages of AD. There was an increased amyloid load in MCI patients and progressive metabolic impairment in AD patients. The authors opined that [(18)F]FDDNP was less useful for examining disease progression.

To estimate the diagnostic accuracy of FDG-PET and PIB-PET for prediction of short-term conversion to AD in patients with MCI, Zhang [111] and co-workers performed a meta-analysis undertaken with a random-effects model. Overall diagnostic accuracy determined for both FDG-PET and PIB-PET suggests that they are potentially valuable techniques for prediction of progression in patients with MCI. Both have their advantages and their combined use is a promising option.

Villain et al recently published a longitudinal PIB study (testing conducted 18 months apart), showing a significant increase in amyloid-β accumulation in both PIB-positive and negative subjects (significantly higher in PIB-positive individuals) with a bimodal distribution of individual rates of neocortical amyloid- β accumulation [112].

5.3. Summary

MRI volumetry and brain atrophy rates have fairly good diagnostic and predictive value in MCI subjects. Longitudinal data on brain atrophy rates with disease progression are available and hence, can be used for monitoring disease progression in clinical trials. The limitations of structural neuroimaging as a biomarker include problems with the accurate delineation of regions of interest and lack of standardization of imaging and measurement techniques, making it difficult to compare data across the different institutions out of Europe, North America and Australia (all of which have their unified imaging consortiums). The advent of automated data-driven innovations for structural imaging holds promise. FDG-PET appears to be the leading candidate among the functional neuroimaging modalities, with available evidence for MCI diagnosis, prediction of MCI-converters and longitudinal data in monitoring serial progression. To date, [(11)C] PIB is the most extensively studied PET amyloid tracer, although 18F florbetapir proves to be an attractive alternative given the longer half-life. There is emerging evidence for amyloid imaging in the diagnosis of preclinical AD. From the standpoint of clinical trials of anti-amyloid therapy, in-vivo amyloid imaging pre-treatment allows selection of patients with demonstrable cerebral $A\beta$ loads; repeated imaging during ongoing treatment allows detection of decrease in insoluble $A\beta$ load in response to amyloid-clearing drugs such as immunotherapy. Amyloid imaging needs to be more practically accessible and affordable before it can be transferable to the clinical diagnostic routine.

6. Combinational biomarkers

Many of the aforementioned biomarker modalities are not separate discrete entities but have an effect on each other. For example, the association of hypertension with CSF tau and ptau-181, was found to be modified by APOEε4 phenotype, where hypertension is directly related to tau pathology (and not Aβ42) in APOEε4 homozygous carriers [113]. Elevated CSF t-tau and p-tau in presence of APOEε4/ε4 genotype has also been shown to influence faster AD progression in MCI subjects [114].

For the identification of MCI-converters, various literature showing combination biomarkers have been published. They include looking at clinical measures (such as cognitive or neuropsychological tests) in combination with CSF biomarkers [115], neuroimaging measures [116, 117], or in combination with both CSF and neuroimaging measures [118-119].

A combination of CSF and neuroimaging biomarkers [120-4] has found improved predictive accuracy of MCI-converters, supported by slope analyses of annual cognitive decline [120]. Okamura showed that a high ratio between cerebrospinal fluid (CSF) tau and posterior cingulate perfusion on SPECT is useful in identifying MCI converters [125]. Using a machine-learning approach (support vector machines), Furney et al examined the utility of adding cytokine and neuroimaging biomarkers to conventional measures, and found that the combination of cytokine and neuroimaging with clinical and APOEε4 genotype improved accuracy [126]. Recent studies have also looked at multimodal neuroimaging techniques to predict MCI progression [127-129].

Other recent studies have used endophenotype-based approach and found single nucleotide polymorphism (SNP) such as rs1868402 to have strong, replicable association with CSFptau$_{181}$ association with rate of AD progression [130].

7. Conclusion and future directions

Clinical criteria alone, often subjective and dependent on clinical judgment, are insufficient to identify the pre-clinical stages of AD accurately. This has prompted the past decade-long intensive research into the use of more objective neuroimaging and biochemical markers to either replace, or complement, clinical approaches to facilitate an early and accurate diagnosis of the illness [131,132]. The chapter thus far details the rationale (most evident from Table 1) for the combined approach of clinical measures with other biomarkers in predicting AD progression; but in the earlier stages (prodromal and especially preclinical AD stages), biomarkers would play an increasingly important role. Combination biomarker approaches appear to be superior to a single biomarker approach, with the recent focus of researchers being

Subjects	Follow-up (years)	Biomarker	Results
MCI (n=8) NC (n=10) [70]	1	CSF p-tau231 CSF Aβ40 CSF Aβ42	MCI: 5.0; NC: 3.0 * MCI: 4.0; NC: 8.0 MCI: 4.0; NC: 2.0
MCI (n=7) NC (n=9) [71]	2	CSF p-tau231 CSF Aβ40 CSFAβ42	MCI: 2.0; NC: 20.0 * MCI: 0.5; NC: 3.5 MCI: 0.35; NC: 1.5
MCI (n=62) AD (n=68) NC (n=24) [72]	2	CSF isoprostane CSF neurofilaments light CSF Aβ40 No change in Aβ42 or p-tau 181.	NC:-1.9; MCI:-0.4; AD: 5.0 ** NC:-0.18; MCI:-0.79; AD: -0.96 NC: 0.61; MCI:0.28; AD:0.43
MCI (n=57) AD (n=56) [65] NC (n=8)	3	CSF Aβ42 CSF tau CSFp-tau CSFAβ42/tau CSFAβ42/ptau	MCI(stable): 3.42, MCI (converters):0.78, AD:-11.9** MCI(stable):19.7, MCI(converters):17.4, AD: 0.55 MCI(stable):1.24, MCI(converters):-0.21, AD: -2.2 MCI(stable):-0.54.MCI(converters):-0.4,AD: -0.008 MCI(stable):-0.19, MCI(converters):-0.07,AD:0.18
NC (n=55) MCI (n=41) AD (n=64) [99]	1.2-2.4	Hippocampus* Entorhinal cortex Whole brain Ventricle	MCI (stable):-4.4,MCI(converters):-7.8, AD slow -9.4, AD fast -15.4 MCI(stable):-15.9, MCI(converters):-16.0, AD slow-20.5, AD fast -22.7 MCI (stable):-0.8, MCI (converters):-2.5, AD slow -2.4, AD fast -3.6 MCI (stable):0.8, MCI(converters):1.8, AD slow -6.5, AD fast 1.9
MCI (n=131) [101]	3	Hippocampus * Entorhinal cortex Whole brain Ventricle	MCI (converters) -6.78; MCI (non-converters) -3.86 MCI (converters) -15.08 ; MCI (non-converters) -8.32 MCI (converters) -0.88 ; MCI (non-converters) -0.36 MCI (converters) 5.66 ; MCI (non-converters) 3.33
MCI (n=72) [104]	1-2	Hippocampus * Entorhinal cortex Whole brain Ventricle	-3.3 (2.7) -7.0 (4.3) -0.7 (1.0) 3.3 (2.3)
AD (n=32) MCI (n=49) NC (n=103) [116]	1.5	PiB-PET (neocortical PiB rate of change) (SuVR_pons/year) *	AD: PiB-(acc) +0.06; PiB+(acc) +0.05; PiB (non-acc) -0.01 MCI: PiB-(acc) +0.04; PiB-(non-acc) -0.001; PiB+ (acc) +0.04; PiB (non-acc) -0.01 HC: PiB-(acc)+0.03; PiB- (non-acc) -0.01; PiB+(acc) +0.04; PiB+ (non-acc) -0.004
NC (n=210) MCI (n=357) AD (n=162) [135]	2	CSF Aβ42 CSF tau PiB FDG-PET Hippocampus Ventricles ADAS-Cog total MMSE CDR-SB RAVLT (5 trial total)	NC: -0.94; MCI: -1.4; AD: -0.1 * NC: 3.45; MCI: 2.34; AD: 1.24 NC: 0.098; MCI: -0.008; AD: -0.004 NC: -177; MCI: 752; AD: 2993 NC: -40; MCI: -80; AD: -116 NC: 848; MCI: 1551; AD: 2540 NC: -0.54; MCI: 1.05; AD: 4.37 NC: 0.0095; MCI:-0.64; AD: -2.4 NC: 0.07; MCI 0.63; AD: 1.62 NC: 0.29; MCI: -1.37; AD: -3.62

* expressed as % change per year compared to baseline values

** expressed as annual change β

MCI = Mild Cognitive Impairment

NC = Normal Controls

AD = Alzheimer's Disease

CSF = Cerebrospinal fluid

PIB = Pittsburgh Compound B

FDG-PET = Fluorodeoxyglucose (18F)-Positron Emission Tomography

MMSE = Mini Mental State Examination

CDR-SB = Clinical Dementia Rating – Sum of Boxes

RAVLT = Rey Auditory Verbal Learning Tes

Table 5. Longitudinal biomarker studies

on multimodal approach using various systems biology and multivariate modeling methods. Additionally, multi-site prospective studies, such as the Alzheimer's Disease Neuroimaging Initiative (ADNI), allow for global summary of results and patterns of change observed in clinical measures and candidate biomarkers [133] (Table 5). It must also be highlighted that some of the heterogeneity of biomarker findings thus far is related to the different periods of follow-up and hence AD conversion rates in MCI subjects.

The dynamic biomarker model, in the AD pathological cascade first proposed by Jack in 2010 [134], has been an area of intense interest. However, this inverse relationship between fibrillar amyloid plaque burden (on PIB imaging) and corresponding decrease in CSF Aβ42 and elevated tau, has led to the simplistic interpretation that the AD pathological cascade is purely driven by the amyloid cascade (Figure 1). This is partly due to extrapolation from cross-sectional studies, where in fact, longitudinal studies are required to determine the temporal order of the appearance of various pathogenic processes involved in this complex disease. Storandt et al [135] has recently demonstrated in a community cohort that CSF Aβ42 and tau were minimally correlated, suggesting that they represent independent processes. Additionally, they accounted for only 60% of variance on PIB imaging, suggesting that a third process may be related to brain atrophy or plaque formation [136].

In addition, understanding longitudinal biomarker change allows its potential inclusion in clinical trials, with recent studies advocating the use of neuroimaging biomarkers [137,138], CSF biomarkers [139] and/or combination biomarkers [137,140] to boost the power of clinical trials and decrease sample size in MCI trials. An integrated analyses approach using patient (age) severity- and disease-related (severe baseline cognitive, global or behavioural status) factors in established AD has been shown, with the potential of symptomatic AD therapy, to decrease likelihood of faster decline [141].

Further work on biomarkers is important because of their multiple potential roles. Biomarkers have the potential to be used as a prognostic tool for the prediction of AD conversion in MCI subjects and rapid AD progression, with translation into clinical practice by using a most practical algorithm, and as a diagnostic tool in prodromal/ preclinical stages of AD. Biomarkers may also lead to a deeper understanding of the complex pathogenesis of AD disease – including stage-specific and stage-independent processes. There is also currently an unfulfil-led potential in biomarker-enriched clinical trials and the use of biomarkers in preclinical AD, especially in the advent of newer therapeutic targets. Finally there is also potential to extrap-olate biomarker findings 'backwards' into the earliest stages of disease so that we may be able to identify those at risk and consider instituting interventions. This would enable earliest therapeutic intervention for at-risk subjects most amenable to disease-modifying treatments, and exclude those for whom the possible risks from investigational treatment would be more difficult to justify. At the very least, it would identify those who might benefit most from intensive monitoring and management of clinical factors, e.g. blood pressure, diabetes and lipids, and also non-invasive interventions, e.g. cognitive training. This vital work can only been done through multi-center studies and standardized evaluation techniques using various systems biology and statistical modeling approaches.

Author details

Mei Sian Chong[1] and Tih-Shih Lee[2]

1 Department of Geriatric Medicine, Tan Tock Seng Hospital, Singapore

2 Duke University Medical School, USA

References

[1] Wimo A, Winbald B, Aguero Torres H, von Strauss E. The magnitude of dementia occurrence in the world. Alz Dis Assoc Disord 2003; 17: 63-67.

[2] Price JL, Morris JC. Tangles and plaques in nondemented aging and preclinical Alzheimer disease. Ann Neurol 1999; 45:358-68.

[3] Bateman RJ, Xiong C, Benzinger TL, Fagan AM, Goate A, Fox NC, Marcus DS, Cairns NJ, Xie X, Blazey TM, Holtzman DM, Santacruz A, Buckles V, Oliver A, Moulder K, Aisen PS, Ghetti B, Klunk WE, McDade E, Martins RN, Masters CL, Mayeux R, Ringman JM, Rossor MN, Schofield PR, Sperling RA, Salloway S, Morris JC; the Dominantly Inherited Alzheimer Network. Clinical and Biomarker Changes in Dominantly Inherited Alzheimer's Disease. N Engl J Med. 2012 Jul 11.

[4] Jack CR Jr, Albert MS, Knopman DS, McKhann GM, Sperling RA, Carrillo MC, Thies B, Phelps CH. Introduction to the recommendations from the National Institute on Aging-Alzheimer's Association workgroups on diagnostic guidelines for Alzheimer's disease. Alzheimers Dement. 2011 May;7(3):257-62. Epub 2011 Apr 21.

[5] Cores F, Nourhashemi F, Guerin O et al. Prognosis of Alzheimer's disease today : a two-year prospective study in 686 patients from the REAL-FR Study. Alzheimers Dement 2008; 4(1): 22-29.

[6] Roselli F, Tartaglione B, Federico F, Lepore V, Defazio G, Livrea P. Rate of MMSE score change in Alzheimer's disease: Influence of education and vascular risk factors. Clin Neurol Neurosurg 2009; 111(4):327-30.

[7] Soto ME, Anrieu S, Cantet C, Reynish E et al. Predictive value of rapid decline in Mini Mental State Examination in clinical practice for prognosis in Alzheimer's disease. Dement Geriatr Cogn Disord 2008; 26(2): 109-16.

[8] de la Monte SM. Contributions of Brain Insulin Resistance and Deficiency in Amyloid-Related Neurodegeneration in Alzheimer's disease. Drugs 2012; 73(1):49-66.

[9] Janson J, Laedtke T, Parisi JE, O/Brien P et al. Increased risk of type 2 diabetes in Alzheimer disease. Diabetes 2004; 53:474-481.

[10] Francis GJ, Martinez JA, Liu WQ, Xu K, Ayer A, Fine J, Tuor UI, Glazner G, Hanson, LR, Frey WH 2nd, Toth C. Intranasal insulin prevents cognitive decline, cerebral

atrophy and white matter changes in murine type I diabetic encephalopathy. Brain 2008;131(Pt 12):3311-34.

[11] Xu E, Caracciolo B, Wang H, Winblad B et a. Accelerated progression from Mild Cognitive Impairment to Dementia in People with Diabetes. Diabetes 2010; 59:2928-2935.

[12] Cole AR, Astell A, Green C, Sutherland C. Molecular connexions between dementia and diabetes. Neurosci Biobehav Rev 2007; 31:1046-63.

[13] Schenider P, Buerger K, Teipel S, Uspenskaya O, Harmann O et al. Antihypertension Therapy is associated with reduced rate of conversion to Alzheimer's disease in midregional proatrial natriuretic peptide strateified subjects with mild cognitive impairment. Biol Psy 2011; 70:145-51.

[14] Siuda J, Gorzkowska A, Patalong-Ogiewa M, Krzystanek E, Czech E et al. From mild cognitive impairment to Alzheimer's disease - influence of homocysteine, vitamin B12 and folate on cognition over time: results from one-year follow-up. Neurol Neurochir Pol. 2009 Jul-Aug;43(4):321-9.

[15] Solfrizzi V, Panza F, Colacicco Am, D'Introno A et al. Vascular risk factors, incidence of MCI, and rates of progression to dementia. Neurology 2004; 63(10): 1882-91.

[16] Mielke MM, Rosenberg PB, Tschanz J et al. Vascular factors predict rate of progression in Alzheimer disease. Neurology 2007; 69:1850-58.

[17] Musicco M, Palmer K, Salamone G, Lupo F, Perri R et al. Predictors of progression of cognitive decline in Alzheimer's disease: the role of vascular and sociodemographic factors." J Neurol. 2009 Aug;256(8):1288-95.

[18] Bellew KM, Pigeon JG, Fleischman W, Gardner RM, Baker WW. Hypertension and the Rate of Cognitive Decline in Patients with Dementia of the Alzheimer Type. Alzheimer Dis Assoc Disord 2004; 18(4): 208-213.

[19] Regan C, Katona C, Walker Z, Hooper J, Donovan J et al. Relationship of vascular risk to the progression of Alzheimer disease. Neurology 2006; 67:1357-62.

[20] Helzner EP, Luchsinger JA, Scarmeas N et al. Contribution of vascular risk factors to disease progressionn in Alzheimer's Disease. Arch Neurol 2009; 66(3):343-48.

[21] Li J, Wang YJ, Zhang M, Xu ZQ et al. Vascular risk factors promote conversion from mild cognitive impairment to Alzheimer disease. Neurology 2011; 76:1485-91.

[22] Li L, Wang Y, Yan J, Chen Y, Zhou R et al. Clinical predictors of cognitive decline in patients with mild cognitive impairment: the Chongqing aging study. J Neurol 2012; 259:1303-1311.

[23] Solfrizzi V, Scafato E, Capurso C, D'Introno A, Colacicco AM, Frisardi V,Vendemiale G, Baldereschi M, Crepaldi G, Di Carlo A, Galluzzo L, Gandin C,Inzitari D, Maggi S, Capurso A, Panza F; Italian Longitudinal Study on Aging Working Group.Metabolic

syndrome, mild cognitive impairment, and progression to dementia. The Italian Longitudinal Study on Aging. Neurobiol Aging 2011;32(11):1932-41.

[24] Forlenza OV, Diniz BS, Talib LL, Radanovic M et al. Clinical and biologic predictors of Alzheimer's disease in patients with amnestic mild cognitive impairment. Revista Brasilerira de Psiquiatria 2010; 32(3):216-22.

[25] Wilkosz PA, Seltman HJ, Devlin B, Weamer EA, Lopez OL et al. Trajectories of Cognitive Decline in Alzheimer's disease. Int Psychogeriatr 2010; 22(2):281-90.

[26] Gomeni R, Simeoni M, Zvartau-Hind M, Irizarry MC, Austin D, Gold M. Modeling Alzheimer's disease progression using the disease system analysis approach. Alz Dement 2012; 8:39-50.

[27] Lopez OL, Schwam E, Cummings J, Gauthier S, Jones R, Wilkinson D et al. Predicting cognitive decline in Alzheimer's disease: An integrated analysis. Alz Dement 2010; 6:431-39.

[28] Hall CB, Derby C, LeValley A, Katz MH, Verghese J, Lipton RB. Education delays accelerated decline on a memory test in persons who develop dementia. Neurology 2007; 69:1657-64.

[29] Doody RS, Pavlik V, Massman P, Rountree S et al. Predicting progression of Alzheimer's disease. Alzheimer's Res Therapy 2010;2:2.

[30] Buccione I, Perri R, Carlesimo GA, Fadda L et al. Cognitive and behavioural predictors of progression rates in Alzheimer's disease. Eur J Neurology 2007; 14:440-6.

[31] Palmer K, Lupo F, Perri R, Salamone G et al. Predicting Disease progression in Alzheimer's disease: The role of Neuropsychiatric syndromes on functional and cognitive decline. J Alz Dis 2011; 24:35-45.

[32] De Jaeger CA, Hoegevorst E, Combrinck M, Budge MM. Sensitivity and specificity of neuropsychological tests for mild cognitive impairment, vascular cognitive impairment and Alzheimer's disease. Psychological Medicine 2003; 33:1039–50.

[33] Albert M, Blacker D, Moss MB, Tanzi R, McArdle JJ. Longitudinal change in cognitive performance among individuals with mild cognitive impairment. Neuropsychology 2007; 21(2):158-69.

[34] Pozueta A, Rodriguez-Rodriguez E, Vazquez-Higuera J, Mateo I et al. Detection of early Alzheimer's disease in MCI patients by combination of MMSE and an episodic memory test. BMC Neurology 2011; 11:78.

[35] Gavett BE, Ozonoff A, Doktor V, Palmisano J et al. Predicting cognitive decine and conversion to Alzheimer's disease in older adults using the NAB List Learning test. J Int Neuropsychol Soc 2010; 16(4): 651-60.

[36] PJ Nestor, P Scheltens, JR Hodges. Advances in the early detection of Alzheimer's disease. Nat Med. 2004 Jul;10 Suppl:S34–41. Review.

[37] Fowler KS, Salling MM, Conway El, Semple JM, Louis WJ. Paired associate performance in the early detection of DAT. J Int Neuropsychol Soc 2002; 8(1):58-71.

[38] DeCarli C, Mungas D, Harvey D, Reed B, Weiner M, Chui H, Jagust WC. Memory
impairment, but not cerebrovascular disease, predicts progression of MCI to dementia.
Neurology 2004; 63:220–7.

[39] Amieva H, Letenneur L, Dartigues JF, Rouch-Leroyer I, Sourgen C, D Alchee-Biree F,
Dib M, Barbeger-Gateau P, Orgogozo JM, Fabrigoule C. Annual Rate and Predictors of
Conversion to Dementia in Subjects Presenting Mild Cognitive Impairment Criteria
Defined according to a Population-Based Study. Dement Geriatr Cogn Disord 2004;
18:87–93.

[40] Dickerson BC, Sperling RA, Hyman BT, Albert MS, Blacker D. Clinical Prediction of
Alzheimer Disease Dementia across the spectrum of mild cognitive impairment. Arch
Gen Psychiatry 2007; 64(12):1443-50.

[41] Guarch J, Marcos T, Salamero M, Blesa R. Neuropsychological markers of dementia in
patients with memory complaints. Int J Geriatr Psychiatry 2004; 19:352–58.

[42] Chapman RM, Mapstone M, McCrary JW, Gardner MN, Porsteinnson AP et al.
Predicting conversion from Mild Cognitive Impairment to Alzheimer's disease using
neuropsychological tests and multivariate methods. J Clin Exp Neuropsychol 2011;
33(2): 187-99.

[43] Chan Y, Bondi MW, Fennema-Notestine C, McEvoy LK et al. Brain substrates of
learning and retention in mild cognitive impairment diagnosis and progression to
Alzheimer's disease. Neuropsychologia 2010; 48(5):1237-47.

[44] Dierckx E, Engelborghs S, De Raedt R, Van Buggenhout M, De Deyn PP et al. Verba;
cued recall as a predictor of conversion to Alzheimer's disease in Mild Cognitive
Impairment. Int J Geriatr Psy 2009;24:1094-1100.

[45] Musicco M, Salamone G, Caltagirone C, Cravello L et al. Neuropsychological Predictors
of Rapidly Progressing Patients with Alzheimer's disease. Dement Geriatr Cogn Disord
2010; 30:219-28.

[46] Backman L, Small BJ, Fratiglioni L. Stability of the preclinical memory deficit in
Alzheimer's disease. Brain 2001; 124:96-102.

[47] Bennett DA, Wilson RS, Schneider JA, Evans DA et al. Natural history of mild cognitive
impairment in older persons. Neurology 2002; 59:198-205.

[48] Blennow K, Hampal H. CSF markers for incipient Alzheimer's disease. Lancet Neurol
2003; 2:605-13.

[49] Fagan AM, Shaw LM, Xiong C, Vanderstichele H et al. Comparison of Analytical
Platforms for cerebrospinal fluid measures of β-amyloid 1-42, total tau, and P-tau$_{181}$ for
identifying Alzheimer Disease Amyloid Plaque Pathology. Arch neurol doi:10.1001/
archneurol.2011.105

[50] Shaw LM, Vanderstichele H, Knapik-Czajka M et al. Qualification of the analytical and clinical performance of CSF biomarker analyses in ADNI. Acta Neuropathol 2011; 121:597-609.

[51] Arai H, Nakagawa T, Kosaka Y et al. Elevated cerebrospinal fluid tau protein as a predictor of dementia in memory-impaired patients. Alzheimer's Res 1997; 3:211-3.

[52] Andreasen N, Vanmechelen E, Vanderstichele H, Davidsson P, Blennow K. Cerebrospinal fluid levels of total-tau, phosphor-tau and Aβ42 predicts development of Alzheimer's disease in patients with mild cognitive impairment. Acta Neurol Scand 2003; 107(suppl 179):47-51.

[53] Hampel H, Teipel SJ, Fuchsberger T, Andreasen N, Wiltfang J, Otto M, Shen Y, Dodel R, u Y, Farlow M, Moller HJ et al. Value of CSF beta-amyloid1-42 and tau as predictors of Alzheimer's disease in patients with mild cognitive impairment. Mol Psychiatry 2004; 9:705-10.

[54] Maruyama M, Arai H, Sugita M, Tanji H, Higuchi M, Okamura N, Matsui T, Higuchi S, Matsushita S, Yoshida H, Sasaki H. Cerebrospinal fluid amyloid β_{1-42} in the mild cognitive impairment stage of Alzheimer's disease. Exp Neurol 2001; 172:433-6.

[55] Mattson N et al. CSF biomarkers and incipient Alzheimer disease in patients with mild cognitive impairment. JAMA 2009; 302:485-93.

[56] Visser PJ et al. Prevalence and prognostic value of CSF markers of Alzheimer's disease pathology in patients with subjective cognitive impairment or mild cognitive impairment in the DESCRIPA study: a prospective cohort study. Lancet Neurol 2009; 8:619-27.

[57] Arai H, Idhiguro K, Ohno H, Moriyama M, Itoh N, Okamura N, Matsui T, Morikawa Y, Horikawa E, Kohno H, Sasaki H et al. CSF phosphorylated tau protein and mild cognitive impairment: a prospective study. Exp Neurol 2000; 1666:201-3.

[58] Buerger K, Teipel SJ, Zinkoiwski R, Blennow K, Arai H, Engel R, Hofmann-Keiffer K, McCulloch C, Ptok U, Heun R, Andreasen N et al. CST tau protein phosphorylated at threonine 231 correlates with cognitive decline in MCI subjects. Neurology 2002; 59:627-9.

[59] Riemenscheneider M, Lautenschlager N, Wagenpfeil S, Diehl J, Drzezga A, Kurz A. Cerebrospinal fluid tau and beta-amyloid 42 proteins identify Alzheimer disease in subjects with mild cognitive impairment. Arch Neurol 2002; 59:1729-34.

[60] Andreasen N, Minthon L, Vanmechelen E, Vanderstichele H, Davidsson P, Winblad B, Blennow K. Cerebrospinal fluid tau and Aβ42 as predictors of development of Alzheimer's disease in patients with mild cognitive impairment. Neurosci Letters 1999; 273:5-8.

[61] Herruka S, Hallikainen M, Soininen H, Pirttila T. CSF Aβ42 and tau or phosphorylated tau and prediction of progressive mild cognitive impairment. Neurology 2005; 64:1294-7.

[62] Zetterberg H, Wahlund LO, Blennow K. Cerebrospinal fluid markers for prediction of Alzheimer's disease. Neurosci Letters 2003; 352: 67-9.

[63] Parnetti L, Lanari A, Silvestrelli G, Saggese E, Reboldi P. Diagnosing prodromal Alzheimer's disease: Role of CSF biochemical markers. Mechan Ageing Dev 2005 [EPub]

[64] Hansson O, Zetterberg H, Buchhave P, Londos E, Blennow K, Minthon L. Association between CSF biomarkers and incipient Alzheimer's disease in patients with mild cognitive impairment: a follow-up study. Lancet Neurol 2006:5:228-34.

[65] Seppala TT, Koivisto AM, Hartikainen P et al. Longitudinal changes of CSF Biomarkers in Alzheimer's disease. J Alz Iis 2011; 24:583-94.

[66] Samgard K, Zetterberg H, Blennow K, Hansson O et al. Cerebrospinal fluid total tau as a marker of Alzheimer's disease intensity. Int J Geriatr Psy 2010: 25:403-10.

[67] Ravaglia S, Bini P, Sinforiani E, Franciotta D et al. Cerebrospinal fluid levels of tau phosphrylated at threonine 181 in patients with Alzheimer's disease and vascular dementia. Neurol Sci 2008; 29:417-23.

[68] Vlachos GSm Oarasjevas GP, Naoumis D, Kapaki E. Cerebrospinal fluid β-amyloid$_{1-42}$ correlates with rate of progression in Alzheimer's disease. J Neural Transm 2012; 119:799-804.

[69] Wallin AK, Blennow K, Zetterberg J, Londos E et al. CSF biomarkers predict a more malignant course in Alzheimer disease. Neurology 2010; 74(19): 1531-7.

[70] deLeon MJ, Segal S, Tarshish CY, DeSanti S, Zinkowski R, Mehta PD, Convit A, Caraos C, Rusinek H, Tsui W, Saint Louis LA et al. Longitudinal cerebrospinal fluid tau load increases in mild cognitive impairment. Neurosci Letters 2002; 333:183-6.

[71] Leon MJ, Desanti S, Zinkowski R, Mehta PD, Pratico D, Segal S, Rusinek H, Li J, Tsui W, Saint Louis LA, Clark CM et al. Longitudinal CSF and MRI biomarkers improve the diagnosis of mild cognitive impairment. Neurobiol Aging. 2005 Aug 25.

[72] Kester ML, Scheffer PG, Koel-Simmelink MJ, Twaalfhoven H et al. Serial CSF sampling in Alzheimer's disease: specific versus non-specific markers. Neurobiol Aging 2012; 33:1591-98.

[73] Rosun D, Schuff N, Shaw LM, Trojanowski JQ, Weiner MW et al. Relationship between CSF biomarkers of Alzheimer's disease and Rates of Regional Cortical Thinning in ADNI data. J Alzheimer's Dis 2011; 26:77-90.

[74] Perrin RJ, Craig-Schapiro R, Malone JP, Shah AR, Gilmore P et al. Identification and Validation of Novel Cerebrospinal fluid biomarkers for staging early Alzheimer's Disease. PLOS One 2011; 6(1):e16032.

[75] Georganopoulou DG, Chang L, Nam J, Thaxton CS et al. Nanoparticle-based detection in cerebral spinal fluid of a soluble pathogenic biomarker for Alzheimer's disease. PNAS 2005; 102(7):2273-6.

[76] Craig-Scharpiro R, Kuhn M, Xiong C, Pickering Eh et al. Multiplexed Immunoassay Panel identified Novel CSF Biomarkers for Alzheimer's Disease Diagnosis and Prognosis. PLOS One 2011; 6(4):e18850.

[77] Glabe CG, Kayed R. Common structure and toxic function of amyloid oligomers implies a common mechanism of pathogenesis. Neurology 2006; 66(Suppl 1): S74-78.

[78] Lemere CA, Maier M, Jiang L, Peng Y, Seabrook TJ. Amyloid-Beta Immunotherapy for the Prevention and Treatment of Alzheimer Disease: Lessons from mice, monkeys and humans. Rejuvenation Res 2006; 9(1): 77-84.

[79] Olsson A et al. Simultaneous measurement of β-amyloid$_{(1-42)}$, total tau, and phosphorylated tau (Thr^{181}) in cerebrospinal fluid by xMAP technology. Lin Chem 2005; 51:336-345.

[80] Mattsson N, Zetterberg H, Blennow K. Lessons from multicenter studies on CSF biomarkers for Alzheimer's disease. Int J Alz Dis 2010. doi:10.4061/2010/610613.

[81] Lee TS, Chua SM, Ly P, Song W. Genomic and molecular characterization of Alzheimer Disease. Current Psych Reviews, 2010, 6, 104-113.

[82] Hansson O, Zetterberg H, Vanmechelen E, Vanderstichele H, Andreasson U, Londos E, Wallin A, Minthon L, Blennow K. Evaluation of plasma Abeta(40) and Abeta(42) as predictors of conversion to Alzheimer's disease in patients with mild cognitive impairment. Neurobiol Aging. 2010 Mar;31(3):357-67. Epub 2008 May 19.

[83] Mayeux R, Schupf N.Mayeux Blood-based biomarkers for Alzheimer's disease: plasma Aβ40 and Aβ42, and genetic variants. Neurobiol Aging. 2011 Dec;32 Suppl 1:S10-9. Review.

[84] Koyama A, Okereke OI, Yang T, Blacker D, Selkoe DJ, Grodstein F. Plasma Amyloid-β as a Predictor of Dementia and Cognitive Decline: A Systematic Review and Meta-analysis.Arch Neurol. 2012 Mar 26.

[85] Borroni B, Colciaghi F, Archetti S, Marcello E, Caimi L, Di Luca M, Padovani A. Predicting cognitive decline in Alzheimer disease. Role of platelet amyloid precursor protein. Alzheimer Dis Assoc Disord. 2004 Jan-Mar;18(1):32-4.

[86] Xu G, Zhou Z, Zhu W, Fan X, Liu X. Plasma C-reactive protein (CRP) is related to cognitive deterioration and dementia in patients with mild cognitive impairment (Xu 2009) Neurol Sci. 2009 Sep 15;284(1-2):77-80. Epub 2009

[87] Locascio JJ, Fukumoto H, Yap L, Bottiglieri T, Growdon JH, Hyman BT, Irizarry MC. Plasma amyloid beta-protein and C-reactive protein in relation to the rate of progression of Alzheimer disease. Arch Neurol. 2008 Jun;65(6):776-85

[88] Thambisetty M, An Y, Kinsey A, Koka D, Saleem M, Güntert A, Kraut M, Ferrucci L, Davatzikos C, Lovestone S, Resnick SM. Plasma clusterin concentration is associated with longitudinal brain atrophy in mild cognitive impairment. Neuroimage. 2012 Jan 2;59(1):212-7. Epub 2011 Jul 28.

[89] Mielke MM, Haughey NJ, Bandaru VV, Weinberg DD, Darby E, Zaidi N, Pavlik V, Doody RS, Lyketsos CG. Plasma sphingomyelins are associated with cognitive progression in Alzheimer's disease. J Alzheimers Dis. 2011;27(2):259-69.

[90] Elias-Sonnenschein LS, Viechtbauer W, Ramakers IH, Verhey FR, Visser PJ. Predictive value of APOE-ε4 allele for progression from MCI to AD-type dementia: a meta-analysis. J Neurol Neurosurg Psychiatry. 2011 Oct;82(10):1149-56. Epub 2011 Apr 14.

[91] Martins CA, Oulhaj A, de Jager CA, Williams JH. APOE alleles predict the rate of cognitive decline in Alzheimer disease: a nonlinear model. Neurology. 2005 Dec 27;65(12):1888-93.

[92] Cosentino S, Scarmeas N, Helzner E, Glymour MM, Brandt J, Albert M, Blacker D, Stern Y. APOE epsilon 4 allele predicts faster cognitive decline in mild Alzheimer disease. Neurology. 2008 May 6;70(19 Pt 2):1842-9. Epub 2008 Apr 9

[93] Lee TS, Goh L, Chong MS, Chua SM, Chen GB, Feng L, Lim WS, Chan M, Ng TP, Krishnan KR. Downregulation of TOMM40 expression in the blood of Alzheimer disease subjects compared with matched controls. J Psychiatr Res. 2012 Jun;46(6): 828-30. Epub 2012 Apr 1.

[94] Ray S, Britschgi M, Herbert C, Takeda-Uchimura Y, Boxer A, Blennow K, Friedman LF, Galasko DR, Jutel M, Karydas A, Kaye JA, Leszek J, Miller BL, Minthon L, Quinn JF, Rabinovici GD, Robinson WH, Sabbagh MN, So YT, Sparks DL, Tabaton M, Tinklenberg J, Yesavage JA, Tibshirani R, Wyss-Coray T. Nat Med. Classification and prediction of clinical Alzheimer's diagnosis based on plasma signaling proteins. 2007 Nov; 13(11):1359-62. Epub 2007 Oct 14.

[95] Soares HD, Chen Y, Sabbagh M, Roher A, Schrijvers E, Breteler M. Identifying early markers of Alzheimer's disease using quantitative multiplex proteomic immunoassay panels. Ann N Y Acad Sci. 2009 Oct;1180:56-67.

[96] Jack CR Jr, Shiung MM, Gunter JL, O'Brien PC, Weigand SD, Knopman DS, Boeve BF, Ivnik RJ, Smith GE, Cha RH, Tangalos EG, Petersen RC. Comparison of different MRI brain atrophy rate measures with clinical disease progression in AD. Neurology. 2004 Feb 24;62(4):591-600.

[97] Jack CR Jr, Petersen RC, Grundman M, Jin S, Gamst A, Ward CP, Sencakova D, Doody RS, Thal LJ; Members of the Alzheimer's Disease Cooperative Study (ADCS). Longitudinal MRI findings from the vitamin E and donepezil treatment study for MCI. Neurobiol Aging. 2008 Sep;29(9):1285-95. Epub 2007 Apr 23.

[98] Jack CR Jr, Shiung MM, Weigand SD, O'Brien PC, Gunter JL, Boeve BF, Knopman DS, Smith GE, Ivnik RJ, Tangalos EG, Petersen RC. Brain atrophy rates predict subsequent clinical conversion in normal elderly and amnestic MCI. Neurology. 2005 Oct 25;65(8): 1227-31.

[99] Apostolova LG, Dutton RA, Dinov ID, Hayashi KM, Toga AW, Cummings JL, Thompson PM Conversion of mild cognitive impairment to Alzheimer disease predicted by hippocampal atrophy maps. Arch Neurol. 2006 May;63(5):693-9.

[100] Thompson PM, Hayashi KM, de Zubicaray G, Janke AL, Rose SE, Semple J, Herman D, Hong MS, Dittmer SS, Doddrell DM, Toga AW. Dynamics of gray matter loss in Alzheimer's disease. J Neurosci. 2003 Feb 1;23(3):994-1005.

[101] Risacher SL, Saykin AJ, West JD, Shen L, Firpi HA, McDonald BC; Alzheimer's Disease Neuroimaging Initiative (ADNI). Baseline MRI predictors of conversion from MCI to probable AD in the ADNI cohort. Curr Alzheimer Res. 2009 Aug;6(4):347-61.

[102] Kinkingnéhun S, Sarazin M, Lehéricy S, Guichart-Gomez E, Hergueta T, Dubois B.VBM anticipates the rate of progression of Alzheimer disease: a 3-year longitudinal study. Neurology. 2008 Jun 3;70(23):2201-11. Epub 2008 Apr 30.

[103] Querbes O, Aubry F, Pariente J, Lotterie JA, Démonet JF, Duret V, Puel M, Berry I, Fort JC, Celsis P; Alzheimer's Disease Neuroimaging Initiative. Early diagnosis of Alzheimer's disease using cortical thickness: impact of cognitive reserve. Brain. 2009 Aug;132(Pt 8):2036-47. Epub 2009 May 12.

[104] Silverman DH, Small GW, Chang CY, Lu CS, Kung De Aburto MA, Chen W, Czernin J, Rapoport SI, Pietrini P, Alexander GE, Schapiro MB, Jagust WJ, Hoffman JM, Welsh-Bohmer KA, Alavi A, Clark CM, Salmon E, de Leon MJ, Mielke R, Cummings JL, Kowell AP, Gambhir SS, Hoh CK, Phelps ME. Positron emission tomography in evaluation of dementia: Regional brain metabolism and long-term outcome. JAMA. 2001 Nov 7;286(17):2120-7.

[105] Lo RY, Hubbard AE, Shaw LM, Trojanowski JQ, Petersen RC, Aisen PS, Weiner MW, Jagust WJ; Alzheimer's Disease Neuroimaging Initiative. Longitudinal change of biomarkers in cognitive decline. Arch Neurol. 2011 Oct;68(10):1257-66. Epub 2011 Jun 13.

[106] Okello A, Koivunen J, Edison P, Archer HA, Turkheimer FE, Någren K, Bullock R, Walker Z, Kennedy A, Fox NC, Rossor MN, Rinne JO, Brooks DJ. Conversion of amyloid positive and negative MCI to AD over 3 years: an 11C-PIB PET study. Neurology. 2009 Sep 8;73(10):754-60. Epub 2009 Jul 8.

[107] Koivunen J, Scheinin N, Virta JR, Aalto S, Vahlberg T, Någren K, Helin S, Parkkola R, Viitanen M, Rinne JO. Amyloid PET imaging in patients with mild cognitive impairment: a 2-year follow-up study. Neurology. 2011 Mar 22;76(12):1085-90. Epub 2011 Feb 16.

[108] Small GW, Siddarth P, Kepe V, Ercoli LM, Burggren AC, Bookheimer SY, Miller KJ, Kim J, Lavretsky H, Huang SC, Barrio JR.Prediction of cognitive decline by positron emission tomography of brain amyloid and tau. Arch Neurol. 2012 Feb;69(2):215-22.

[109] Doraiswamy PM, Sperling RA, Coleman RE, Johnson KA, Reiman EM, Davis MD, Grundman M, Sabbagh MN, Sadowsky CH, Fleisher AS, Carpenter A, Clark CM, Joshi

AD, Mintun MA, Skovronsky DM, Pontecorvo MJ; For the AV45-A11 Study Group. Amyloid-β assessed by florbetapir F 18 PET and 18-month cognitive decline: A multicenter study. Neurology. 2012 Aug 1.

[110] Ossenkoppele R, Tolboom N, Foster-Dingley JC, Adriaanse SF, Boellaard R, Yaqub M, Windhorst AD, Barkhof F, Lammertsma AA, Scheltens P, van der Flier WM, van Berckel BN. Longitudinal imaging of Alzheimer pathology using [11C]PIB, [18F]FDDNP and [18F]FDG PET. Eur J Nucl Med Mol Imaging. 2012 Jun;39(6):990-1000. Epub 2012 Mar 23.

[111] Zhang S, Han D, Tan X, Feng J, Guo Y, Ding Y. Diagnostic accuracy of 18 F-FDG and 11 C-PIB-PET for prediction of short-term conversion to Alzheimer's disease in subjects with mild cognitive impairment. Int J Clin Pract. 2012 Feb;66(2):185-98. doi: 10.1111/j.1742-1241.2011.02845.x.

[112] Villain N, Chetelat G, Grassiot B, Bourgeat P et al. Regional dynamics of amyloid- β deposition in healthy elderly, mild cognitive impairment and Alzheimer's disease: a voxelwise PiB-PET longitudinal study. Brain 2012; doi:10.1093/brain/aws125.

[113] Kester MI, van der Lier WM, Mandic G, Blankenstein MA et al. Joint effect of hypertension and APOE genotype on CSF biomarkers for Alzheimer's disease. J Alz IDis 2010;20:1083-90.

[114] Blom ES, Gledraitis V, Zetterberg H, Fukumoto H et al. Rapid progression from mild cognitive impairment to Alzheimer's Disease in subjects with elevated levels of tau in cerebrospinal fluid and the APOE e4/e4 genotype. Dement Geriatr Cogn Disord 2009; 27:458-464.

[115] Palmqvist S, Hertze J, Minthon L, Wattmo C et al. Comparison of Brief Cognitive Tests and CSF biomarkers in prediciting Alzheimer's disease in mild cognitive impairment: Six-year follow-up study. PLOS one 2012; 7(6):e38639

[116] Ewers M, Walsh C, Trojanowski JQ, Shaw LM et al. Prediction of conversion from mild cognitive impairment to Alzheimer's disease dementia based upon biomarkers and neuropsychological test performance. Neurobiol Aging 2012; 33(7):1203-14.

[117] Cui Y, Liu B, Luo S, Zhen X et al. Identification of Conversion from mild cognitive impairment to Alzheimer's disease using multivariate predictors. PLOS One 2011; 6(7):e21896.

[118] El Fakhri G, Kijewski MF, Johnson KA, Syrkin G, Killany RJ, Becker JA, Zimmerman RE, Albert MS. MRI-guided SPECT perfusion measures and volumetric MRI in Prodromal Alzheimer Disease. Arch Neurol 2003; 60:1066-72.

[119] Huang C, Wahlund LO, Almkvist O, Elehu D, Svensson L, Jonsson T, Winblad B, Julin P. Voxel- and VOI-based analysis of SPECT CBF in relation to clinical and psychological heterogeneity of mild cognitive impairment. Neuroimage. 2003 Jul;19(3):1137-44.

[120] Stephanie V, van Rossum I, Burns L, KNol D et al. Test sequence of CSF and MRI biomarkers for prediction of AD in subjects with MCI. Neurobiol Aging 2012; 33:2272-81.

[121] Vemuri P, Wiste HJ, Weigand SD, Shaw LM et al. MRI and CSF biomarkers in normal, MCI and AD subjects. Neurology 2009;73:294-301.

[122] Eckerstrom C, Andreasson U, Olsson E, Rolstad S, Blennow K et al. Combination of hippocampal volume and cerebrospinal fluid biomarkers improves predictive value in mild cognitive impairment. Dement Geriatr Cogn Disord 2010; 29:294-300.

[123] Davatzikos C, Bhatt P, Shaw LM, Batmanghelich KN, Trojanowski JQ. Prediction of MCI to AD conversion, via MRI, CSF biomarkers and pattern classification. Neurobiol Aging 2011; 2322.e19-2322.e27

[124] Hansson O, Buchhave P, Zetterberg H, Blennow K et al. Combined rCBF and CSF biomarkers predict preogression from mild cognitive impairment to Alzheimer's disease. Neurobiol Aging 2009;30:165-173.

[125] Okamura N, Arai H, Maruyama M et al. Combined analysis of CSF tau levels and [(123)I]Iodoamphetamine SPECT in mild cognitive impairment: implications for a novel predictor of Alzheimer's disease. Am J Psychiatry 2002; 159:474-76.

[126] Furney SJ, Kronenberg D, Simmons A, Guntert A, Dobson RJ et al. Combinatorial markers of mild cognitive impairment conversion to Alzheimer's disease – cytokines and MRI measures together predict disease progression. J Alz Dis 2011; 26:395-405.

[127] Zhang D, Shen D, Alzheimer's Disease Neuroimaging Initiative. Predicting future clinical changes of MCI patients using Longitudinal and Multimodal Biomarkers. PLOS One 2012; 7(3):e33182.

[128] Zhang D, Wang Y, Zhou L, Yuan H et al. Multimodal classification of Alzheimer's disease and mild cognitive impairment. Neuroimage 2011; 55:856-67.

[129] Hinrichs C, Singh V, Xu G, Johnson SC et al. Predictive markers for AD in a multi-modality Framework: An Analysis of MCI progression in the ADNI population. Neuroimage 2011; 55(2): 574-89.

[130] Cruchaga C, Kauwe JSK, Mayo K, Spiegel N et al. SNPs associated with cerebrospinal fluid phosphor-tau levels influence rate of decline in Alzheimer Disease. PLOS Genetics 2010; 6(9):e1001101.

[131] Chong MS, Sahadevan S. Preclinical Alzheimer's disease: diagnosis and prediction of progression. Lancet Neurol 2005; 4: 576-79.

[132] Chong MS, Lim WS, Sahadevan S. Biomarkers in prediction of progression of preclinical Alzheimer's disease. Current Opinion in Investigational Drugs 2006: 7(7): 600-607.

[133] Beckett LA, Harvey DJ, Gamst A, Donohue M et al. The Alzheimer's Disease Neuroimaging Initiative: Annual Change in Biomarkers and Clinical Outcomes. Alz Dement 2010; 6(3): 257-64.

[134] Jack CR, Knopman DS, Jagust WJ, et al. Hypothetical model of dynamic biomarkers of the Alzheimer's pathological cascade. Lancet Neurol 2010; 9:119-28

[135] Storandt M, Head D, Fagan AM, Holtzman DM, Morris JC. Toward a multifactorial model of Alzheimer disease. Neurobiol Aging 2012; 33:2262-71.

[136] Rowe CC, Ellisa KA, Rimajova M, Bourgeat P et al. Amyloid imaging results from the Australian Imaging, Biomarkers and Lifestyle (AIBL) study of aging. Neurobiol Aging 2010; 31:1275-83.

[137] Kohannim O, HUa X, Hibar DP, Lee S, Chou U, Toga AW et al. Boosting power for clinical trials using classifiers based on multiple biomarkers. Neurobiol Aging 2010; 31:1429-42.

[138] Lorenzi M, Donohue M, Paternico D, Scarpazza C et al. Enrichment through biomarkers in clinical trials of Alzheimer's drugs in patients with mild cognitive impairment. Neurobiol Aging 2010; 31:1443-51.

[139] van Rossum IA, Vos S, Handels R, Visser PJ. Biomarkers as Predictors for Conversion from Mild Cognitive Impairment to Alzheimer-Type Dementia: Implications for Trial Design. J Alz Dis 2010; 20:881-91.

[140] Yu P, Dean RA, Hall SD, Qi Y et al. Enriching Amnestic Mild Cognitive Impairment Populations for Clinical Trials: Optimal Combination of Biomarkers to Predict Conversion to Dementia. J Alz Dis; doi 10.3233/JAD-2012-120832.

[141] Lopez OL, Schqam E, Cummings J, Gautheir S, Jones R et al. Predicting cognitive decline in Alzheimer's diseae: An integrated analysis. Alz Dement 2010; 6:431-9.

Chapter 7

Prevention of Alzheimer's Disease: Intervention Studies

Francesca Mangialasche, Weili Xu and
Miia Kivipelto

Additional information is available at the end of the chapter

1. Introduction

The aging of the population is a worldwide phenomenon, and studying age-related diseases has become a relevant issue from both a scientific and a public health perspective. Dementia is a syndrome characterised by loss of cognitive abilities in multiple domains that results in impairment in normal activities of daily living and loss of independence [1]. Both prevalence and incidence of dementia rise exponentially with advancing age, and 70% of all dementia cases occur in people aged 75+ years [2]. The worldwide increase in the number of older adults, more pronounced in the 80+ age group, explains the epidemic proportions assumed by dementia. According to the World Alzheimer Report, there were 35.6 million people living with dementia worldwide in 2010, a number that will increase to 65.7 million by 2030 and 115.4 million by 2050 unless effective means reducing the disease incidence are introduced [3]. Dementia is a major cause of disability and institutionalization of elderly people and because of its increased prevalence this disorder is becoming an emerging public health issue not only in developed countries but also in less developed regions of the world. The total estimated worldwide costs of dementia were US$604 billion in 2010, including the costs of informal care (unpaid care provided by family and others), direct costs of social care (provided by community care professionals, and in residential home settings) and the direct costs of medical care (the costs of treating dementia and other conditions in primary and secondary care) [3].

Alzheimer's disease (AD) is considered the most common cause of dementia, accounting for 60–70% of all dementia cases. The hallmarks of AD neuropathology in the brain are the presence of extracellular plaques composed of amyloid-β (Aβ) and intracellular neurofibrillary tangles (NFTs) composed of hyperphosphorylated aggregates of the microtubule-associated tau protein [4].

Vascular dementia (VaD), mainly due to cerebrovascular diseases (CVD), is the second most frequent type of dementia [5, 6]. This current classification of dementia types is being reconsidered in light of recent neuropathological and neuroimaging studies, which have shown a range of dementia-associated brain abnormalities from pure vascular lesions at one end to pure AD pathologies at the other, with most dementia cases being attributable to both CVD and AD. In fact, AD and CVD-related changes often coexist in the brain of older adults with dementia and mild cognitive impairment (MCI) [7, 8]. Also, both types of lesions are detected in the brain of cognitively normal elderly people, highlighting the importance of mixed pathologies in increasing the risk of late-life dementia [9]. The co-occurrence of AD and CVD is consistent with the evidence that AD and VaD share several risk and protective factors, including cardiovascular and lifestyle related factors. Overall, this implies that dementia syndrome is a valid target for prevention, especially from the public health perspective.

Prevention is traditionally divided into three levels: primary, secondary, and tertiary prevention. Primary prevention aims to reduce the incidence of the disease by eliminating or treating specific risk factors, which may decrease or delay the development of dementia. Secondary prevention aims to early detection of the disease, before any symptom has emerged, when treatment could stop its progression. Tertiary prevention aims to reduce the impact of complications and disability of long-term diseases.

Regarding primary prevention, both observational and interventional epidemiological studies have been conducted for dementia and AD. On the other hand, in the field of AD the development of pharmacological interventions has been mainly limited to a tertiary prevention level, since the diagnostic criteria currently in use for AD (National Institute of Neurological and Communicative Disorders and Stroke-Alzheimer's Disease and Related Disorders Association, NINCDS-ADRDA - criteria) identify the presence of the disease only when AD is severe enough to cause a dementia syndrome [10]. Thus, the majority of anti-AD drugs have been tested in subjects already in the symptomatic stage of the disease, and so far no drug has shown the ability to stop the disease progression (i.e. disease-modifying effect) [11]. However, several studies have shown that the pathophysiological process of AD begins years, if not decades, before the diagnosis of Alzheimer's dementia and individuals generally experience a gradual impairment of cognitive functions, which can progress to a dementia syndrome [12-14].

Recent advances in neuroimaging, cerebrospinal fluid (CSF) assays, and other techniques now provide the ability to detect evidence of the AD pathophysiological process in vivo, but the diagnostic criteria currently in use do not take into account these biomarkers. Three international workgroups promoted by the American National Institute of Aging (NIA) and the American Alzheimer's Association recently proposed new diagnostic guidelines to identify dementia due to AD, MCI due to AD, and preclinical AD [15-17]. These new criteria formalize the different clinical stages of AD and incorporate biomarkers (genetic, biochemical, neuroimaging) that can be detected in vivo and are believed to reflect AD pathology. These diagnostic criteria are now being validated and can be revised as long as new findings from research on biomarkers in AD will clarify the link between AD pathophysiology and the AD clinical syndrome. These criteria offer the opportunity to identify subjects who can be target of secondary prevention in order to halt the progression of the brain damage and prevent or delay the onset of cognitive symptoms. A step in this direction has been done by planning randomized controlled trials (RCTs) testing anti-amyloid drugs in older adults with evidence of brain amyloid accumulation. The same type of intervention will also be tested in subjects at risk of early onset AD due to genetic mutations associated with familial AD.

This chapter summarizes the major findings concerning primary prevention of late onset dementia and AD, based on current epidemiological evidence from observational and interventional studies. Preventive strategies for early onset AD are also mentioned. Although many aspects of the dementias are still unclear, some risk and protective factors have been identified. It is also possible to delineate some preventative strategies. Ongoing interventional studies testing the effect of preventive measures for dementia and AD are discussed, and methodological challenges in designing dementia prevention trials are summarized.

2. Observational studies

Several community-based prospective studies of aging and health have been carried out in different countries since the 80s'. These studies have provided relevant information on the aetiology of dementia and AD, and have led to the identification of possible preventive strategies. Evidence from these observational studies has shown that dementia is a multifactorial disorder caused by several interrelated mechanisms in which the interaction of genetic and environmental factors plays the major role (Table 1). The pathways that lead from different risk factors to dementia are not fully understood, but several etiological hypotheses have been proposed: the vascular hypothesis, inflammatory hypothesis, oxidative-stress hypothesis, toxic hypothesis and psychosocial hypothesis [18, 19]. These theories highlight potential links of various risk factors to both the vascular and the neurodegenerative brain pathologies that can cause dementia, supporting the validity of dementia syndrome as target for prevention [6, 20].

2.1. Non-modifiable risk factors for Alzheimer's disease

Both modifiable and non-modifiable risk factors have been identified for dementia and AD, and while for some factors the scientific evidence is quite robust, for others the results are still inconclusive.

2.1.1. Age

Increasing age is a well-established risk factor for dementia, which is a common disorders after 75 years of age, but rare before age 60. The incidence rates of dementia increase exponentially with advancing age. In Europe, approximately two per 1,000 person-years become demented among people aged 65-69 years, and the incidence increases to 70 to 80 per 1,000 person-years for people 90 years or over [21, 22]. It is still unclear if the incidence of dementia continues to increase even in the oldest old or reaches a plateau at a certain age. The Cache County Study found that the incidence of dementia increased with age, peaked, and then started to decline at extreme old ages for both men and women. However, some meta-analyses and large-scale studies in Europe provided no evidence for the potential decline in the incidence of dementia among the oldest old [21, 22].

Risk factors	Protective factors	Combined effects
Age	**Genetic**	**Increased risk**
	APP	*Genetic and environmental factors in midlife*
Genetic		
Familial aggregation	**Psychosocial factors**	APOEε4 magnifies the effect of high alcohol intake, smoking, physical inactivity and high intake of saturate fat
APOE ε4	High education and SES	
APP	High work complexity	
GSK3β	Rich social network and social engagement	*Vascular factors in midlife*
DYRK1A		Hypertension, obesity, hypercholesterolemia and physical inactivity have an additive effect when they co-occur
Tau	Mentally stimulating activity	
CLU		
TOMM40	**Lifestyle**	
PICALM	Physical activity	
CR1		*Vascular factors/diseases in late-life*
	Diet	Higher risk in individuals with brain hypoperfusion profile: chronic heart failure, low pulse pressure, low diastolic pressure
Vascular	Mediterranean diet	
Cerebrovascular lesions	Polyunsaturated (PUFA) and fish-related fats	
Cardiovascular diseases		
Diabetes mellitus and pre-diabetes	Vitamin B$_6$, B$_{12}$, folate	Higher risk in individuals with atherosclerosis profile: high systolic pressure, diabetes mellitus or prediabetes, stroke
	Antioxidant vitamins (A, C, E)	
Midlife positive association but late-life negative association	Vitamin D	
Hypertension		
High BMI (overweight and obesity)	**Drugs**	**Decreased risk**
High serum cholesterol	Statins	*Genetic and environmental factors in midlife*
	Antihypertensive drugs	High education reduces the negative effect of *APOEε4*
Lifestyle	HRT	
Smoking	NSAIDs	Physical activity counteracts the risk due to *APOEε4*
High alcohol intake		
Diet		*Environmental factors in midlife*
Saturated fats		High work complexity modulates the increased dementia risk due to low education
Homocysteine		
Others		*Genetic and environmental factors in late-life*
Depression		
Occupational exposure		Active leisure activities or absence of vascular risk factors reduces the risk due to *APOEε4*
Traumatic brain injury		
Infective agents (Herpes Simplex Virus Type I, Clamydophila pneumoniae, Spirochetes)		

APOE: apolipoprotein E. BMI: body mass index. *CLU*: clusterin. *CR1*: complement component receptor 1. *DYRK1A*: dual-specificity tyrosine-(Y)-phosphorylation regulated kinase 1A. *GSK3β*: glycogen synthase kinase-3beta. HRT: hormone replacement therapy. NSAIDs: nonsteroidal anti-inflammatory drugs. *PICALM*: phosphatidylinositol binding clathrin assembly protein. PUFA: polyunsaturated fatty acid. SES: socioeconomic status. *TOMM40*: translocase of outer mitochondrial membrane 40 homolog.

Table 1. Proposed risk and protective factors for dementia and Alzheimer's disease

2.1.2. Familial aggregation

Familial aggregation is another important risk factor for late life dementia and AD. First-degree relatives of AD patients have a higher lifetime risk for developing AD than relatives of non-demented people or the general population (Table 1) [21, 22]. It is likely that shared genetic and environmental factors contribute to the familial aggregation. The amount of risk of AD that is attributable to genetics is estimated to be around 70% [25].

2.1.3. Genes

The Apolipoprotein E *(APOE)* ε4 allele is the only established genetic risk factor for both early- and late-onset AD; it is a susceptibility gene, being neither necessary nor sufficient for the development of AD. The risk of AD increases with increasing number of the ε4 alleles in a dose-dependent manner, but the risk effect decreases with increasing age. Individuals with two *APOE* ε4 alleles have a more than seven times increased risk of developing AD compared with those with *APOE* ε3 alleles and approximately 15 to 20 percent of AD cases are attributable to the *APOE* ε4 allele [25-28].

Other genes have been related to increased risk of late life AD, but the association is less consistent. These are mainly genes involved in the metabolism and processing of the amyloid precursor protein (APP) and Aβ, as well as tau protein, including the *GSK3β*, *DYRK1A, Tau,* and *CLU* genes [25]. Until now, mutations in APP have not been implicated in the late-onset form of AD, with the exception of the rare variant, N660Y, which was recently identified in one case from a late-onset AD family [29]. A recent study identified a mutation in the *APP* gene that can be protective against AD and age-related cognitive decline. This mutation is associated with a reduced production of amyloidogenic peptides [30]. Other genes that have been associated with increased risk of AD are *TOMM40*, *CR1* and *PICALM*. The *TOMM40* gene is located in a region of chromosome 19, which is in linkage disequilibrium with *APOE*, and its polymorphism affects the age on onset of AD in subjects with an *APOE* genotype [31]. *CR1* is involved in the complement cascade, while *PICALM* encodes a protein that is involved in clathrin-mediated endocytosis, an essential step in the intracellular trafficking of proteins and lipids such as nutrients, growth factors and neurotransmitters [32].

Several aspects challenge the identification of genetic risk factors for late life AD, including the fact that risk conferred by a single gene is generally small, and for some genes is the combination of risk alleles that is relevant for a significant change of the overall risk. Also, the heterogeneous and mixed nature of brain pathology causing dementia, particularly coexisting CVD, makes it more difficult to identify genetic risk factors for AD. Nevertheless, the identification of genetic risk factors for late onset AD can have implication for preventive and therapeutic strategies. In fact, it has been shown that the *APOE* ε4 allele can modulate the effect of lifestyle related risk factors [33] and influence the effect of pharmacological treatment for AD [34]. It is thus possible that future preventive and therapeutic measures will be tailored according to specific genetic risk profiles.

2.2. Modifiable risk and protective factors for Alzheimer's disease

Different modifiable factors have been proposed to play a role in late life dementia and AD, including nutritional factors (i.e., diet and nutritional supplements), social or economic factors, medical conditions and lifestyle related factors (e.g., smoking habit, physical activity, etc.) (Table 1). A report commissioned by the National institute of Health (NIH) to the Agency for Healthcare Research and Quality (AHRQ) was published in 2010, and concluded that current research evidence on many risk and protective factors for cognitive decline and AD is not of sufficient strength, thus recommendations for preventing these conditions cannot be made [35, 36]. Another previous review yielded similar conclusions [37]. These negative perspectives have been criticized, since there is consistent and robust epidemiological evidence that use of antihypertensive medications, cessation of smoking and increasing physical activity produces cognitive benefits in older adults [38]. Furthermore, the analytical strategy used in the Evidence Based Review carried out by the AHRQ did not take into account the life-course perspective [39]. Observational longitudinal studies have shown that the risk of late-life dementia and AD is determined by exposures to multiple factors experienced over the life-span and that the effect of specific risk/protective factors largely depends on age [39]. Thus, a life-course perspective is relevant for chronic disorders with a long latent period (such as dementia). It allows the identification of time windows when exposures have their greatest effect on outcome and assessment of whether cumulative exposures could have multiplicative or additive effects over the life course [40]. Age-dependent associations with AD have been suggested for several aging-related medical conditions. For example, elevated blood pressure, body mass index (BMI) and total cholesterol levels at a young age and in middle age (<65 years) have been associated with an increased risk of dementia and AD, whereas having lower values in late life (age >75 years) has been also associated with subsequent development of dementia/AD [41-46].

2.2.1. Risk factors

1. **Vascular risk factors and disorders**: An association of elevated blood pressure in midlife with an increased risk of dementia and AD later in life has been reported in several population-based studies [41, 47], while follow-up studies of late-life blood pressure and risk of dementia yield mixed results, largely depending on the length of follow-up. The short-term follow-up studies (e.g., less than 3 years) often found no association or even an inverse association between blood pressure and risk of dementia and AD [41]. However, studies of very old people (i.e., 75 + years) with a longer follow-up period (i.e., more than 6 years) also revealed an increased risk of dementia associated with low blood pressure [48], suggesting that among very old people low blood pressure may also contribute to the development of dementia, possibly by influencing cerebral blood perfusion.

   For BMI, the bidirectional association with dementia and AD has been shown in several studies, and longitudinal studies of elderly people have associated accelerated decline in BMI with subsequent development of dementia. This implies that low BMI and weight loss in advanced age can be interpreted as markers for preclinical dementia [45, 46, 49-55].

Regarding serum total cholesterol, the importance of the pattern of change in cholesterol levels after midlife has been shown by two studies with a long follow-up, reporting that a decline in plasma total cholesterol after midlife may be associated with the risk of cognitive decline, dementia and AD in late life [56, 57]. These findings suggest that high total serum cholesterol in midlife seems to be a risk factor for dementia and AD in advanced age, while decreasing serum cholesterol after midlife may reflect ongoing disease processes and represent a marker of early stages in the development of dementia and AD. The use of statins (cholesterol-lowering drugs) in relation to dementia has been investigated in several community studies, with mixed findings. Some observational studies suggest a protective effect, while others did not, and clinical trials using statins for prevention of cognitive decline or dementia mainly reported no effects [6, 58]. Diabetes mellitus has been associated with increased risk of dementia and AD over adult life, but the risk is stronger when diabetes occurs in mid-life than in late-life [59]. Also pre-diabetes, impaired glucose regulation, and impaired insulin secretion have been associated with and increased risk of dementia and AD [60].

Cerebrovascular lesions and cardiovascular diseases have been shown to be risk factors for dementia and AD. Several population-based studies reveal an approximately two- to four-fold increased risk of incident dementia associated with clinical stroke (post-stroke dementia) [61, 62]. It is probable that an association of clinical stroke with AD is rarely reported due to the fact that a history of stroke is part of the current criteria for excluding the diagnosis of AD. However, asymptomatic cerebrovascular lesions such as silent brain infarcts and white matter lesions have been associated with an increased risk of dementia and AD [63, 64], although the association with AD is likely to be due to the inclusion of mixed dementia cases. The Cardiovascular Health Study found that cardiovascular disease was associated with an increased incidence of dementia, with the highest risk seen among people with peripheral arterial disease, suggesting that extensive peripheral atherosclerosis is a risk factor for dementia [65]. Atrial fibrillation, heart failure, and severe atherosclerosis measured with ankle-to-brachial index are also associated with the increased risk of dementia and AD [66-69].

2. **Environmental and other factors:** Current smoking is another major risk factor for dementia and AD, and based on the worldwide prevalence of smoking, about 14% of all AD cases are potentially attributable to this risk factor [70]. Although it is not entirely clear whether depression is a risk factor for or a preclinical symptom of dementia, studies with long-term follow-up support the risk-factor hypothesis [71]. Other conditions have been proposed as risk factors for dementia and AD, but the evidence is still sparse. These include occupational exposure, traumatic brain injury and infections. Occupational exposure to heavy metals such as aluminum and mercury has been suggested to be a risk factor for AD; even high consumption of aluminum from drinking water has been associated with an elevated risk of AD and dementia [6, 72]. In addition, occupational exposure to extremely-low-frequency electromagnetic fields (ELF-EMFs) has been related to an increased risk of dementia and AD [73, 74].

Traumatic brain injury has been extensively investigated as a possible risk factor for AD. The meta-analysis of case-control studies supported an association between a history of head injury and the increased risk of AD [75]. In contrast, some longitudinal studies found that AD was not associated with head trauma or only associated with severe traumatic head injury [76]. The role of viral and bacterial organisms in the development of chronic neurodegeneration is long established. Thus, Treponema pallidum and HIV, in particular, have been associated with the development of dementia. Other infections in the central nervous system (CNS), particularly Herpes Simplex Virus Type 1, Chlamydophila pneumoniae and several types of Spirochetes, have been suggested as possible aetiological agents in the development of sporadic AD, but with little consistent evidence. It has also been suggested that peripheral infections may have a role in accelerating neurodegeneration in AD by activating already primed microglial cells within the CNS [77].

2.2.2. Protective factors

1. **Psychosocial factors**: Protective factors for dementia and AD have also been identified, including high education and socioeconomic status (SES) in early life as well as a number of factors in adult life: high work complexity, rich social network, social engagement, mentally-stimulating activity, non-smoking and regular physical exercise [6, 78, 79]. Living with a partner during mid-life has been associated with reduced risk of cognitive impairment and dementia later in life, suggesting that being in a relationship entails cognitive and social challenges that can increase the cognitive reserve [80]. Even at old ages the active engagement in mental, physical and social activities may postpone the onset of dementia, possibly by increasing the cognitive reserve [81].

2. **Lifestyle and diet**: In addition, several follow-up studies reported a decreased risk of dementia and AD associated with healthy dietary patterns and nutritional factors, such as high adherence to a Mediterranean diet or dietary intake of antioxidants (e.g., vitamins E and C) and ω-3 polyunsaturated fatty acid (PUFA, often measured as fish consumption) [82-86], although some negative results have been also reported [87-90]. Light-to-moderate alcohol intake (e.g., 1-3 drinks per day) has been associated to a reduced incidence of dementia and AD [6, 91, 92], while heavy alcohol consumption at midlife has been associated to an increased risk of dementia/AD, especially among APOE ε4 carriers [93]. Alcohol may have beneficial influences on several cardiovascular factors, including lipid and lipoprotein levels, inflammatory and hemostatic factors. Indeed, moderate alcohol drinking has been related to a reduced risk of cardiovascular diseases, and may be associated with fewer brain infarcts [6]. However, it has been also suggested that the apparent cognitive benefits of light-to-moderate alcohol intake could be due to potential biases that result from methodological limitations of the observational studies such as information bias, confounding of socioeconomic status and healthy lifestyles, and inconsistent approaches of alcohol assessments [6].

3. **Vitamins**: The micronutrient vitamin E is the main lipid-soluble, chain-breaking, non-enzymatic antioxidant in the human body [94], and is essential for normal neurological functions [95]. Vitamin E includes eight natural congeners: four tocopherols and four

tocotrienols, named as α, β, γ, and δ [96]. Each congener shows different biological properties potentially relevant for neuroprotection. These include antioxidant and anti-inflammatory activity and modulation of signaling pathways involved in neurodegeneration [96, 97]. Most investigation of vitamin E in relation to dementia and AD has focused primarily only on α-tocopherol, with conflicting findings. Overall, studies investigating vitamin E intake only from supplements found no association with dementia/AD risk [89, 98-101], or a reduced incidence was found only for the combined use of vitamin E and C supplements [102, 103]. On the other hand, studies examining vitamin E dietary intake consistently report a reduced risk of dementia/AD in individuals with high vitamin E intake [84, 85, 104-106]. This might be explained by the fact that while vitamin E supplements contain only α-tocopherol, dietary intake can provide a balanced combination of different forms of vitamin E, which can be more relevant for neuroprotection. Recent studies seem to support this hypothesis: a multicenter European study found that both AD and MCI were associated with low plasma tocopherols and tocotrienols levels [107]. Further, in the Swedish Kungsholmen Project a decreased AD risk was found in subjects with high plasma levels of total tocopherols and total tocotrienols [108].

Vitamin B12 and folate are essential micronutrients that are part of the homocysteine metabolic cycle, and both vitamin B12 and folate deficiencies can result in increased total homocysteine levels, which may lead to a variety of disorders including cardiovascular and cerebrovascular conditions. Several studies reported and increased risk of dementia/AD, worse cognitive functioning and structural brain changes in individuals with low levels of vitamin B12, holotranscobalamin (the biologically active fraction of vitamin B12) or folate, or high levels of total homocysteine [109-115]. Other studies did not confirm these findings, but methodological differences (e.g., different follow-up duration, implementing the study after mandatory folic acid fortification, etc.) could account for the discrepancy [116-119]. Reviews of RCTs concluded that supplementations of folic acid and vitamin B12 had no benefits on cognition in healthy or cognitively impaired older people, although they were effective in reducing serum homocysteine levels [120, 121]. A more recent RCT testing the efficacy of B vitamins (B6, B12, folate) in subjects with MCI reported beneficial effects of the supplementation, in terms of reduced rate of brain atrophy and cognitive decline, which were more evident in subjects with elevated homocysteine levels [122, 123].

Vitamin D is a secosteroid hormone that is suggested to have neuroprotective effects that include regulation of neuronal calcium homeostasis, as well as antioxidant, neurotrophic and anti-inflammatory properties. Few recent longitudinal studies found a reduced risk of cognitive decline or AD in subjects with higher blood levels or higher dietary intake of vitamin D [124-126]. Despite the epidemiological evidence is still weak vitamin D is already being tested as a therapeutic agent in AD [127].

2.2.3. Combined effect

Cumulative and combined exposure to different risk factors can lead to modified effects on dementia/AD risk (Table 1). In the Finnish Cardiovascular Risk Factors, Aging, and Dementia study (CAIDE), the risk of dementia has been evaluated in relation to a score (CAIDE Dementia Risk Score) combining mid-life risk factors, including low education and cardiovascular factors (i.e., hypertension, obesity, hypercholesterolemia, physical inactivity). The risk of dementia increased as the score increased in a dose-response trend, making it possible to identify individuals who can greatly benefit from preventive intervention that targets vascular risk factors [128]. Similar findings have been reported for late-life exposures: in the Swedish Kungsholmen Project, the cumulative effect of vascular risk factors and vascular diseases on dementia/AD risk has been investigated in people aged 75+ years. These factors were aggregated according to two pathophysiological hypotheses: the brain hypoperfusion profile, defined by chronic heart failure, low pulse pressure, and low diastolic pressure, and the atherosclerosis profile, which included high systolic pressure, diabetes mellitus or prediabetes, and stroke. In both profiles, dementia/AD risk increased with increasing scores in a dose-response manner, suggesting a synergy of vascular risk factors in promoting dementia/AD also in advanced age [129]. The American Cardiovascular Health Cognition Study developed a Late-life Dementia Risk Index, and also its brief version, which groups older adults in the three categories of low, moderate, and high risk of developing dementia. Both versions of the index support the cumulative effect of different factors in determining the risk of dementia after the age of 65 years. These indices include information from different domains, including demographic factors (age), genetic (presence of the *APOE* ε4 allele), lifestyle (BMI<18.5, lack of alcohol consumption), comorbid vascular conditions (internal carotid artery thickening, angina, coronary artery by-pass surgery, stroke, peripheral artery disease), evidence of brain abnormalities showed by magnetic resonance imaging (MRI) (white matter diseases or enlarged ventricles), cognitive test scores and physical performances [130, 131].

The combined effect of genetic-environmental or environmental-environmental joint exposures may also lead to the attenuation of the dementia risk. Population-based studies suggest an effect modification for the *APOE* ε4 allele, the most important genetic risk factor for sporadic AD. *APOE* ε4 carriers seem more vulnerable to risk factors like alcohol drinking, smoking, physical inactivity and high intake of saturate fat, indicating that people with genetic susceptibility may reduce their initial AD risk by lifestyle interventions (i.e., physical activity, sufficient intake of PUFA, and avoiding excess alcohol drinking and smoking) [33]. The protective effect of lifestyle in *APOE* ε4 carriers seem to be present also in advanced age: in the Swedish Kungsholmen Project, subjects aged 75+ years who were *APOE* ε4 carriers, but with high education, active leisure activities, or good vascular health (i.e., absence of vascular risk factors), had a reduced risk of dementia and AD, as well as a delayed time of onset of the disease [132]. Further, it has been shown that high education may reduce dementia risk among *APOE* ε4 allele carriers [133].

Regarding the interactions among modifiable risk factors, results from the Kungsholmen Project suggested that complexity of work with data and people was related to a decreased dementia risk and that the highest level of work complexity may modulate the increased dementia risk due to low education [78].

In conclusion, even though the evidence for some risk and protective factors in dementia and AD is still scarce, and their role needs to be further clarified, findings from observational studies points at different modifiable factors that can be managed in order to prevent or delay dementia onset. Moreover, epidemiological findings strongly suggest that the life-course approach model and the multifactorial nature of dementia and AD should be considered when planning any preventive strategy.

3. Interventional studies

3.1. Current evidence

Different medications, including statins, antihypertensive drugs, estrogens alone or in combination with progestin (hormone replacement therapy, HRT), nonsteroidal anti-inflammatory drugs (NSAIDs), and nutraceuticals (vitamin B12, C, E, folate, Ginkgo biloba) have been tested as primary or secondary prevention measures for dementia and AD in subjects with normal cognition or MCI. In general, for all these compounds the protective effects suggested by observational studies have not been confirmed in RCTs, the results of which are inconsistent or even suggest a detrimental effect on cognition (e.g., NSAIDs, HRT) [120, 134-136]. Few interventional studies implementing non-pharmacological approaches have been carried out. Among them some RCTs on cognitive training and physical activity provided encouraging results, which need further confirmation [134, 137]. It is possible that the negative results from the RCTs done so far reflect the real inefficacy of the tested strategies in preventing dementia and AD. However, the apparent contradiction of results from observational and interventional studies could be explained by several factors:

1.   The intervention was done outside the time-window when management of a risk factor would reduce dementia risk: several risk factors exert their effect mainly during mid-life, whereas RCTs have been done in older adults. This is the case for vascular risk factors, which seem to be more relevant when the exposure occurs during mid-life. Moreover, the HRT research suggests that estrogens may have beneficial, neutral, or detrimental effects on the brain depending on age at treatment, type of menopause (natural versus medically or surgically induced) or stage of menopause [138]. This concept, called the "window of opportunity hypothesis" is in agreement with the life-course approach model. There is evidence of neuroprotective effects of estrogens in women before the age of natural menopause and in the early postmenopausal stage (50-60 years), while estrogens initiated in late postmenopause (65-79 years) increase the risk of cognitive impairment and dementia [138-142]. The large-scale RCT of the Women's Health Initiative Memory Study (WHI-MS) showed that estrogens therapy alone or in combination with progestin was associated with a two-fold increased risk for dementia and MCI [139, 140]. The WHI-MS study enrolled women aged 65-79 years, who were given the HRT many years after the onset of natural or surgical menopause. In contrast, the Kronos Early Estrogen Prevention Study (KEEPS) tested the HRT in recently menopausal women (mean age 53 years; enrolment within three years after menopause), reporting beneficial effects [141]. In fact, the use of the HRT in the KEEPS participants has been associated with the improvement of markers of cardiovascular risk, anxiety and depression, without adverse effects on

cognition [141]. Overall these results suggest that the role of the HRT in age-related cognition and dementia needs to be further investigated, taking into account the time-window when the treatment is administered.

2. Short treatment and follow-up: many studies were of relatively short length. Thus, interventions have been implemented for a period that is not long enough to determine a neuroprotective effect, and the limited follow-up duration of many RCTs would not allow detection of differences in dementia incidence.

3. The statistical power was inadequate, since some RCTs had small samples and dementia has been considered a secondary endpoint in most clinical trials (e.g., antihypertensive therapy), in which clear benefits for primary endpoints (e.g., coronary heart disease and stroke) are shown usually in a short period of observation.

4. The choice of compounds tested in RCTs using nutraceuticals was not optimal: although several products have been tested, supplements composition is still a debated issue. For instance, whereas observational studies suggested that a balanced intake of different forms of vitamin E can be important for reducing dementia/AD risk, only one form (α-tocopherol) has been tested in RCTs, with conflicting findings [84, 85, 107, 108, 143]. Moreover, intake of high doses of α-tocopherol supplements has been associated with increased hemorrhagic stroke and mortality risk [144]. Regarding the studies on vitamins B, while the majority of RCTs done so far did not find evidence of benefit [120, 121], a recent RCT reported favourable effects in subjects with MCI, especially individuals with elevated homocysteine levels. In this latter RCT supplementation was done using a combination of vitamins B (B6, B12, folate) at high doses, suggesting that refining the type of supplements (i.e. composition, concentration) might increases the possibility to achieve beneficial effects in selected populations [122, 123].

5. Despite the multifactorial nature of dementia and the importance of combined risk exposures, most studies were based on a mono-intervention approach, almost always testing single agents or lifestyle interventions. In multifactorial conditions, a small reduction in multiple risk factors can substantially decrease overall risk.

In conclusion, despite the discrepancies between findings of observational and interventional studies and the disappointing results of intervention studies on dementia and AD, methodological issues of the RCTs carried out thus far suggest that a valid evaluation of the efficacy of preventive measures has yet to be undertaken.

3.2. Ongoing multidomain intervention studies

The disappointing results of previous trials, testing the effects of mono-intervention strategies in cognitively normal elderly or already cognitively impaired persons, have pointed out some key issues: i) timing – starting earlier may lead to better effects; ii) target group – a healthy, young population would require long follow-up times, large sample sizes and considerable financial resources; iii) lack of consistent and uniformly applied definitions of MCI has lead to enrolment of heterogeneous groups underpowering the studies; iv) outcome measures – cognitive impairment may be a better endpoint than conversion to dementia; v) ethical issues are also important, as placebo-controlled trials for high blood pressure and cholesterol are not possible due to their known protective effects regarding cardio- and cerebrovascular disease. Furthermore, a critical aspect that needs to be taken into account when planning preventive measures for dementia and AD, is the multifactorial nature of these disorders, which require multiple prevention approaches. Intervention studies combining several different approaches have not been conducted for AD so far, and the knowledge derived from the previously described observational and interventional studies has paved the way for some ongoing RCTs on prevention of cognitive decline and dementia. In Europe there are three large ongoing RCTs: FINGER, MAPT and PreDIVA [145, 146] (Table 2). The common denominator of these studies is the multidomain approach, which aims to target simultaneously several risk factors for dementia and AD in older adults, mainly by promoting lifestyle changes and adherence to medical treatments for vascular risk factors and vascular diseases. All RCTs exclude individuals with dementia or substantial cognitive decline, and use clinical evaluation and neuropsychological tests to detect cognitive changes and dementia incidence as main outcomes. Further, secondary outcomes include functional status, mood disorders, quality of life, adherence to the intervention programs and health resources utilization. These two latter aspects are essential from a public health perspective, since they provide information on feasibility and cost effectiveness of prevention strategies. Additionally, both FINGER and MAPT include ancillary studies on neuroimaging (morphological and functional), CSF and blood markers related to AD pathophysiology in order to investigate the effect of the interventions on brain morphology and metabolism, clarify mechanisms underlying preventive measures and identify biomarkers that can be used to monitor effects of interventions.

The Finnish Geriatric Intervention Study to Prevent Cognitive Impairment and Disability (FINGER, NCT01041989) is a multicenter RCT aiming to prevent cognitive impairment, dementia and disability in 60-77 year-old people. The study population is represented by 1282 individuals at increased risk of dementia, selected according to the CAIDE Dementia Risk Score and the CERAD neuropsychological test battery [128, 145]. The 2-year multidomain intervention includes nutritional guidance, physical activity, cognitive training, increased social activity and intensive monitoring and management of metabolic and vascular risk factors (hypertension, dyslipidemia, obesity, impaired glucose tolerance). Individuals in the reference group are given general public health advice on lifestyle and vascular risk factors. FINGER participants are recruited from previous population-based observational surveys (i.e., FINRISK, FIN-D2D) with detailed retrospective information on lifestyle and vascular factors [145]. Thus, differences in these variables can be taken into account, which is normally not possible in RCTs. The primary outcome is cognitive decline measured by a sensitive Neuropsychological Test Battery (NTB) and the Stroop and Trail Making tests, which can depict early cognitive impairment typical for AD and VaD. The planned 7-year extended follow-up will allow detection of differences in dementia/AD incidence. Two earlier intervention trials in Finland were important sources of inspiration for the FINGER study. The Diabetes Prevention Study (now completed) is a landmark RCT showing the effectiveness and feasibility of physical exercise and dietary interventions as preventive measures in people with impaired glucose tolerance. In this RCT lifestyle intervention in people at high risk for type 2 diabetes resulted in sustained lifestyle changes and a reduction in diabetes incidence, which remained after the individual lifestyle counselling was stopped [147, 148]. The four-year exercise and dietary intervention study Dose-Responses to Exercise Training (DRs EXTRA) had a drop-out rate of only 8% after two years, and preliminary results suggested a potential benefit of higher physical fitness on cognition [149].

RCT	FINGER	MAPT	Pre-DIVA
Country	Finland	France	Netherlands
Sample size	1282	1680	3534
Main inclusion criteria	Dementia Risk Score >6 and mild degree of cognitive impairment	Frail elderly people (subjective memory complaint, slow walking speed, limitation in IADL)	All elderly within GP practices, non demented (MMSE >23)
Age at enrolment, yrs	60 -77	≥ 70	70-78
Study design	Multi-center, randomized, single-blind, parallel-group	Multi-center, randomized, controlled trial	Multi-site, open, cluster-randomized parallel group
Multi-domain intervention	Nutritional guidance, physical activity, cognitive training, increased social activity and intensive monitoring and management of metabolic and vascular risk factors	Vascular care, nutritional advice, exercise advice, cognitive training, and/or DHA 800 mg/day	Nurse-led vascular care including medical treatment of risk factors, diet advice, exercise advice
Intervention period	2 yrs	3 yrs	6 yrs
Follow-up period	7 yrs	5 ysr	6 yrs
Primary outcome	Neuropsychological test battery, Trail Making test, Stroop test, Dementia	Change in cognitive function (Grober and Buschke memory test)	Dementia, Disability
Study Completion	2013	2013	2016

DHA: docosahexaenoic acid acid. IADL: Instrumental Activities of Daily Living. MMSE: Mini Mental State Examination

Table 2. Ongoing multi-domain prevention RCTs on dementia

The Multidomain Alzheimer Preventive Trial (MAPT, NCT00672685) is a French multicenter RCT evaluating the efficacy of isolated supplementation with ω-3 fatty acid, isolated multidomain intervention, or their combination in the prevention of cognitive decline in frail individuals aged ≥70 years. 1680 community-dwelling participants have been enrolled, using a definition of frailty that includes three components: presence of memory complaints, limitation in one instrumental activity of daily living (IADL) and slow walking speed. The 3-year multidomain intervention consists of group training sessions (physical exercise, cognitive training and nutritional advice) and yearly personalized preventive consultations that aim to identify dementia and frailty risk factors (vascular risk factors, nutritional problems, sensory deficits, mood disorders, walking difficulties) and promote their management in collaboration with the general practitioner. Follow-up is 5 years, and the main outcome measure is the 3-year change in cognitive function assessed with a neuropsychological test (Grober and Buschke) [145, 150].

The Prevention of Dementia by Intensive Vascular Care (PreDIVA) study is a Dutch multi-center, open, cluster-RCT comparing standard and intensive care of cardiovascular risk factors in preventing dementia and disability in elderly people. The study includes 3534 community-dwellers aged 70-78 years, recruited from primary care practices. The standard care is based on guidelines for Dutch general practice, while the multi-component intensive vascular care addresses hypertension, hypercholesterolemia, smoking habits, overweight, physical inactivity and diabetes mellitus, which are strictly controlled with medication and lifestyle interventions. Study duration is 6 years, and primary outcomes are incident dementia assessed according to standard criteria and disability as measured with the AMC Linear Disability Scale (ALDS) [146].

Researchers involved in these large European trials (FINGER, MAPT and PreDIVA) recently started the European Dementia Prevention Initiative (EDPI), an international collaboration to improve preventive strategies against dementia [151]. Collaboration and data sharing within the EDPI will allow refining methodological aspects of prevention trials, including identification of target populations; improvement of intervention methods (i.e., type, intensity, duration); and development and standardization of relevant outcome measures and prognostic and monitoring tools that can be easily implemented in large populations. This will help planning larger and international prevention trials able to provide robust evidence on dementia/AD prevention.

3.3. Presymptomatic Alzheimer's disease treatment: Anti-amyloid drugs

Presymptomatic (or preclinical) AD treatments have been defined as "those interventions that are initiated before apparent cognitive decline and are intended to reduce the chance of developing AD-related symptoms" [152]. The proposed term refers to an intervention whether it is started before or after biological evidence of the underlying disease, and whether it postpones the onset, partially reduces the risk of, or completely prevents symptomatic AD [153]. The progress on the knowledge about the AD phenotype, particularly on the biomarkers which have been incorporated in the new diagnostic criteria for dementia and MCI due AD, as well preclinical AD, has provided the basis for intervention studies evaluating pharmacological interventions in asymptomatic subjects who are at risk of AD, because of an established biomarker burden or a specific genetic profile. Three RCTs are planned to start in 2013 to verify safety and efficacy of anti-amyloid drugs as preventive measure in AD (Table 3). The Alzheimer's Prevention Initiative (API) and the Dominantly Inherited Alzheimer's Network (DIAN) studies will enrol subjects who carry genetic mutations for dominantly inherited AD: mutations in the *APP*, presenilin-1 (*PSEN1*), and presenilin-2 (*PSEN2*) genes can cause early-onset familial AD that accounts for no more than 5 percent of all cases [154].

Data from the DIAN study have shown that different phenotypic changes can be detected several years before the onset of cognitive symptoms in individual with autosomal dominant AD: it has been shown that CSF levels of Aβ42 decline 25 years before expected symptom onset, and brain deposition of Aβ can be detected 15 years before. Further, increased concentrations of tau protein in the CSF and brain atrophy are visible 15 years before expected symptom onset, while cerebral hypometabolism can be observed 10 years before [155]. The API RCT will focus on the world largest early-onset AD kindred in Antioquia, Columbia. Of about 5000 individuals in this kindred, approximately 1500 carry a mutation in the *PSEN1* gene (E280A) causing early onset AD (mean age of onset: 45 years) [156, 157]. The trial will also include a small number of individuals in the United States, recruited in collaboration with researchers from the DIAN study [158]. The drug used in the API study is the anti-amyloid antibody crenezumab, which has been chosen based on the evidence of its ability to remove from the brain different forms of Aβ and its safety profile (low risk of cerebral vasogenic oedema and microhaemorrhages) [157]. The trial within the DIAN cohort will include people with mutations in any of the three genes linked to early-onset AD: *PSEN1*, *PSEN2*, and *APP*. Three different anti-amyloid compounds will be evaluated in the first phase of the study (2 years): the beta-secretase inhibitor LY2886721, which limits the production of Aβ; and two anti-amyloid antibodies (Gantenerumab, Solanezumab) which promote Aβ removal from the brain. The more effective drug(s) will be further tested in a 3 years extension phase of the study. A third trial, the Anti-Amyloid Treatment of Asymptomatic Alzheimer's (A4) RTC, aims to prevent sporadic AD and will evaluate the effect of an anti-amyloid compound in older adults with evidence of brain amyloid accumulation at neuroimaging evaluation. The study is sponsored by the Alzheimer's Disease Cooperative Study, and also in this case the drug candidate still needs to be identified among anti-amyloid compounds. The study is expected to detect differences in the rate of cognitive decline, while it has not enough statistical power to detect a difference in dementia incidence. The A4 study will also include an ethics arm examining the psychological impact of disclosing information to individuals about their risk of developing AD [157].

Overall, these studies provide the opportunity to test the efficacy of AD-modifying treatments in an earlier stage of AD compared to the pharmacological RCTs done so far. While testing these compounds in young, healthy individuals would require enormous financial resources and too long follow up, the recruitment strategies implemented in these studies allow testing the benefit of anti-amyloid drugs earlier than otherwise possible. This approach provides also the opportunity to further verify the amyloid hypothesis, which has been reconsidered many times over the past decades and criticized in light of the recent failures of RCTs testing anti-amyloid drugs in subjects with mild-to-moderate AD. A possible interpretation of these failures is that the anti-amyloid therapies have missed their "window of opportunity", since they have been provided too late. The preventive RCTs on anti-amyloid drugs are based on the assumption that an earlier interference on amyloid accumulation, before irreversible brain damage occurs, would exert a significant disease-modifying effect. These prevention studies will also allow determining the ability of different biomarkers to predict a clinical benefit, information needed to help qualify biomarker endpoints for use in prevention trials. These studies offer great hope, but also safety concerns, since anti-amyloid compounds will be tested in subjects with no cognitive problems and the long-term risk associated with the use of anti-amyloid drugs is yet unknown.

RCT	API Alzheimer's Prevention Initiative	DIAN Dominantly Inherited Alzheimer Network	A4 Anti-Amyloid Treatment of Asymptomatic AD
Sample size	300 members of Colombian families. A small number of individuals from USA (collaboration with the DIAN network) will also be included	240 members of families with early-onset AD	1500 older adults with no cognitive impairment
Main inclusion criteria	Carriers of a mutated *PSEN1* gene. Non-carriers will also be included, to ensure double-blinding about the genetic status	Carriers of mutation in *PSEN1*, or *PSEN2*, or *APP*. Non-carriers will also be included, to ensure double-blinding about the genetic status	Evidence of brain amyloid accumulation. Subject with no evidence of amyloid burden will also be included
Age at enrolment, yrs	≥ 30	NA	≥ 70
Study design	Randomized, double blind, placebo controlled trial	Randomized, double blind, placebo controlled trial	Randomized, double blind, placebo controlled trial
Intervention	Anti-amyloid antibody Crenezumab (Genentech)	Three anti-amyloid therapies: the beta-secretase inhibitor LY2886721 (Lilly), and the anti-amyloid antibodies Gantenerumab (Roche) and Solanezumab (Lilly)	One anti-amyloid therapy (to be determined)
Duration	5 yrs, (interim analysis at 2 yrs)	2 yrs + 3 yrs extension	3 yrs + 2 yrs extension
Outcomes	Primary: cognitive function Secondary: biomarkers, including brain amyloid load and brain atrophy	Initial phase (2 yrs): biomarkers analysis, to identify the most promising drug candidate Follow-up phase (3 yrs): cognitive function	Primary: cognitive function Secondary: biomarkers

APP: amyloid precursor protein. *PSEN1*: presenilin 1. *PSEN2*: presenilin 1

Table 3. Alzheimer's prevention trials based on anti-amyloid treatments

4. Conclusion

Prevention is a newer area in dementia/AD research, and the shift from observation to action has occurred only in the last decade, with several intervention studies now ongoing, and other RCTs starting soon. Although the pathogenesis of dementia is not fully elucidated, primary prevention seems possible, as most factors involved in dementia onset and progression are modifiable or amenable to management. The recent AHRQ/NIH report shows that development of successful preventive strategies requires a more refined knowledge on risk and protective factors for dementia and AD, as well as a validation of the observational studies with large intervention studies [19]. AD and VaD share several risk factors, and most dementia cases are attributable to both vascular and neurodegenerative brain damage. Furthermore, population-based neuropathological studies have shown that both subclinical neurodegenerative (amyloid plaques, neurofibrillary tangles, Lewy bodies) and vascular lesions are common in the brains of cognitively normal elderly individuals, as is their co-occurrence [9]. In light of this, preventive strategies aiming to postpone the onset of dementia syndrome have great potential.

Epidemiological research suggests that the most effective strategy may be to encourage the implementation of multiple preventive measures throughout the life course, including high educational attainment in childhood and early adulthood; active control of vascular factors and disorders over adulthood; and maintenance of mentally, physically, and socially active lifestyles during middle age and later in life. It has been estimated that half of AD cases worldwide are potentially attributable to modifiable risk factors, and a 10-25% reduction in these factors could potentially prevent 3 million AD cases worldwide, with a reduction in all risk factors having the greatest impact on dementia prevalence [70]. However, RCTs are indispensable to confirm the effect of risk reduction strategies targeting multiple risk factors. Multidomain interventional RCTs are now ongoing and will provide new insights into prevention of cognitive impairment and dementia. Full implementation of the life-course approach is more challenging, due to the difficulties of carrying out RCTs over many decades. Such long-term studies would require very large sample sizes and huge financial resources, and a pragmatic way to assess the effect of long-term interventions within a RCT has not yet been established. Furthermore, several risk and protective factors are not appropriate for intervention trials, due to unethical reasons, thus evidence about these factors rely on conducting rigorous observational studies (e.g., placebo-controlled trials for high blood pressure or cholesterol are not possible because such treatments are known to protect against cardio/ cerebrovascular diseases) [35]. Methodological alternatives to RCTs have been proposed to obtain robust evidence on AD and dementia prevention [37, 159].

Platforms for early intervention could be established by incorporating the classical clinical trial approach to disease into a public health model, with long-term longitudinal databases including large populations. Establishing comprehensive databases for studies on aging can create the opportunity to formulate and validate tools for early detection of people who are at increased risk of late-life cognitive impairment, to identify important targets (risk factors) for preventive interventions, and to test such interventions in RCTs.

The first initiatives with an international perspective have already been established, for example the Leon Thal Symposia [160], Prevent Alzheimer's Disease by 2020 (PAD2020, http://www.pad2020.org), and the European Dementia Prevention Initiative (EDPI, http://www.edpi.org). It has been suggested that a worldwide database could be built by integrating and expanding already existing cohorts and registries [160].

The ongoing RTCs on dementia prevention will have to take into account the "window of opportunity hypothesis" when evaluating the results of interventions. In fact, efficacy of preventive actions may vary by age. Thus, implementation of interventions at the appropriate time in the life course is crucial for successful prevention. Refining of prognostic tools, which can be used for early detection of subjects at risk of dementia in the general population, will also help to better plan intervention studies. Also, when targeting elderly individuals, the frequent coexistence of chronic diseases needs to be considered, since it can negatively impact cognitive performance and limit adherence to preventive interventions. On the other hand, appropriate management of morbidity can help improve cognitive performance and delay dementia onset. For instance, although stroke is a known risk factor for dementia, it has been recently reported that about 25% of stroke patients discontinued one or more of their prescribed secondary prevention medications within 3 months of hospitalization for acute stroke [161-163]. Improving long-term adherence to post-stroke treatment can prevent recurrent cerebrovascular diseases and contribute to preventing or delaying clinical expression of dementia syndrome. Additionally, there is evidence of inadequate management of hypertension and hypercholesterolemia in the older adults [146]. Similar situations exist for heart failure, which increases the risk of dementia among older adults [68], and diabetes mellitus, which accelerates the progression from mild cognitive impairment to dementia by more than 3 years [164]. Preliminary results from the PreDIVA study showed that 87% of the study participants have at least one modifiable risk factor amenable to intervention, proving the presence of a window of opportunity for improved risk management [146].

In conclusion, prevention of dementia is now moving from observational to interventional studies to verify hypotheses and define tools that can be applied in the general population. Epidemiological and preclinical studies will continue to provide new information on risk/protective factors and pathological mechanisms. The international collaboration among research teams involved in ongoing multidomain RCTs will allow the sharing of experiences and discussions on methodological aspects of these studies. This can help in interpretation of results, identification and solution of problems related to intervention strategies, and refinement of preventative approaches. The multidomain intervention RCTs are at one end of the current spectrum of intervention trials in AD/cognitive impairment. At the other end are RCTs testing disease-modifying drugs (i.e. anti-amyloid therapy) in genetically at-risk groups or those with established biomarker burden. The shift towards pre-symptomatic and pre-dementia stages of AD has brought prevention and treatment RCTs much closer to each other than before. Since a cure for dementia is not yet available, finding effective preventive strategies is essential for a sustainable society in an aging world. As dementia, cardiovascular diseases, stroke and diabetes mellitus – all major public health problems – share several risk factors, public health efforts promoting healthier lifestyle have the potential to enhance health status in advanced age.

Acknowledgements

This work has been supported by: the Swedish Research Council for Medical Research; Academy of Finland; La Carita Foundation, Finland; Alzheimer's Association (USA); the Swedish Foundations Ragnhild och Einar Lundströms-Minne-Lindhés, Stohnes-Stiftelse and Gamla-Tjänarinnor.

Author details

Francesca Mangialasche[1,2*], Weili Xu[1,3] and Miia Kivipelto[1,4]

*Address all correspondence to: francesca.mangialasche@ki.se

1 Aging Research Center, Karolinska Institutet-Stockholm University, Stockholm, Sweden

2 Institute of Gerontology and Geriatrics, Department of Clinical and Experimental Medicine, University of Perugia, Perugia, Italy

3 Department of Epidemiology, Tianjin Medical University, Tianjin, P.R., China

4 Department of Neurology, University of Eastern Finland, Kuopio, Finland

References

[1] American Psychiatric AssociationDiagnostic and statistic manual of mental disorders 3rd ed., revised (DSM-III-R). Association AP, editor. Washington D.C.(1987).

[2] Fratiglioni, L, Launer, L. J, Andersen, K, Breteler, M. M, Copeland, J. R, Dartigues, J. F, et al. Incidence of dementia and major subtypes in Europe: A collaborative study of population-based cohorts. Neurologic Diseases in the Elderly Research Group. Neurology. (2000). Suppl 5):S, 10-5.

[3] Alzheimer's Disease International, World Alzheimer Report. The Global Economic Impact of Dementia. 2010; Available from: http://www.alz.co.uk/research/files/WorldAlzheimerReport2010ExecutiveSummary.pdf.

[4] Jack, C. R. Jr., Albert MS, Knopman DS, McKhann GM, Sperling RA, Carrillo MC, et al. Introduction to the recommendations from the National Institute on Aging-Alz-

heimer's Association workgroups on diagnostic guidelines for Alzheimer's disease. Alzheimers Dement. (2011). May;, 7(3), 257-62.

[5] Fratiglioni, L, & Qiu, C. Prevention of common neurodegenerative disorders in the elderly. Experimental gerontology. (2009). Jan-Feb;44(1-2):46-50.

[6] Qiu, C, Kivipelto, M, & Von Strauss, E. Epidemiology of Alzheimer's disease: occurrence, determinants, and strategies toward intervention. Dialogues in clinical neuroscience. (2009). , 11(2), 111-28.

[7] Stephan, B. C, Matthews, F. E, Ma, B, Muniz, G, Hunter, S, Davis, D, et al. Alzheimer and vascular neuropathological changes associated with different cognitive States in a non-demented sample. J Alzheimers Dis. (2012). , 29(2), 309-18.

[8] Schneider, J. A, Arvanitakis, Z, Bang, W, & Bennett, D. A. Mixed brain pathologies account for most dementia cases in community-dwelling older persons. Neurology. (2007). Dec 11;, 69(24), 2197-204.

[9] Sonnen, J. A. Santa Cruz K, Hemmy LS, Woltjer R, Leverenz JB, Montine KS, et al. Ecology of the aging human brain. Archives of neurology. (2011). Aug;, 68(8), 1049-56.

[10] Mckhann, G, Drachman, D, Folstein, M, Katzman, R, Price, D, & Stadlan, E. M. Clinical diagnosis of Alzheimer's disease: report of the NINCDS-ADRDA Work Group under the auspices of Department of Health and Human Services Task Force on Alzheimer's Disease. Neurology. (1984). Jul;, 34(7), 939-44.

[11] Mangialasche, F, Solomon, A, Winblad, B, Mecocci, P, & Kivipelto, M. Alzheimer's disease: clinical trials and drug development. Lancet neurology. (2010). Jul;, 9(7), 702-16.

[12] Morris, J. C. Early-stage and preclinical Alzheimer disease. Alzheimer disease and associated disorders. (2005). Jul-Sep;, 19(3), 163-5.

[13] Petersen, R. C, Doody, R, Kurz, A, Mohs, R. C, Morris, J. C, Rabins, P. V, et al. Current concepts in mild cognitive impairment. Arch Neurol. (2001). Dec;, 58(12), 1985-92.

[14] Harvey, R, Fox, N, & Rossor, M. Dementia Handbook. London: Martin Dunitz; (1999).

[15] Albert, M. S, Dekosky, S. T, Dickson, D, Dubois, B, Feldman, H. H, Fox, N. C, et al. The diagnosis of mild cognitive impairment due to Alzheimer's disease: recommendations from the National Institute on Aging-Alzheimer's Association workgroups on diagnostic guidelines for Alzheimer's disease. Alzheimers Dement. (2011). May;, 7(3), 270-9.

[16] Mckhann, G. M, Knopman, D. S, Chertkow, H, Hyman, B. T, & Jack, C. R. Jr., Kawas CH, et al. The diagnosis of dementia due to Alzheimer's disease: recommendations from the National Institute on Aging-Alzheimer's Association workgroups on diag-

nostic guidelines for Alzheimer's disease. Alzheimers Dement. (2011). May;, 7(3), 263-9.

[17]   Sperling, R. A, Aisen, P. S, Beckett, L. A, Bennett, D. A, Craft, S, Fagan, A. M, et al. Toward defining the preclinical stages of Alzheimer's disease: recommendations from the National Institute on Aging-Alzheimer's Association workgroups on diagnostic guidelines for Alzheimer's disease. Alzheimers Dement. (2011). May;, 7(3), 280-92.

[18]   Qiu, C, & Fratiglioni, L. Epidemiology of the dementias. In: McNamara P, editor. Dementia History and Incidence. Santa Barbara, CA: ABC-CLIO PRESS, INC; (2011).

[19]   Fratiglioni, L, & Qiu, C. Prevention of cognitive decline in ageing: dementia as the target, delayed onset as the goal. Lancet neurology. (2011). Sep;, 10(9), 778-9.

[20]   Kivipelto, M, & Solomon, A. Preventive neurology: on the way from knowledge to action. Neurology. (2009). Jul 21;, 73(3), 168-9.

[21]   Fratiglioni, L, Von Strauss, E, & Qiu, C. Epidemiology of the dementias of old age. In: Dening T, R. Jacoby, C. Oppenheimer, and A. Thomas., editor. The Oxford Textbook of Old Age Psychiatry. London: Oxford University Press; (2008). , 391-406.

[22]   Matthews, F, & Brayne, C. The incidence of dementia in England and Wales: findings from the five identical sites of the MRC CFA Study. PLoS medicine. (2005). Aug; 2(8):e193.

[23]   Green, R. C, Cupples, L. A, Go, R, Benke, K. S, Edeki, T, Griffith, P. A, et al. Risk of dementia among white and African American relatives of patients with Alzheimer disease. Jama. (2002). Jan 16;, 287(3), 329-36.

[24]   Seshadri, S, & Wolf, P. A. Lifetime risk of stroke and dementia: current concepts, and estimates from the Framingham Study. Lancet neurology. (2007). Dec;, 6(12), 1106-14.

[25]   Ballard, C, Gauthier, S, Corbett, A, Brayne, C, Aarsland, D, & Jones, E. Alzheimer's disease. Lancet. [Research Support, Non-U.S. Gov't Review]. (2011). Mar 19;, 377(9770), 1019-31.

[26]   Qiu, C, Kivipelto, M, Aguero-torres, H, Winblad, B, & Fratiglioni, L. Risk and protective effects of the APOE gene towards Alzheimer's disease in the Kungsholmen project: variation by age and sex. J Neurol Neurosurg Psychiatry. (2004). Jun;, 75(6), 828-33.

[27]   Slooter, A. J, Cruts, M, Kalmijn, S, Hofman, A, Breteler, M. M, Van Broeckhoven, C, et al. Risk estimates of dementia by apolipoprotein E genotypes from a population-based incidence study: the Rotterdam Study. Archives of neurology. (1998). Jul;, 55(7), 964-8.

[28]   Corder, E. H, Saunders, A. M, Strittmatter, W. J, Schmechel, D. E, Gaskell, P. C, Small, G. W, et al. Gene dose of apolipoprotein E type 4 allele and the risk of Alz-

heimer's disease in late onset families. Science (New York, NY. (1993). Aug 13;, 261(5123), 921-3.

[29] Cruchaga, C, Haller, G, Chakraverty, S, Mayo, K, Vallania, F. L, Mitra, R. D, et al. Rare variants in APP, PSEN1 and PSEN2 increase risk for AD in late-onset Alzheimer's disease families. PloS one. (2012). e31039.

[30] Jonsson, T, Atwal, J. K, Steinberg, S, Snaedal, J, Jonsson, P. V, Bjornsson, S, et al. A mutation in APP protects against Alzheimer's disease and age-related cognitive decline. Nature. (2012). Aug 2;, 488(7409), 96-9.

[31] Roses, A. D, Lutz, M. W, Amrine-madsen, H, Saunders, A. M, Crenshaw, D. G, Sundseth, S. S, et al. A TOMM40 variable-length polymorphism predicts the age of late-onset Alzheimer's disease. The pharmacogenomics journal. Oct;, 10(5), 375-84.

[32] Harold, D, Abraham, R, Hollingworth, P, Sims, R, Gerrish, A, Hamshere, M. L, et al. Genome-wide association study identifies variants at CLU and PICALM associated with Alzheimer's disease. Nature genetics. (2009). Oct;, 41(10), 1088-93.

[33] Kivipelto, M, Rovio, S, Ngandu, T, Kareholt, I, Eskelinen, M, Winblad, B, et al. Apolipoprotein E epsilon4 magnifies lifestyle risks for dementia: a population-based study. Journal of cellular and molecular medicine. (2008). Dec;12(6B):, 2762-71.

[34] Salloway, S, Sperling, R, Gilman, S, Fox, N. C, Blennow, K, Raskind, M, et al. A phase 2 multiple ascending dose trial of bapineuzumab in mild to moderate Alzheimer disease. Neurology. (2009). Dec 15;, 73(24), 2061-70.

[35] Williams, J. W, Plassman, B. L, Burke, J, Holsinger, T, & Benjamin, S. Preventing Alzheimer's Disease and Cognitive Decline. Evidence Report/Technology Assessment Prepared by the Duke Evidence-based Practice Center under Contract No. HHSA 290-(2007). I.). Rockville, MD: Agency for Healthcare Research and Quality.: AHRQ Publication No. E0052010.(193), 10.

[36] NIHConsensus Development Conference Statement on Preventing Alzheimer's Disease and Cognitive Decline. Bethesda, MD (2010).

[37] Hughes, T. F, & Ganguli, M. Modifiable Midlife Risk Factors for Late-Life Cognitive Impairment and Dementia. Current psychiatry reviews. (2009). May 1;, 5(2), 73-92.

[38] Flicker, L, Liu-ambrose, T, & Kramer, A. F. Why so negative about preventing cognitive decline and dementia? The jury has already come to the verdict for physical activity and smoking cessation. British journal of sports medicine. (2010). May;, 45(6), 465-7.

[39] Qiu, C, Kivipelto, M, & Fratiglioni, L. Preventing Alzheimer disease and cognitive decline. Annals of internal medicine. (2011). Feb 1;154(3):211; author reply , 2-3.

[40] Whalley, L. J, Dick, F. D, & Mcneill, G. A life-course approach to the aetiology of late-onset dementias. Lancet Neurol. (2006). Jan;, 5(1), 87-96.

[41] Qiu, C, Winblad, B, & Fratiglioni, L. The age-dependent relation of blood pressure to cognitive function and dementia. Lancet Neurol. (2005). Aug;, 4(8), 487-99.

[42] Qiu, C, Xu, W, & Fratiglioni, L. Vascular and psychosocial factors in Alzheimer's disease: epidemiological evidence toward intervention. J Alzheimers Dis. (2010). , 20(3), 689-97.

[43] Kivipelto, M, Helkala, E. L, Laakso, M. P, Hanninen, T, Hallikainen, M, Alhainen, K, et al. Apolipoprotein E epsilon4 allele, elevated midlife total cholesterol level, and high midlife systolic blood pressure are independent risk factors for late-life Alzheimer disease. Annals of internal medicine. (2002). Aug 6;, 137(3), 149-55.

[44] Mielke, M. M, Zandi, P. P, Sjogren, M, Gustafson, D, Ostling, S, Steen, B, et al. High total cholesterol levels in late life associated with a reduced risk of dementia. Neurology. (2005). May 24;, 64(10), 1689-95.

[45] Atti, A. R, Palmer, K, Volpato, S, Winblad, B, De Ronchi, D, & Fratiglioni, L. Late-life body mass index and dementia incidence: nine-year follow-up data from the Kungsholmen Project. J Am Geriatr Soc. (2008). Jan;, 56(1), 111-6.

[46] Kivipelto, M, Ngandu, T, Fratiglioni, L, Viitanen, M, Kareholt, I, Winblad, B, et al. Obesity and vascular risk factors at midlife and the risk of dementia and Alzheimer disease. Arch Neurol. (2005). Oct;, 62(10), 1556-60.

[47] Alonso, A, & Mosley, T. H. Jr., Gottesman RF, Catellier D, Sharrett AR, Coresh J. Risk of dementia hospitalisation associated with cardiovascular risk factors in midlife and older age: the Atherosclerosis Risk in Communities (ARIC) study. Journal of neurology, neurosurgery, and psychiatry. (2009). Nov;, 80(11), 1194-201.

[48] Qiu, C, Winblad, B, & Fratiglioni, L. Low diastolic pressure and risk of dementia in very old people: a longitudinal study. Dementia and geriatric cognitive disorders. (2009). , 28(3), 213-9.

[49] Dahl, A. K, Lopponen, M, Isoaho, R, Berg, S, & Kivela, S. L. Overweight and obesity in old age are not associated with greater dementia risk. Journal of the American Geriatrics Society. (2008). Dec;, 56(12), 2261-6.

[50] West, N. A, & Haan, M. N. Body adiposity in late life and risk of dementia or cognitive impairment in a longitudinal community-based study. The journals of gerontology. (2009). Jan;, 64(1), 103-9.

[51] Hughes, T. F, Borenstein, A. R, Schofield, E, Wu, Y, & Larson, E. B. Association between late-life body mass index and dementia: The Kame Project. Neurology. (2009). May 19;, 72(20), 1741-6.

[52] Fitzpatrick, A. L, Kuller, L. H, Lopez, O. L, Diehr, P, Meara, O, Longstreth, E. S, Jr, W. T, et al. Midlife and late-life obesity and the risk of dementia: cardiovascular health study. Archives of neurology. (2009). Mar;, 66(3), 336-42.

[53] Rosengren, A, Skoog, I, Gustafson, D, & Wilhelmsen, L. Body mass index, other cardiovascular risk factors, and hospitalization for dementia. Archives of internal medicine. (2005). Feb 14;, 165(3), 321-6.

[54] Whitmer, R. A, Gunderson, E. P, Barrett-connor, E, & Quesenberry, C. P. Jr., Yaffe K. Obesity in middle age and future risk of dementia: a 27 year longitudinal population based study. BMJ (Clinical research ed. (2005). Jun 11;330(7504):1360.

[55] Hassing, L. B, Dahl, A. K, Thorvaldsson, V, Berg, S, Gatz, M, Pedersen, N. L, et al. Overweight in midlife and risk of dementia: a 40-year follow-up study. International journal of obesity ((2005). Aug;, 33(8), 893-8.

[56] Solomon, A, Kareholt, I, Ngandu, T, Winblad, B, Nissinen, A, Tuomilehto, J, et al. Serum cholesterol changes after midlife and late-life cognition: twenty-one-year follow-up study. Neurology. (2007). Mar 6;, 68(10), 751-6.

[57] Stewart, R, White, L. R, Xue, Q. L, & Launer, L. J. Twenty-six-year change in total cholesterol levels and incident dementia: the Honolulu-Asia Aging Study. Arch Neurol. (2007). Jan;, 64(1), 103-7.

[58] Cramer, C, Haan, M. N, Galea, S, Langa, K. M, & Kalbfleisch, J. D. Use of statins and incidence of dementia and cognitive impairment without dementia in a cohort study. Neurology. (2008). Jul 29;, 71(5), 344-50.

[59] Xu, W, Qiu, C, Gatz, M, Pedersen, N. L, Johansson, B, & Fratiglioni, L. Mid- and late-life diabetes in relation to the risk of dementia: a population-based twin study. Diabetes. (2009). Jan;, 58(1), 71-7.

[60] Xu, W, Qiu, C, Winblad, B, & Fratiglioni, L. The effect of borderline diabetes on the risk of dementia and Alzheimer's disease. Diabetes. (2007). Jan;, 56(1), 211-6.

[61] Pendlebury, S. T, & Rothwell, P. M. Prevalence, incidence, and factors associated with pre-stroke and post-stroke dementia: a systematic review and meta-analysis. Lancet neurology. (2009). Nov;, 8(11), 1006-18.

[62] Savva, G. M, & Stephan, B. C. Epidemiological studies of the effect of stroke on incident dementia: a systematic review. Stroke; a journal of cerebral circulation. (2010). Jan;41(1):e, 41-6.

[63] Troncoso, J. C, Zonderman, A. B, Resnick, S. M, Crain, B, Pletnikova, O, & Brien, O. RJ. Effect of infarcts on dementia in the Baltimore longitudinal study of aging. Annals of neurology. (2008). Aug;, 64(2), 168-76.

[64] Vermeer, S. E, & Prins, N. D. den Heijer T, Hofman A, Koudstaal PJ, Breteler MM. Silent brain infarcts and the risk of dementia and cognitive decline. N Engl J Med. (2003). Mar 27;, 348(13), 1215-22.

[65] Newman, A. B, Fitzpatrick, A. L, Lopez, O, Jackson, S, Lyketsos, C, Jagust, W, et al. Dementia and Alzheimer's disease incidence in relationship to cardiovascular dis-

ease in the Cardiovascular Health Study cohort. J Am Geriatr Soc. (2005). Jul;, 53(7), 1101-7.

[66] Laurin, D, Masaki, K. H, White, L. R, & Launer, L. J. Ankle-to-brachial index and dementia: the Honolulu-Asia Aging Study. Circulation. (2007). Nov 13;, 116(20), 2269-74.

[67] Ott, A, Breteler, M. M, De Bruyne, M. C, Van Harskamp, F, Grobbee, D. E, & Hofman, A. Atrial fibrillation and dementia in a population-based study. The Rotterdam Study. Stroke; a journal of cerebral circulation. (1997). Feb;, 28(2), 316-21.

[68] Qiu, C, Winblad, B, Marengoni, A, Klarin, I, Fastbom, J, & Fratiglioni, L. Heart failure and risk of dementia and Alzheimer disease: a population-based cohort study. Arch Intern Med. (2006). May 8;, 166(9), 1003-8.

[69] Van Oijen, M, De Jong, F. J, Witteman, J. C, Hofman, A, Koudstaal, P. J, & Breteler, M. M. Atherosclerosis and risk for dementia. Annals of neurology. (2007). May;, 61(5), 403-10.

[70] Barnes, D. E, & Yaffe, K. The projected effect of risk factor reduction on Alzheimer's disease prevalence. Lancet neurology. (2011). Sep;, 10(9), 819-28.

[71] Ownby, R. L, Crocco, E, Acevedo, A, John, V, & Loewenstein, D. Depression and risk for Alzheimer disease: systematic review, meta-analysis, and metaregression analysis. Archives of general psychiatry. (2006). May;, 63(5), 530-8.

[72] Rondeau, V, Jacqmin-gadda, H, Commenges, D, Helmer, C, & Dartigues, J. F. Aluminum and silica in drinking water and the risk of Alzheimer's disease or cognitive decline: findings from 15-year follow-up of the PAQUID cohort. American journal of epidemiology. (2009). Feb 15;, 169(4), 489-96.

[73] Feychting, M, Jonsson, F, Pedersen, N. L, & Ahlbom, A. Occupational magnetic field exposure and neurodegenerative disease. Epidemiology. [Research Support, Non-U.S. Gov't]. (2003). Jul;discussion 27-8., 14(4), 413-9.

[74] Garcia, A. M, Sisternas, A, & Hoyos, S. P. Occupational exposure to extremely low frequency electric and magnetic fields and Alzheimer disease: a meta-analysis. International journal of epidemiology. (2008). Apr;, 37(2), 329-40.

[75] Fleminger, S, Oliver, D. L, Lovestone, S, Rabe-hesketh, S, & Giora, A. Head injury as a risk factor for Alzheimer's disease: the evidence 10 years on; a partial replication. Journal of neurology, neurosurgery, and psychiatry. (2003). Jul;, 74(7), 857-62.

[76] Himanen, L, Portin, R, Isoniemi, H, Helenius, H, Kurki, T, & Tenovuo, O. Longitudinal cognitive changes in traumatic brain injury: a 30-year follow-up study. Neurology. (2006). Jan 24;, 66(2), 187-92.

[77] Holmes, C, & Cotterell, D. Role of infection in the pathogenesis of Alzheimer's disease: implications for treatment. CNS drugs. (2009). Dec;, 23(12), 993-1002.

[78] Karp, A, Andel, R, Parker, M. G, Wang, H. X, Winblad, B, & Fratiglioni, L. Mentally stimulating activities at work during midlife and dementia risk after age 75: follow-up study from the Kungsholmen Project. Am J Geriatr Psychiatry. (2009). Mar;, 17(3), 227-36.

[79] Rovio, S, Kareholt, I, Helkala, E. L, Viitanen, M, Winblad, B, Tuomilehto, J, et al. Lei-sure-time physical activity at midlife and the risk of dementia and Alzheimer's disease. Lancet neurology. (2005). Nov;, 4(11), 705-11.

[80] Hakansson, K, Rovio, S, Helkala, E. L, Vilska, A. R, Winblad, B, Soininen, H, et al. Association between mid-life marital status and cognitive function in later life: population based cohort study. BMJ (Clinical research ed. (2009). b2462.

[81] Paillard-borg, S, Fratiglioni, L, Winblad, B, & Wang, H. X. Leisure activities in late life in relation to dementia risk: principal component analysis. Dementia and geriatric cognitive disorders. (2009). , 28(2), 136-44.

[82] Barberger-gateau, P, Raffaitin, C, Letenneur, L, Berr, C, Tzourio, C, Dartigues, J. F, et al. Dietary patterns and risk of dementia: the Three-City cohort study. Neurology. (2007). Nov 13;, 69(20), 1921-30.

[83] Morris, M. C, Evans, D. A, Bienias, J. L, Tangney, C. C, Bennett, D. A, Aggarwal, N, et al. Dietary fats and the risk of incident Alzheimer disease. Arch Neurol. (2003). Feb;, 60(2), 194-200.

[84] Devore, E. E, Grodstein, F, Van Rooij, F. J, Hofman, A, Stampfer, M. J, Witteman, J. C, et al. Dietary antioxidants and long-term risk of dementia. Archives of neurology. (2010). Jul;, 67(7), 819-25.

[85] Morris, M. C, Evans, D. A, Tangney, C. C, Bienias, J. L, Wilson, R. S, Aggarwal, N. T, et al. Relation of the tocopherol forms to incident Alzheimer disease and to cognitive change. The American journal of clinical nutrition. (2005). Feb;, 81(2), 508-14.

[86] Scarmeas, N, Stern, Y, Tang, M. X, Mayeux, R, & Luchsinger, J. A. Mediterranean diet and risk for Alzheimer's disease. Annals of neurology. (2006). Jun;, 59(6), 912-21.

[87] Devore, E. E, Grodstein, F, Van Rooij, F. J, Hofman, A, Rosner, B, Stampfer, M. J, et al. Dietary intake of fish and omega-3 fatty acids in relation to long-term dementia risk. The American journal of clinical nutrition. (2009). Jul;, 90(1), 170-6.

[88] Kroger, E, Verreault, R, Carmichael, P. H, Lindsay, J, Julien, P, Dewailly, E, et al. Omega-3 fatty acids and risk of dementia: the Canadian Study of Health and Aging. The American journal of clinical nutrition. (2009). Jul;, 90(1), 184-92.

[89] Gray, S. L, Anderson, M. L, Crane, P. K, Breitner, J. C, Mccormick, W, Bowen, J. D, et al. Antioxidant vitamin supplement use and risk of dementia or Alzheimer's disease in older adults. Journal of the American Geriatrics Society. (2008). Feb;, 56(2), 291-5.

[90] Feart, C, Samieri, C, Rondeau, V, Amieva, H, Portet, F, Dartigues, J. F, et al. Adherence to a Mediterranean diet, cognitive decline, and risk of dementia. Jama. (2009). Aug 12;, 302(6), 638-48.

[91] Anstey, K. J, Mack, H. A, & Cherbuin, N. Alcohol consumption as a risk factor for dementia and cognitive decline: meta-analysis of prospective studies. Am J Geriatr Psychiatry. (2009). Jul;, 17(7), 542-55.

[92] Peters, R, Peters, J, Warner, J, Beckett, N, & Bulpitt, C. Alcohol, dementia and cognitive decline in the elderly: a systematic review. Age and ageing. (2008). Sep;, 37(5), 505-12.

[93] Anttila, T, Helkala, E. L, Viitanen, M, Kareholt, I, Fratiglioni, L, Winblad, B, et al. Alcohol drinking in middle age and subsequent risk of mild cognitive impairment and dementia in old age: a prospective population based study. Bmj. (2004). Sep 4;329(7465):539.

[94] Parks, E, & Traber, M. G. Mechanisms of vitamin E regulation: research over the past decade and focus on the future. Antioxidants & redox signaling. (2000). Fall;, 2(3), 405-12.

[95] Muller, D. P, & Goss-sampson, M. A. Neurochemical, neurophysiological, and neuropathological studies in vitamin E deficiency. Critical reviews in neurobiology. (1990). , 5(3), 239-63.

[96] Reiter, E, Jiang, Q, & Christen, S. Anti-inflammatory properties of alpha- and gamma-tocopherol. Molecular aspects of medicine. (2007). Oct-Dec;28(5-6):668-91.

[97] Sen, C. K, Khanna, S, Rink, C, & Roy, S. Tocotrienols: the emerging face of natural vitamin E. Vitamins and hormones. (2007). , 76, 203-61.

[98] Luchsinger, J. A, Tang, M. X, Shea, S, & Mayeux, R. Antioxidant vitamin intake and risk of Alzheimer disease. Archives of neurology. (2003). Feb;, 60(2), 203-8.

[99] Laurin, D, Foley, D. J, Masaki, K. H, White, L. R, Launer, L. J, Vitamin, E, & Supplements, C. and risk of dementia. Jama. (2002). Nov 13;, 288(18), 2266-8.

[100] Fillenbaum, G. G, Kuchibhatla, M. N, Hanlon, J. T, Artz, M. B, Pieper, C. F, Schmader, K. E, et al. Dementia and Alzheimer's disease in community-dwelling elders taking vitamin C and/or vitamin E. The Annals of pharmacotherapy. (2005). Dec;, 39(12), 2009-14.

[101] Maxwell, C. J, Hicks, M. S, Hogan, D. B, Basran, J, & Ebly, E. M. Supplemental use of antioxidant vitamins and subsequent risk of cognitive decline and dementia. Dement Geriatr Cogn Disord. (2005). , 20(1), 45-51.

[102] Zandi, P. P, Anthony, J. C, Khachaturian, A. S, Stone, S. V, Gustafson, D, Tschanz, J. T, et al. Reduced risk of Alzheimer disease in users of antioxidant vitamin supplements: the Cache County Study. Archives of neurology. (2004). Jan;, 61(1), 82-8.

[103] Masaki, K. H, Losonczy, K. G, Izmirlian, G, Foley, D. J, Ross, G. W, Petrovitch, H, et al. Association of vitamin E and C supplement use with cognitive function and dementia in elderly men. Neurology. (2000). Mar 28;, 54(6), 1265-72.

[104] Engelhart, M. J, Geerlings, M. I, Ruitenberg, A, Van Swieten, J. C, Hofman, A, Witteman, J. C, et al. Dietary intake of antioxidants and risk of Alzheimer disease. Jama. (2002). Jun 26;, 287(24), 3223-9.

[105] Corrada, M. M, Kawas, C. H, Hallfrisch, J, Muller, D, & Brookmeyer, R. Reduced risk of Alzheimer's disease with high folate intake: the Baltimore Longitudinal Study of Aging. Alzheimers Dement. (2005). Jul;, 1(1), 11-8.

[106] Li, F. J, Shen, L, & Ji, H. F. Dietary Intakes of Vitamin E, Vitamin C, and beta-Carotene and Risk of Alzheimer's Disease: A Meta-Analysis. J Alzheimers Dis. (2012). Apr 27.

[107] Mangialasche, F, Xu, W, Kivipelto, M, Costanzi, E, Ercolani, S, Pigliautile, M, et al. Tocopherols and tocotrienols plasma levels are associated with cognitive impairment. Neurobiology of aging. (2012). Oct;, 33(10), 2282-90.

[108] Mangialasche, F, Kivipelto, M, Mecocci, P, Rizzuto, D, Palmer, K, Winblad, B, et al. High plasma levels of vitamin E forms and reduced Alzheimer's disease risk in advanced age. J Alzheimers Dis. (2010). , 20(4), 1029-37.

[109] Hooshmand, B, Solomon, A, Kareholt, I, Leiviska, J, Rusanen, M, Ahtiluoto, S, et al. Homocysteine and holotranscobalamin and the risk of Alzheimer disease: a longitudinal study. Neurology. (2011). Oct 19;, 75(16), 1408-14.

[110] Hooshmand, B, Solomon, A, Kareholt, I, Rusanen, M, Hanninen, T, Leiviska, J, et al. Associations between serum homocysteine, holotranscobalamin, folate and cognition in the elderly: a longitudinal study. Journal of internal medicine. (2010). Feb;, 271(2), 204-12.

[111] Dufouil, C, Alperovitch, A, Ducros, V, & Tzourio, C. Homocysteine, white matter hyperintensities, and cognition in healthy elderly people. Annals of neurology. (2003). Feb;, 53(2), 214-21.

[112] Garcia, A, Haron, Y, Pulman, K, Hua, L, & Freedman, M. Increases in homocysteine are related to worsening of stroop scores in healthy elderly persons: a prospective follow-up study. The journals of gerontology. (2004). Dec;, 59(12), 1323-7.

[113] Nurk, E, Refsum, H, Tell, G. S, Engedal, K, Vollset, S. E, Ueland, P. M, et al. Plasma total homocysteine and memory in the elderly: the Hordaland Homocysteine Study. Annals of neurology. (2005). Dec;, 58(6), 847-57.

[114] Seshadri, S, Beiser, A, Selhub, J, Jacques, P. F, Rosenberg, I. H, & Agostino, D. RB, et al. Plasma homocysteine as a risk factor for dementia and Alzheimer's disease. The New England journal of medicine. (2002). Feb 14;, 346(7), 476-83.

[115] Wang, H. X, Wahlin, A, Basun, H, Fastbom, J, Winblad, B, Fratiglioni, L, & Vitamin, B. and folate in relation to the development of Alzheimer's disease. Neurology. (2001). May 8;, 56(9), 1188-94.

[116] Kado, D. M, Karlamangla, A. S, Huang, M. H, Troen, A, Rowe, J. W, Selhub, J, et al. Homocysteine versus the vitamins folate, B6, and B12 as predictors of cognitive function and decline in older high-functioning adults: MacArthur Studies of Successful Aging. The American journal of medicine. (2005). Feb;, 118(2), 161-7.

[117] Kang, J. H, Irizarry, M. C, & Grodstein, F. Prospective study of plasma folate, vitamin B12, and cognitive function and decline. Epidemiology (Cambridge, Mass. (2006). Nov;, 17(6), 650-7.

[118] Mooijaart, S. P, Gussekloo, J, Frolich, M, Jolles, J, Stott, D. J, Westendorp, R. G, et al. Homocysteine, vitamin B-12, and folic acid and the risk of cognitive decline in old age: the Leiden 85-Plus study. The American journal of clinical nutrition. (2005). Oct;, 82(4), 866-71.

[119] Tangney, C. C, Tang, Y, Evans, D. A, & Morris, M. C. Biochemical indicators of vitamin B12 and folate insufficiency and cognitive decline. Neurology. (2009). Jan 27;, 72(4), 361-7.

[120] Malouf, R. Grimley Evans J. Folic acid with or without vitamin B12 for the prevention and treatment of healthy elderly and demented people. Cochrane database of systematic reviews (Online). (2008). CD004514.

[121] Dangour, A. D, Whitehouse, P. J, Rafferty, K, Mitchell, S. A, Smith, L, Hawkesworth, S, et al. B-vitamins and fatty acids in the prevention and treatment of Alzheimer's disease and dementia: a systematic review. J Alzheimers Dis. (2010). , 22(1), 205-24.

[122] De Jager, C. A, Oulhaj, A, Jacoby, R, Refsum, H, & Smith, A. D. Cognitive and clinical outcomes of homocysteine-lowering B-vitamin treatment in mild cognitive impairment: a randomized controlled trial. International journal of geriatric psychiatry. (2011). Jun;, 27(6), 592-600.

[123] Smith, A. D, Smith, S. M, De Jager, C. A, Whitbread, P, Johnston, C, Agacinski, G, et al. Homocysteine-lowering by B vitamins slows the rate of accelerated brain atrophy in mild cognitive impairment: a randomized controlled trial. PloS one. (2010). e12244.

[124] Slinin, Y, Paudel, M. L, Taylor, B. C, Fink, H. A, Ishani, A, Canales, M. T, et al. Hydroxyvitamin D levels and cognitive performance and decline in elderly men. Neurology. (2010). Jan 5;, 74(1), 33-41.

[125] Annweiler, C, Rolland, Y, Schott, A. M, Blain, H, Vellas, B, Herrmann, F. R, et al. Higher Vitamin D Dietary Intake Is Associated With Lower Risk of Alzheimer's Disease: A Year Follow-up. The journals of gerontology. (2012). Apr 13., 7.

[126] Llewellyn, D. J, Lang, I. A, Langa, K. M, Muniz-terrera, G, Phillips, C. L, Cherubini, A, et al. Vitamin D and risk of cognitive decline in elderly persons. Archives of internal medicine. (2010). Jul 12;, 170(13), 1135-41.

[127] Annweiler, C, & Beauchet, O. Possibility of a new anti-alzheimer's disease pharmaceutical composition combining memantine and vitamin D. Drugs & aging. (2012). Feb 1;, 29(2), 81-91.

[128] Kivipelto, M, Ngandu, T, Laatikainen, T, Winblad, B, Soininen, H, & Tuomilehto, J. Risk score for the prediction of dementia risk in 20 years among middle aged people: a longitudinal, population-based study. Lancet neurology. (2006). Sep;, 5(9), 735-41.

[129] Qiu, C, Xu, W, Winblad, B, & Fratiglioni, L. Vascular risk profiles for dementia and Alzheimer's disease in very old people: a population-based longitudinal study. J Alzheimers Dis. (2010). , 20(1), 293-300.

[130] Barnes, D. E, Covinsky, K. E, Whitmer, R. A, Kuller, L. H, Lopez, O. L, & Yaffe, K. Predicting risk of dementia in older adults: The late-life dementia risk index. Neurology. (2009). Jul 21;, 73(3), 173-9.

[131] Barnes, D. E, Covinsky, K. E, Whitmer, R. A, Kuller, L. H, Lopez, O. L, & Yaffe, K. Commentary on "Developing a national strategy to prevent dementia: Leon Thal Symposium 2009." Dementia risk indices: A framework for identifying individuals with a high dementia risk. Alzheimers Dement. (2010). Mar;, 6(2), 138-41.

[132] Ferrari, C, Xu, W. L, Wang, H. X, Winblad, B, Sorbi, S, Qiu, C, et al. How can elderly apolipoprotein E epsilon4 carriers remain free from dementia? Neurobiol Aging. (2012). Apr 11.

[133] Wang, H. X, Gustafson, D, Kivipelto, M, Pedersen, N. L, Skoog, I, Winblad, B, et al. Education halves the risk of dementia due to apolipoprotein ε4 allele: a collaborative study from the Swedish Brain Power initiative. Neurobiol Aging. (2012). May; 33(5): 1007.e1-7.

[134] Daviglus, M. L, Bell, C. C, Berrettini, W, Bowen, P. E, & Connolly, E. S. Jr., Cox NJ, et al. National Institutes of Health State-of-the-Science Conference statement: preventing alzheimer disease and cognitive decline. Annals of internal medicine. (2011). Aug 3;, 153(3), 176-81.

[135] Solomon, A, & Kivipelto, M. Cholesterol-modifying strategies for Alzheimer's disease. Expert review of neurotherapeutics. (2009). May;, 9(5), 695-709.

[136] Wald, D. S, Kasturiratne, A, & Simmonds, M. Effect of folic acid, with or without other B vitamins, on cognitive decline: meta-analysis of randomized trials. The American journal of medicine. (2010). Jun;e2., 123(6), 522-7.

[137] Komulainen, P, Kivipelto, M, Lakka, T. A, Savonen, K, Hassinen, M, Kiviniemi, V, et al. Exercise, fitness and cognition- A randomised controlled trial in older individuals: The DR's EXTRA study. European Geriatric Medicine. (2010). , 1(5), 266-72.

[138] Rocca, W. A, Grossardt, B. R, & Shuster, L. T. Oophorectomy, menopause, estrogen treatment, and cognitive aging: clinical evidence for a window of opportunity. Brain research. (2011). Mar 16;, 1379, 188-98.

[139] Shumaker, S. A, Legault, C, Kuller, L, Rapp, S. R, Thal, L, Lane, D. S, et al. Conjugated equine estrogens and incidence of probable dementia and mild cognitive impairment in postmenopausal women: Women's Health Initiative Memory Study. Jama. (2004). Jun 23;, 291(24), 2947-58.

[140] Shumaker, S. A, Legault, C, Rapp, S. R, Thal, L, Wallace, R. B, Ockene, J. K, et al. Estrogen plus progestin and the incidence of dementia and mild cognitive impairment in postmenopausal women: the Women's Health Initiative Memory Study: a randomized controlled trial. Jama. (2003). May 28;, 289(20), 2651-62.

[141] Kronos Longevity Research Institute. Hormone Therapy Has Many Favorable Effects in Newly Menopausal Women: Initial Findings of the Kronos Early Estrogen Prevention Study (KEEPS). (2012). October 3, 2012]; Available from: http://www.menopause.org/docs/agm/general-release.pdf?sfvrsn=0.

[142] Whitmer, R. A, Quesenberry, C. P, Zhou, J, & Yaffe, K. Timing of hormone therapy and dementia: the critical window theory revisited. Annals of neurology. (2011). Jan;, 69(1), 163-9.

[143] Isaac, M. G, Quinn, R, & Tabet, N. Vitamin E for Alzheimer's disease and mild cognitive impairment. Cochrane database of systematic reviews (Online). (2008). CD002854.

[144] Schurks, M, Glynn, R. J, Rist, P. M, Tzourio, C, & Kurth, T. Effects of vitamin E on stroke subtypes: meta-analysis of randomised controlled trials. BMJ (Clinical research ed. (2010). c5702.

[145] Andrieu, S, Aboderin, I, Baeyens, J. P, Beard, J, Benetos, A, Berrut, G, et al. IAGG Workshop: Health Promotion Program on Prevention of Late Onset Dementia. The journal of nutrition, health & aging. (2011). , 15(7), 562-75.

[146] Richard, E. Van den Heuvel E, Moll van Charante EP, Achthoven L, Vermeulen M, Bindels PJ, et al. Prevention of dementia by intensive vascular care (PreDIVA): a cluster-randomized trial in progress. Alzheimer disease and associated disorders. (2009). Jul-Sep;, 23(3), 198-204.

[147] Lindstrom, J, Ilanne-parikka, P, Peltonen, M, Aunola, S, Eriksson, J. G, Hemio, K, et al. Sustained reduction in the incidence of type 2 diabetes by lifestyle intervention: follow-up of the Finnish Diabetes Prevention Study. Lancet. (2006). Nov 11;, 368(9548), 1673-9.

[148] Tuomilehto, J, Lindstrom, J, Eriksson, J. G, Valle, T. T, Hamalainen, H, Ilanne-parikka, P, et al. Prevention of type 2 diabetes mellitus by changes in lifestyle among subjects with impaired glucose tolerance. N Engl J Med. (2001). May 3;, 344(18), 1343-50.

[149] Komulainen, P, Kivipelto, M, Lakka, T. A, Savonen, K, Hassinen, M, Kiviniemi, V, et al. Exercise, fitness and cognition- A randomised controlled trial in older individuals: The DR's EXTRA study. European Geriatric Medicine (2012). , 1(2), 266-72.

[150] Gillette-guyonnet, S, Andrieu, S, Dantoine, T, Dartigues, J. F, Touchon, J, & Vellas, B. Commentary on "A roadmap for the prevention of dementia II. Leon Thal Symposium 2008." The Multidomain Alzheimer Preventive Trial (MAPT): a new approach to the prevention of Alzheimer's disease. Alzheimers Dement. (2009). Mar;, 5(2), 114-21.

[151] Richard, E, Andrieu, S, Solomon, A, Mangialasche, F, Ahtiluoto, S, Moll van Charante, et al. Methodological challenges in designing dementia prevention trials - the European Dementia Prevention Initiative (EDPI). J Neurol Sci. (2012). Nov 15;322(1-2):64-70.

[152] Reiman, E. M, Langbaum, J. B, & Tariot, P. N. Alzheimer's prevention initiative: a proposal to evaluate presymptomatic treatments as quickly as possible. Biomarkers in medicine. (2010). Feb;, 4(1), 3-14.

[153] Reiman, E. M, Langbaum, J. B, Fleisher, A. S, Caselli, R. J, Chen, K, Ayutyanont, N, et al. Alzheimer's Prevention Initiative: a plan to accelerate the evaluation of presymptomatic treatments. J Alzheimers Dis. (2011). Suppl , 3, 321-9.

[154] Blennow, K, De Leon, M. J, & Zetterberg, H. Alzheimer's disease. Lancet. (2006). Jul 29;, 368(9533), 387-403.

[155] Bateman, R. J, Xiong, C, Benzinger, T. L, Fagan, A. M, Goate, A, Fox, N. C, et al. Clinical and biomarker changes in dominantly inherited Alzheimer's disease. The New England journal of medicine. (2012). Aug 30;, 367(9), 795-804.

[156] Lopera, F, Ardilla, A, Martinez, A, Madrigal, L, Arango-viana, J. C, Lemere, C. A, et al. Clinical features of early-onset Alzheimer disease in a large kindred with an E280A presenilin-1 mutation. Jama. (1997). Mar 12;, 277(10), 793-9.

[157] Miller, G. Alzheimer's research. Stopping Alzheimer's before it starts. Science (New York, NY. (2012). Aug 17;, 337(6096), 790-2.

[158] Alzheimer's Prevention Initiative, Treatment Trials. (2012). October 2012; Available from: http://endalznow.org/about-api/treatment-trials.aspx.

[159] West, S. G, Duan, N, Pequegnat, W, & Gaist, P. Des Jarlais DC, Holtgrave D, et al. Alternatives to the randomized controlled trial. American journal of public health. (2008). Aug;, 98(8), 1359-66.

[160] Khachaturian, Z. S, Petersen, R. C, Snyder, P. J, Khachaturian, A. S, Aisen, P, De Leon, M, et al. Developing a global strategy to prevent Alzheimer's disease: Leon Thal Symposium 2010. Alzheimers Dement. (2011). Mar;, 7(2), 127-32.

[161] Zhu, L, Fratiglioni, L, Guo, Z, Basun, H, Corder, E. H, Winblad, B, et al. Incidence of dementia in relation to stroke and the apolipoprotein E epsilon4 allele in the very

old. Findings from a population-based longitudinal study. Stroke; a journal of cerebral circulation. (2000). Jan;, 31(1), 53-60.

[162] Honig, L. S, Tang, M. X, Albert, S, Costa, R, Luchsinger, J, Manly, J, et al. Stroke and the risk of Alzheimer disease. Archives of neurology. (2003). Dec;, 60(12), 1707-12.

[163] Bushnell, C. D, Zimmer, L. O, Pan, W, Olson, D. M, Zhao, X, Meteleva, T, et al. Persistence with stroke prevention medications 3 months after hospitalization. Archives of neurology. (2010). Dec;, 67(12), 1456-63.

[164] Xu, W, Caracciolo, B, Wang, HX, Winblad, B, Bäckman, L, Qiu, C, et al. Accelerated progression from mild cognitive impairment to dementia in people with diabetes. Diabetes. 2010 Nov;59(11):2928-35

Permissions

The contributors of this book come from diverse backgrounds, making this book a truly international effort. This book will bring forth new frontiers with its revolutionizing research information and detailed analysis of the nascent developments around the world.

We would like to thank Inga Zerr, MD, for lending her expertise to make the book truly unique. She has played a crucial role in the development of this book. Without her invaluable contribution this book wouldn't have been possible. She has made vital efforts to compile up to date information on the varied aspects of this subject to make this book a valuable addition to the collection of many professionals and students.

This book was conceptualized with the vision of imparting up-to-date information and advanced data in this field. To ensure the same, a matchless editorial board was set up. Every individual on the board went through rigorous rounds of assessment to prove their worth. After which they invested a large part of their time researching and compiling the most relevant data for our readers. Conferences and sessions were held from time to time between the editorial board and the contributing authors to present the data in the most comprehensible form. The editorial team has worked tirelessly to provide valuable and valid information to help people across the globe.

Every chapter published in this book has been scrutinized by our experts. Their significance has been extensively debated. The topics covered herein carry significant findings which will fuel the growth of the discipline. They may even be implemented as practical applications or may be referred to as a beginning point for another development. Chapters in this book were first published by InTech; hereby published with permission under the Creative Commons Attribution License or equivalent.

The editorial board has been involved in producing this book since its inception. They have spent rigorous hours researching and exploring the diverse topics which have resulted in the successful publishing of this book. They have passed on their knowledge of decades through this book. To expedite this challenging task, the publisher supported the team at every step. A small team of assistant editors was also appointed to further simplify the editing procedure and attain best results for the readers.

Our editorial team has been hand-picked from every corner of the world. Their multi-ethnicity adds dynamic inputs to the discussions which result in innovative outcomes. These outcomes are then further discussed with the researchers and contributors who give their valuable feedback and opinion regarding the same. The feedback is then collaborated with the researches and they are edited in a comprehensive manner to aid the understanding of the subject.

Apart from the editorial board, the designing team has also invested a significant amount of their time in understanding the subject and creating the most relevant covers. They scrutinized every image to scout for the most suitable representation of the subject and create an appropriate cover for the book.

The publishing team has been involved in this book since its early stages. They were actively engaged in every process, be it collecting the data, connecting with the contributors or procuring relevant information. The team has been an ardent support to the editorial, designing and production team. Their endless efforts to recruit the best for this project, has resulted in the accomplishment of this book. They are a veteran in the field of academics and their pool of knowledge is as vast as their experience in printing. Their expertise and guidance has proved useful at every step. Their uncompromising quality standards have made this book an exceptional effort. Their encouragement from time to time has been an inspiration for everyone.

The publisher and the editorial board hope that this book will prove to be a valuable piece of knowledge for researchers, students, practitioners and scholars across the globe.

List of Contributors

Sibel Cevizci
Canakkale Onsekiz Mart University, School of Medicine, Department of Public Health, Canakkale, Turkey

Halil Murat Sen
Canakkale Onsekiz Mart University, School of Medicine, Department of Neurology, Canakkale, Turkey

Fahri Güneş
Canakkale Onsekiz Mart University, School of Medicine, Department of Internal Medicine, Canakkale, Turkey

Elif Karaahmet
Canakkale Onsekiz Mart University, School of Medicine, Department of Psychiatry, Canakkale, Turkey

Ester Aso and Isidre Ferrer
Institut de Neuropatologia, Hospital Universitari de Bellvitge, Universitat de Barcelona, CIBERNED, Spain

Weili Xu
Department of Epidemiology, Tianjin Medical University, Tianjin, P.R., China
Aging Research Center, Karolinska Institutet-Stockholm University, Stockholm, Sweden

Camilla Ferrari
Aging Research Center, Karolinska Institutet-Stockholm University, Stockholm, Sweden
Department of Neurological and Psychiatric Sciences, University of Florence, Italy

Hui-Xin Wang
Aging Research Center, Karolinska Institutet-Stockholm University, Stockholm, Sweden

Brent D. Aulston, Zaid Aboud and Gordon W. Glazner
St. Boniface Hospital Research Centre, Winnipeg, MB, Canada
Department of Pharmacology and Therapeutics, University of Manitoba, Winnipeg, MB, Canada

Gary L. Odero
St. Boniface Hospital Research Centre, Winnipeg, MB, Canada

Rita Moretti, Paola Torre, Francesca Esposito, Enrica Barro and Rodolfo M. Antonello
Medicina Clinica, Ambulatorio Complicanze Internistiche Cerebrali, Dipartimento Universitario Clinico di Scienze Mediche Tecnologiche e Traslazionali, Università degli Studi di Trieste, Italy

Paola Tomietto
Reumatologia-Clinica Medica, AOUTS, Ospedale di Cattinara, Italy

Mei Sian Chong
Department of Geriatric Medicine, Tan Tock Seng Hospital, Singapore

Tih-Shih Lee
Duke University Medical School, USA

Francesca Mangialasche
Aging Research Center, Karolinska Institutet-Stockholm University, Stockholm, Sweden
Institute of Gerontology and Geriatrics, Department of Clinical and Experimental Medicine, University of Perugia, Perugia, Italy

Weili Xu
Aging Research Center, Karolinska Institutet-Stockholm University, Stockholm, Sweden
Department of Epidemiology, Tianjin Medical University, Tianjin, P.R., China

Miia Kivipelto
Aging Research Center, Karolinska Institutet-Stockholm University, Stockholm, Sweden
Department of Neurology, University of Eastern Finland, Kuopio, Finland

Printed in the USA
CPSIA information can be obtained
at www.ICGtesting.com
JSHW011428221024
72173JS00004B/717

9 781632 424150